KU-113-992

A PRACTICAL HANDBOOK OF MIDWIFERY AND GYNÆCOLOGY

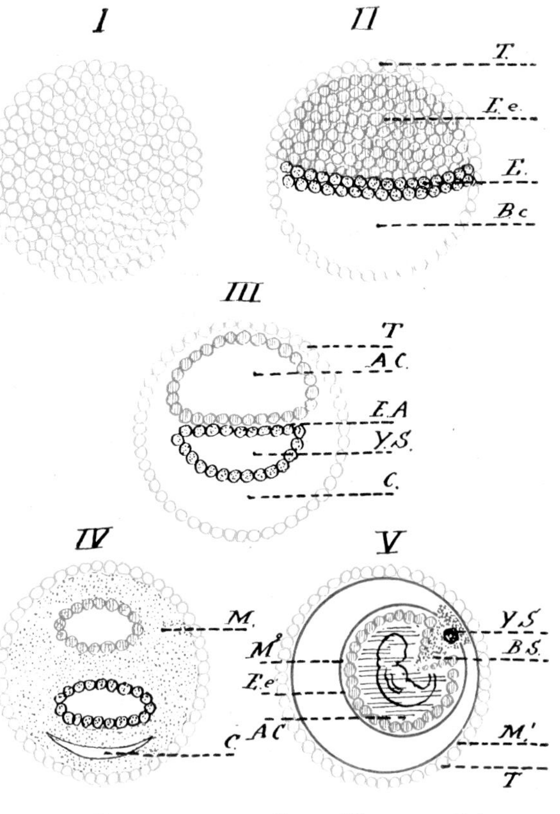

DEVELOPMENT OF OVUM (diagrammatic).

I. Morula Stage.

II. Blastocyst Stage.
T. Trophoblast.
E.e. Embryonic ectoderm.
E. Entoderm.
B.c. Blastocyst cavity.

III. T. Trophoblast.
A.C. Amniotic Cavity.
E.A. Embryonic Area.
Y.S. Yolk Sac.
C. Cœlom.

IV. M. Mesoderm.
C. Cœlom.

V. Y.S. Remains of Yolk Sac.
B.S. Belly Stalk.
M^1. Mesoderm } Chorion.
T. Trophoblast }
M^2. Mesoderm }
E.e. Embryonic ectoderm } Amnion.
A.C. Amniotic Cavity.

Frontispiece

A PRACTICAL HANDBOOK OF MIDWIFERY AND GYNÆCOLOGY

FOR STUDENTS AND PRACTITIONERS

BY

W. F. T. HAULTAIN

O.B.E., M.C., B.A., M.B., B.Ch., F.R.C.P.Ed., F.R.C.S.Ed., F.R.C.O.G.

HON. CONSULTING OBSTETRICIAN AND GYNÆCOLOGIST, ROYAL INFIRMARY, EDINBURGH, AND GYNÆCOLOGIST, LEITH HOSPITAL; CONSULTANT OBSTETRICIAN AND GYNÆCOLOGIST, BANGOUR HOSPITAL AND EASTERN GENERAL HOSPITAL, EDINBURGH; LECTURER IN MIDWIFERY AND GYNÆCOLOGY, EDINBURGH UNIVERSITY; EXAMINER IN MIDWIFERY AND GYNÆCOLOGY, TRIPLE QUALIFICATION AND FELLOWSHIP EXAMINATION, ROYAL COLLEGE OF SURGEONS, EDINBURGH

AND

CLIFFORD KENNEDY

M.B., Ch.B., F.R.C.S.Ed., F.R.C.O.G.

ASSISTANT OBSTETRICIAN AND GYNÆCOLOGIST, ROYAL INFIRMARY, EDINBURGH; HON. CONSULTING GYNÆCOLOGIST, DEACONESS HOSPITAL, EDINBURGH; CONSULTANT GYNÆCOLOGIST, CHALMERS HOSPITAL, EDINBURGH, AND GALASHIELS AND SELKIRK HOSPITALS; LECTURER IN MIDWIFERY AND GYNÆCOLOGY, EDINBURGH UNIVERSITY; EXAMINER MIDWIFERY AND GYNÆCOLOGY, GLASGOW UNIVERSITY, TRIPLE QUALIFICATION AND CENTRAL MIDWIVES (SCOT.) BOARDS AND FELLOWSHIP EXAMINATION, ROYAL COLLEGE OF SURGEONS, EDINBURGH

Including a Section on the

MANAGEMENT OF THE INFANT AND NEO-NATAL CONDITIONS

BY

J. L. HENDERSON

M.D., F.R.C.P.Ed.

PROFESSOR CHILD HEALTH, ST. ANDREWS' UNIVERSITY; LATE CONSULTANT TO ROYAL HOSPITAL FOR SICK CHILDREN, EDINBURGH, AND SIMPSON MEMORIAL MATERNITY PAVILION, EDINBURGH

FOURTH EDITION

E. & S. LIVINGSTONE LTD.
EDINBURGH AND LONDON
1952

This book is protected under the Berne Convention. It may not be reproduced by any means in whole or in part without permission. Application with regard to reproduction should be addressed to the Publishers.

PRINTED IN GREAT BRITAIN BY J. AND J. GRAY, EDINBURGH

PREFACE

ONLY four years have elapsed since this Handbook was thoroughly revised and brought up-to-date, and yet the changes in Midwifery and Gynæcology have been such that a thorough revision has been required. New sections have been entirely re-written on Placenta Prævia, Delayed Labour, Venous Thrombosis and Dysmenorrhœa, whereas other sections have been altered considerably. Once more we have to thank Dr. J. L. Henderson, now Professor of Child Health at St. Andrew's University for undertaking the re-writing of the section on the Infant and on infant feeding, and Dr. R. A. P. Cumming, Director of the Edinburgh Blood Transfusion Service, for a short new section on the difficult and intricate subject of the Rh factor in Midwifery. The sections on Venereology have been entirely re-written by Miss Marjorie Murrell, F.R.C.S.E., one of the consultant Venereologists at the Royal Infirmary, Edinburgh, and to her also we are indeed indebted.

We also acknowledge our gratitude to others who have helped us in previous editions with plates and illustrations, which have again been included in this edition. As previously Messrs. E. & S. Livingstone have given us every assistance in the publication and merit our sincere thanks. We are most grateful to Dr. Donald Irvine for the exacting task of proof reading and to Miss Elizabeth Galloway for her help in compiling the index.

We hope that this book will be of great help to final year students and to general practitioners, in that essential and up-to-date information in the subjects it embraces can be obtained readily and quickly. We feel that it may be especially useful to the graduate who has returned to general practice from the Forces where he has been unavoidably divorced from Midwifery and Gynæcology.

W.F.T.H.
C.K.

September, 1951.

CONTENTS

LIST OF ILLUSTRATIONS

CHAPTER I

ANATOMY, DEVELOPMENT AND PHYSIOLOGY

(*a*) OBSTETRICAL AND GYNÆCOLOGICAL ANATOMY

(A) PELVIS. (From Obstetrical Standpoint)

Bones

1. **Os Innominatum.**—
   - (*a*) Ilium. *Important Landmarks.*
     - (1) Anterior superior spine.
     - (2) Posterior superior spine.
     - (3) Crest.
     - (4) Ilio-pectineal eminence.
     - (5) Ilio-pectineal line.
   - (*b*) Ischium.
     - (1) Tuberosity.
     - (2) Spine.
     - (3) Ridge of bone between spine and ilio-pectineal eminence, which divides ischium into two planes. (This ridge was at one time thought to aid internal rotation of the occiput.)
   - (*c*) Pubis.
     - (1) Symphysis.
     - (2) Pubic arch.
2. **Sacrum.**—Consists of five vertebræ—promontory.
3. **Coccyx.**

Joints

1. **Sacro-iliac Joints.**—Movable joints, the sacral promontory swinging slightly backwards when the hip joint is extended, from which fact Walcher's position is made use of (see p. 68). When the hip joint is flexed the promontory advances slightly and thus diminishes the true conjugate.

2. **Pubic Joint.**—Also mobile, having a small synovial cavity, which was entered in performing symphysiotomy. The strongest ligament is the sub-pubic ligament.

3. **Sacro-coccygeal.**—Softens during latter months of pregnancy and allows coccyx to pass backwards during labour.

The pelvis is divided into a false and true pelvis by the upper margin of symphysis, ilio-pectineal lines, upper margin of sacral alæ and upper anterior margin of promontory. All above this line is the false pelvis, and all below, the true pelvis; the latter is of great importance in obstetrics.

Boundaries of True Pelvis.—

	Anterior.	*Lateral.*	*Posterior.*
Inlet .	Symphysis pubis.	Ilio-pectineal lines.	Promontory sacrum.
Cavity .	Pubic bones.	Ischial bones and sacro-sciatic ligaments.	Sacrum and coccyx.
Outlet .	Inferior rami of pubis.	Ischial tuberosities.	Sacro-sciatic ligaments and coccyx.

Diameters of True Pelvis.—How measured :—

	Antero-posterior.	*Oblique.*	*Transverse.*
Inlet .	From promontory to nearest point on posterior surface of symphysis. **True conjugate.**	From upper margin one sacro-iliac joint to opposite ilio-pectineal eminence. (*N.B.*—The right oblique is measured from the right, and the left from the left sacro-iliac joints.)	Greatest distance between ilio-pectineal lines.
Cavity .	From junction of 2nd and 3rd sacral vertebræ to posterior surface symphysis.	From lower margin sacro-iliac joint to centre of opposite obturator membrane.	Between ridges of ischia.
Outlet .	From tip of coccyx to lower posterior surface of symphysis. (This is increased in labour as coccyx is mobile and is therefore measured obstetrically from lower border of sacrum.)	From middle of sacro-tuberous ligament to opposite junction of rami of ischium and pubis.	Between inner surfaces of ischial tuberosities.

Measurements.—

	Antero-posterior.	*Oblique.*	*Transverse.*
Inlet .	. 4 in. (true conjugate).	4½ in.	5 in.
Cavity .	. 4½ ,,	4½ ,, (approx.).	4½ ,,
Outlet .	. 5 ,, (with coccyx back).	4½ ,, ,,	4 ,,

Sacro-cotyloid diameter (of importance in occipito-posterior cases) is measured from the promontory of the sacrum to the posterior surface of the middle of the acetabulum, and measures 3½ in. (For other measurements of clinical importance, see p. 46.)

Pelvic Planes.—

1. *Imaginary.*—As the sacrum curves backwards the posterior wall of the pelvis is much longer than the anterior and so the passage must be curved. This is shown by drawing numerous lines from the sacrum to corresponding points on the posterior surface of symphysis—promontory to top of symphysis, middle to middle, and tip of coccyx to lower margin, etc. If these lines are all bisected and a line drawn through all the middle points, a curve is formed, which is known as the curve of Carus, and it is by way of such a curve that the centre of the child's head passes during labour.

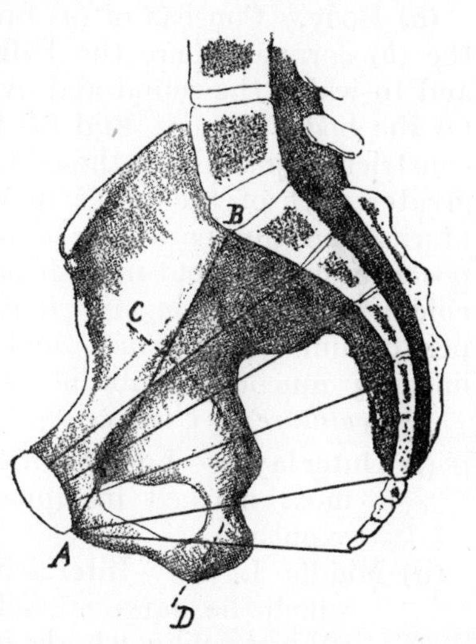

Fig. 1.—Pelvic Planes and Diagonal Conjugate.

A-B, Diagonal conjugate.
C-D, Curve of Carus.

2. *Bony.*—The two planes of ischium receding on each side of the ridge, which may aid internal rotation.

3. *Soft.*—Formed by the muscles of the pelvic floor, a gutter being formed by the muscles coming in from the sides, the gutter becoming broader as it passes anteriorly. It is this formation which is partly the cause of internal rotation (see p. 60). In the upright position the plane of the brim is at an angle of 60 degrees and the plane of the outlet at 10 degrees to the horizontal.

Dynamic Pelvis.—Pelvis complete with soft parts, which encroach more or less into pelvic cavity. At the brim the psoas and iliacus muscles encroach on the transverse diameter, the largest available transverse diameter lying about 1 in. in front of the bony diameter, being sometimes called the obstetrical diameter, 4½ in. In the cavity the pyriformis and obturator internus are found laterally, and the rectum and pelvic colon encroach on the left oblique. The outlet is occupied by the pelvic floor.

(B) INTERNAL GENERATIVE ORGANS

1. Uterus

Length, 3 in.; breadth, 2 in.; thickness, 1 in.; length of cavity, $2\frac{1}{2}$ in. Consists of a body and a cervix, the junction being indicated by the internal os on the inside, and by the isthmus on the outside.

(*a*) **Body.**—Consists of (*a*) fundus, which is the part above the (*b*) cornua, where the Fallopian tubes enter the uterus, and to which the round and ovarian ligaments are attached; (*c*) the body proper; and (*d*) the isthmus, which is a slight constriction just above the cervix, and which goes to form the greater part of the lower uterine segment in the pregnant uterus. In nulliparæ the anterior surface is flat and the posterior convex, but in multiparæ both are convex. Consists chiefly of muscle—*myometrium*, but is covered externally by peritoneum—*perimetrium*, and inside is a potential cavity lined by mucous membrane—*endometrium.*

Musculature of Uterus.—

(i) Outer layer.—Longitudinal, but transverse across fundus; most marked in upper part of body. Muscles of expulsion.

(ii) Middle Layer.—Interlacing fibres in all directions in which lie large vessels, which are surrounded by sphincter-like whorls of muscle fibres. Contraction stops hæmorrhage after separation and expulsion of placenta.

(iii) Inner Layer.—Circular. Sparse at fundus, but greatly increased towards isthmus, forming sphincter at internal os. Acts as inhibitor to expulsion of uterine contents.

Endometrium.—No constant appearance microscopically, as it changes with age, phase of menstrual cycle and individual. Consists of so-called glands, which are not true glands but crypts formed by the surface epithelium penetrating mucosa. These glands are lined by one single row of cells. Boundary between glands and muscle not absolutely precise, and a few glands may encroach into myometrium. The stroma consists of spindle cells, which contain little protoplasm unless just before a menstrual period, or more pronouncedly, during early pregnancy. The stroma becomes more dense the deeper it is. A number of leucocytes are also present. The vessels are delicate capillaries.

(*b*) **Cervix.**—(*a*) Supravaginal portion ; (*b*) vaginal portion. The canal communicates with uterine cavity through the internal os, and with the vagina through the external os. The cavity is lined by columnar epithelium, and the mucosa contains large glands, which secrete a glairy mucus. The surface epithelium and glands are lined by one layer of cells. Stroma is dense connective tissue poorly supplied with cells.

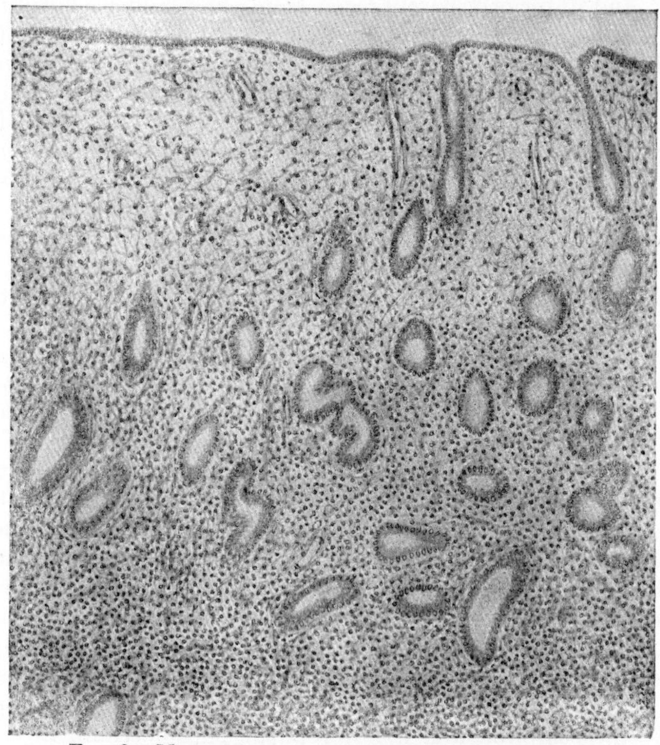

FIG. 2.—MICROSCOPIC APPEARANCE OF ENDOMETRIUM.

The vaginal surface is lined by several layers of squamous epithelium, which pass abruptly at the external os into the columnar type. The cervix consists chiefly of muscle. The cervix and external os differ in nulliparæ and multiparæ, the cervix being hard, cylindrical and cone-shaped in nulliparæ, and having a small rounded os ; whereas in multiparæ it is lacerated, and the os is slit-shaped or patulous.

Normally the uterus lies almost horizontal with woman in upright position, the fundus being level with the upper border of symphysis and the external os at level of ischial spines. The body is normally inclined forward upon the cervix at an angle of 160 degrees (anteversion).

(*c*) **Peritoneum.**—Covers body of the uterus completely anteriorly and posteriorly, and is firmly attached except at isthmus, where it is loosely attached owing to cellular tissue intervening. (An important point in a supravaginal hysterectomy.) The cervix is covered by peritoneum posteriorly only, and anteriorly is separated from the bladder by cellular tissue, the peritoneum being reflected off the uterus on to the bladder at the isthmus, forming the utero-vesical pouch. Laterally, the peritoneum passes to the side walls of the pelvis in two layers, forming the broad ligaments, and thus the uterus is uncovered by peritoneum laterally, the uncovered area being very narrow above, but broad below. Posteriorly the peritoneum is reflected from the upper third of vagina to rectum, forming lowest limit of pouch of Douglas. The uterus normally is freely mobile.

(*d*) **Ligaments.**—Of little importance for keeping a healthy uterus in position.

1. *Broad Ligaments.*—Double folds of peritoneum running laterally and slightly backwards from uterus. Upper border free and contains the tube as far as abdominal ostium, from which point ligament is continued to side wall of pelvis as the *infundibulo-pelvic ligament*; in the upper third run the ovarian vessels. With the normal position of uterus, the anterior surface of broad ligament looks forward and downwards, whereas posterior surface looks upwards and backwards. The two layers separate greatly as they pass downwards, thus the upper half of the ligament has little cellular tissue between the layers, the lower half, however, contains much. Attached to the posterior surface by the mesovarium is the ovary, which divides the ligament into an upper part—mesosalpinx, and a lower part—parametrium, in each of which important structures are found between or attached to layers.

Mesosalpinx :—

(*a*) Fallopian tube.
(*b*) Round ligament.
(*c*) Ovarian ligament.
(*d*) Parovarium (a series of vertical tubules joined by a horizontal tubule—beginning of Gärtner's duct, the whole being vestigial remnants).
(*e*) Branches of ovarian and uterine arteries anastomosing.

Parametrium :—

(*a*) Ureter.
(*b*) Uterine vessels.
(*c*) Gärtner's duct.
(*d*) Lymphatic glands.
(*e*) Abundant cellular tissue.

2. *Round Ligaments.*—Slender cord-like structures corresponding to the gubernaculum in the male, composed of unstriated muscle fibres and connective tissue, which pass from cornua along anterior layer of broad ligament through the internal abdominal ring, inguinal canal and external abdominal ring to the labium majus on each side. (At the cornu the round ligament is most anterior, then the tube, and the ovarian ligament most posterior; whereas from above downwards the structures are tube, round ligament, ovarian ligament.)

3. *Genito-sacral Ligaments.*—Duplications of peritoneum passing from posterior surface of uterus at the level of the internal os to the second and third sacral vertebræ. Thus they commence in close relation to one another, but diverge as they approach the sacrum, forming three pouches, the central being the pouch of Douglas, and the two lateral the pararectal pouches. (*N.B.*—Clinically, the whole is called the pouch of Douglas, but anatomically, this is not strictly correct.) There is " cellular tissue " and unstriate muscle present between the folds of peritoneum—*true utero-sacral ligaments.*

4. *Ovarian Ligament.*—From inner pole of ovary to the cornu running along the posterior layer of the broad ligament.

Supports of Pelvic Viscera.—

1. *Levatores Ani Muscles.*—*Arise* from posterior surface of pubis, white line and ischial spines. Traced towards insertion, fail to meet in middle line exposing a gap in pelvic floor behind symphysis, which is filled by pelvic fascia (superior layer of urogenital diaphragm). *Inserted* into (i) lateral aspect lower end vagina, acting as sphincter; (ii) central point perineum blending together and with transversi perinei and superficial part external sphincter ani behind vagina; (iii) lower end anal canal blending with internal sphincter ani and deep part external sphincter ani; (iv) ano-coccygeal body by blending together behind anal canal and (v) lower lateral border coccyx. Each muscle is ensheathed by pelvic fascia.

2. *Pelvic Fascia* (*Visceral layer*).—Continuous with parietal layer covering pelvic floor and is reflected on to adjacent viscera blending with connective tissue surrounding organs and with its fellow on opposite side round organs. Certain thickened bands act as supports.

(i) Medial pubo-vesical ligament—between body of pubis and bladder.
(ii) Lateral pubo-vesical ligaments—between lateral pelvic walls and bladder.
(iii) Cardinal ligaments of cervix (Mackenrodt's transverse cervical ligaments)—between lateral pelvic walls and supra-vaginal cervix.
(iv) Utero-sacral ligaments—between sacrum and supra-vaginal cervix lying in genito-sacral folds.

N.B.—All these ligaments contain plain muscle fibres amongst cellular tissue.

3. *Parametrium.*—Pelvic cellular tissue lying laterally to vagina and cervix, the connective tissue being thickened around vessels, lymphatics and nerves lying in it.

(*e*) **Vessels.**—

(*a*) *Arteries*

1. *Uterine*, from anterior division of internal iliacs, which pass in the parametrium, crossing anterior to the ureter to supply the upper part of vagina, uterus, and inner part of Fallopian tube, finally anastomosing with the ovarian arteries at the cornua of uterus and in mesosalpinx.

2. *Ovarian*, from aorta, passing down between the layers of infundibulo-pelvic ligament, supplying the ovary and anastomosing with the uterine arteries.

3. *Round Ligament Artery.*—Not always present. Branch of deep epigastric.

(*b*) *Veins*

Run into a plexus consisting of vesical, utero-vaginal and hæmorrhoidal vessels, and these drain into the internal iliac veins.

(*f*) **Nerve Supply.**—

(i) *Inferior hypogastric plexus* (*sympathetic*).—Bilateral continuations of pre-sacral nerve. Sensory. Supply muscles of inhibition (circular) and thus may cause contraction round internal os during labour from fear or anxiety.

(ii) *Nervi Erigentes* (*parasympathetic*).—Motor to muscles of expulsion (longitudinal).

(iii) *Local nerve centres in muscle* (*automatic*) act on longitudinal muscles.

Nerves pass along between sacro-genital ligaments to form a pelvic plexus postero-lateral to isthmus on each side (Frankenhauser's ganglia), which distribute mixed nerves to pelvic organs. Sympathetic impulses tend to inhibit impulses of nervi erigentes, but not those of local nerve centres.

(*g*) **Lymphatic Supply.**—Capillary networks in peritoneum, muscle and mucous membrane send branches to sub-peritoneal network, which gives off collecting trunks, which pass

(*a*) *from cervix to*—

(1) External iliac glands—superior glands of middle chain.

(2) Internal iliac glands—around origin of the uterine and vaginal arteries.

(3) Lateral sacral glands.

(*b*) *from body to*—

(1) Aortic glands—in lumbar region.

(2) External iliac glands—middle chain.

(3) Inguinal glands—via round ligament to upper and internal group.

2. Fallopian Tubes

Attached to cornu of the uterus on each side, the lateral end lying free in the pelvic peritoneal cavity. The length is 4 to 4½ in. Four parts :—

1. *Interstitial.*—½ in., lying in uterine muscle ; lumen very narrow, 1 mm.

2. *Isthmic.*—Inner third. Lumen slightly wider.

3. *Ampulla.*—Curved upwards, backwards and inwards, surrounding upper part of ovary. Lumen widens to 4 to 5 mm. at termination.

4. *Abdominal Ostium.*—Surrounded by fimbriæ, one of which is much larger than the rest, and passes on to ovary—the ovarian fimbria.

The tubes are covered by peritoneum except at the base, which lies between the layers of the broad ligament. They consist of three walls, peritoneum, muscle and mucous membrane, which is ciliated. They are supplied by uterine and ovarian arteries.

3. Ovaries

White oval structures 3 cm. long, 2 cm. wide, and 1 cm. thick, attached by the mesovarium to the posterior layer of the broad ligament, and by the ovarian ligament to the cornu of the uterus. Anatomically, each lies in fossa ovarica close to lateral pelvic wall, between external iliac artery in front and internal iliac artery and ureter behind, being separated by peritoneum from obturator vessels and nerve, which lie lateral to each. Supplied by ovarian arteries from aorta ; veins join on the right side the inferior vena cava, and on the left, the left renal vein.

4. Vagina

Passage joining cervix to vulva, being 4 in. long posteriorly and 3 in. anteriorly. The cervix passes through dome-shaped upper extremity and gives rise to four fornices—anterior, posterior, and two lateral, the posterior being the deepest. The anterior wall is in apposition with bladder and urethra, and has no peritoneal covering.

The posterior wall has peritoneum covering its upper third, separating it from pouch of Douglas, the middle third being in relation to the rectal ampulla and the lower third to the perineal body. Cavity potential, the walls lying in apposition, at right angles to vulva. Mucosa lined by squamous epithelium.

5. Pelvic Cellular Tissue

1. *Traced Antero-posteriorly.*—Continuation of sub-peritoneal layer of anterior abdominal wall—large areolar space between bladder and symphysis (space of Retzius)—along anterior pelvic wall between fascia covering obturator internus and peritoneum—between bladder and cervix and vagina, passing up on to isthmus uteri—in utero-sacral folds to extensive areolar mass between vagina and rectum, continuous with mesentery of pelvic colon. Sides of rectum—thin layer over some parts sacrum.

2. *Traced Laterally.*—Covering fascia iliaca—in infundibulo-pelvic ligament—extensive mass between layers of broad ligament—connected with other side under utero-vesical peritoneum in front and by a thin layer posteriorly.

3. *Traced Caudally.*—Small amount in mesosalpinx—abundant in parametrium — ligamentary attachments of vagina.

Exits.—

(1) To ischio-rectal fossa near exit of obturator internus (very small).
(2) Through external abdominal ring via round ligaments.
(3) Through sacro-sciatic foramen via vascular sheaths.
(4) Through obturator foramen via vascular sheaths.
(5) Through crural canal via vascular sheaths.
(6) Along sheath of ureter to cellular tissue round kidney.
(7) To anterior abdominal wall by direct extension.
(8) To retro-peritoneal tissue by direct extension.

All these exits are of importance, as a pelvic cellulitis, which goes on to suppuration, may track through any of them.

(C) EXTERNAL GENITAL ORGANS

VULVA

1. **Mons Veneris.**—Pad of fat in front of symphysis pubis covered by hair at puberty.

2. **Labia Majora.**—The two outer folds of vulva starting in front at mons and meeting behind at the *posterior commissure.* Two surfaces, the outer covered by hair and the inner with smooth skin.

3. **Labia Minora.**—Two triangular folds of smooth, moist skin found inside the majora. Anteriorly they meet to form the prepuce of the clitoris, whereas posteriorly they are joined by a fine fold known as the *fourchette.*

4. **Vestibule.**—Almond-shaped area bounded by clitoris at apex and the labia minora at either side. It is pierced near the centre by the urethra and posteriorly by the vagina.

5. **Clitoris.**—Analogous to penis and consists of two crura, a glans, a prepuce and a frenulum.

6. **External Urethral Meatus.**—Four-fifths of an inch below clitoris and anterior to vagina. Appears as a soft slit owing to walls being in contact. The female urethra normally measures $1\frac{1}{2}$ to $1\frac{3}{4}$ in., but may be stretched to a length of 6 in. or more during the second stage of labour or by tumours, etc.

7. **Bartholin Glands.**—One on each side, opening by small ducts on each side of vaginal orifice, just below and anterior to hymen.

8. **Vaginal Orifice.**—Below the urinary meatus and bounded on each side and posteriorly by the hymen.

9. **Hymen.**—Fold of connective tissue, which is usually crescentic and is covered by vaginal mucosa. Almost obliterates the vaginal opening in a virgin and may close it absolutely in a condition known as imperforate hymen.

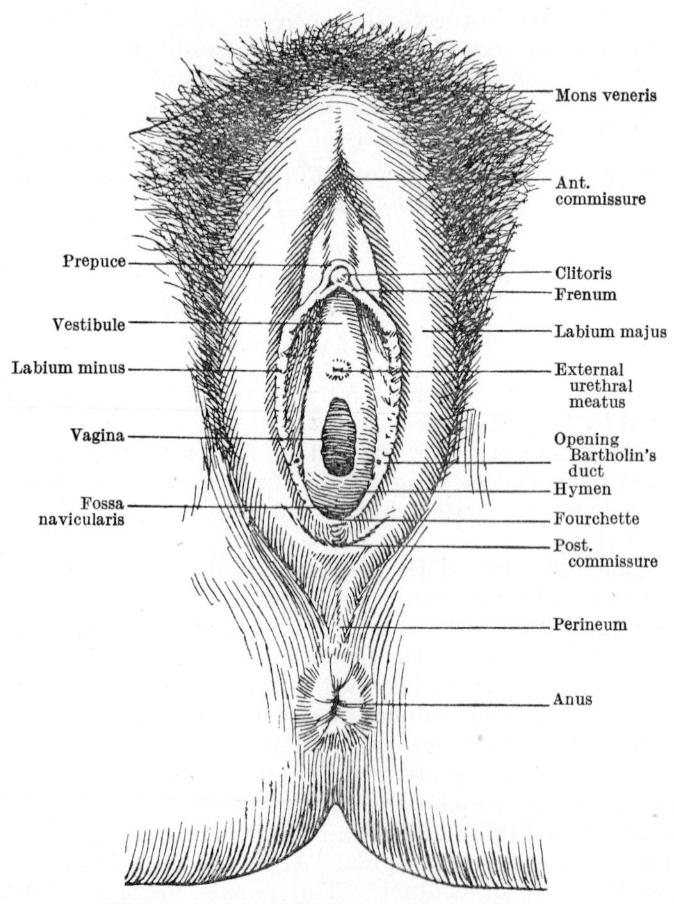

FIG. 3.—FEMALE EXTERNAL GENITAL ORGANS.

This fold is torn at labour and is represented by tags known as carunculæ myrtiformes.

10. **Fossa Navicularis.**—Area between vaginal orifice and fourchette.

11. **Perineum.**—Area between the posterior commissure and anus. Is the base of the perineal body, a triangular

pyramidal mass of strong connective tissue and fat, through which runs a strong raphe, which receives the insertions of the levatores ani.

URETER IN FEMALE

Abdominal Course.—Both rest on the psoas muscle, passing in front of the genito-crural nerve and behind the ovarian vessels. Anterior to the right ureter is the second part of the duodenum and mesentery and anterior to the left ureter is the pelvic colon.

Pelvic Course.—Both enter the pelvis by passing anterior to the bifurcation of the common iliac arteries. Each passes anterior to the internal iliac artery, obturator vessels and nerve, but posterior to the fossa ovarica, and thence in the parametrium, lying about three-fifths of an inch at each side of the external os, at which point each is crossed anteriorly by the uterine artery. The vagina is crossed antero-laterally, the left ureter being more anterior than the right, and then the bladder is pierced obliquely for about three-quarters of an inch. The lower end of the ureter is surrounded by a dense plexus of veins and a nerve cord joining the hypogastric and pelvic plexuses is also in near relation.

(*b*) DEVELOPMENT OF FEMALE GENITAL ORGANS

The internal genital organs come from the intermediate cell area and are derived from the Wolffian ducts, the Wolffian bodies, the Müllerian ducts and the genital ridges.

The Wolffian ducts consist of an outer longitudinal tube with three sets of tubules arising from its medial surface. Those at the cephalic end represent the pronephros. Caudal to this, tubules derived from the upper part of the mesonephros or Wolffian body have an intimate relationship with the genital gland on their ventral and medial aspects. Still more distal are the tubules from the lower part of the mesonephros. The Wolffian duct joins the pronephros to the cloaca.

Most of the Wolffian duct and body atrophy in the female, but remains are to be found as follows :—

(*a*) The Wolffian duct remains as the horizontal duct joining the vertical parovarian tubules, passing down in the parametrium to the side wall of the vagina and perhaps to the depression in the vestibule as Gärtner's duct.

(*b*) The pronephros remains as (1) Kobelt's tubules, which are found medial to Gärtner's duct at its beginning; (2) some tubules in the fimbria ovarica; (3) the hydatid of Morgagni at the fimbriated extremity of the tube.

(*c*) Upper mesonephric tubules remain as the parovarium or tubules of the epoöphoron in the mesosalpinx, the lower tubules persist as the paroöphoron between the ovary and the uterus.

The Müllerian ducts arise from the ventral surface of the mesonephric fold lateral to the Wolffian ducts. As the latter atrophy, the Müllerian ducts develop and approach each other, passing over in front of the Wolffian ducts and fusing in the midline. The upper end communicates with the peritoneal cavity, the lower end with the allantoic division of the cloaca or urogenital sinus between the openings of the Wolffian ducts. The ununited parts form the Fallopian tubes and the fused portion the uterus and vagina.

Septa in fused portions of Müllerian ducts disappear in the cervix at three and a half months, and in the body of the uterus at four and a half months. Failure to disappear and imperfect fusion cause the various forms of uterine malformation, *e.g.* septate, bicornuate, didelphys, etc.

During this stage of development the genital mesentery or gubernaculum becomes folded on itself and attached to the uterine cornu, the cephalic portion forming the ovarian ligament, the caudal portion the round ligament.

The vagina is formed from two solid columns of cells, the lower ends of the Müllerian ducts. These columns, surrounded by mesoderm, grow downwards towards the cloacal membrane, shortening the urogenital sinus in so doing. The mesoderm at the same time forms the bladder base and the posterior wall of the urethra.

Atresia of the vagina is due to failure of the solid columns to canalise; septa may arise from incomplete absorption. Resistance of that part of the cloacal membrane responsible for the development of the hymen results in imperforate hymen.

Ovary.—In the lumbar region, just medial to the intermediate cell mass, is found the genital ridge, which is covered by germinal epithelium. This latter is connected with a tubular system of cells which penetrates the ovarian substance and gives origin to the Graafian follicles.

The descent of the ovary is guided by the gubernaculum, which extends from the lower pole of the ovary to the lower part of the anterior abdominal wall and thence along the inguinal canal to the labium majus.

(c) DEVELOPMENT OF EMBRYO (see Frontispiece)

1. Fertilisation probably takes place in the Fallopian tube, the head and body of the spermatozoon fusing with the ovum.

2. Segmentation of the ovum occurs until a ball of cells—the morula—appears.

3. Some cells in the centre become vacuolated, and a space filled with fluid is formed, the blastocyst. The cells projecting into this space form the embryonic cell mass, while the outer cells lining the cavity make up the trophoblast or extra-embryonic ectoderm, and are destined to form the epithelial part of the chorion.

4. The innermost cells of the embryonic cell mass now split to enclose a cavity, the yolk sac or entoderm cavity; the surrounding cells are destined to become the entoderm.

5. About this time also the outer cells of the embryonic cell mass split to form another cavity, the amniotic cavity; the cells immediately lining this become flattened to form the embryonic ectoderm.

6. The mesoderm now appears at the sides and comes in between ectoderm and entoderm, splitting to line the outside of the yolk sac and the inner side of the trophoblast. The inner lining is called the splanchnopleure, the outer lining the somatopleure.

7. The mesoderm is specially thick between the hind end of the embryonic area and the trophoblast or primitive chorion. This mesodermal thickening is the body stalk, the forerunner of the umbilical cord.

8. The chorion consists of an outer layer of ectoderm or trophoblast and an inner layer of mesoderm, whereas the amnion is made up of an outer layer of mesoderm and an inner layer of ectoderm.

9. The embryonic area is that part where all three germinal layers are in contact, in other words, where the amniotic and entoderm cavities are approximated.

10. Then begins a process of " folding off " of the embryo.

The greater part of the entoderm cavity gradually becomes enclosed within the amniotic cavity by the latter enlarging and dipping down over each end of the embryonic area in the form of a cephalic and caudal fold, and also at each side. Eventually, the ventral surface of the embryo becomes closed except where two diverticula, formed by the part of the entoderm cavity not included, run out in the belly stalk. These diverticula are : (1) the vitelline duct and umbilical vesicle ; (2) allantois. That portion of the entoderm cavity included in the amniotic cavity forms the alimentary tract.

Embedding of Ovum

The ovum, in the blastocyst stage, reaches the uterus seven days after fertilisation. The trophoblast consists of an outer layer of thick undifferentiated and vacuolated protoplasm with no cell outline, and an inner layer of cuboidal epithelium. The former is called the plasmodi-trophoblast, the latter the cyto-trophoblast. The plasmodi-trophoblast has a destructive action on the tissues and eats into the uterine mucosa, thus allowing the ovum to become embedded in the endometrium.

Formation of Decidua

Following on implantation of the fertilised ovum in the uterus, the endometrium undergoes a series of changes to form the decidua. These changes make up the *decidual reaction.* The decidua is composed of two layers : (1) the superficial compact layer consists of gland openings and enlarged oval stroma cells or decidual cells ; (2) the deep spongy layer rests on the muscle and is made up of the deep dilated portions of the uterine glands. The decidua is much thicker than normal endometrium, becomes increasingly vascular and shows large dilated capillaries or decidual sinuses. The glands are much hypertrophied and dilated, interstitial hæmorrhages are present, while there is an appreciable loss of surface epithelium.

The decidua is divided into three parts :—

(1) The part on which the ovum rests, consisting incidentally of the deep spongy layer—*decidua basalis.*
(2) The part surrounding the ovum and between the ovum and the uterine cavity—*decidua capsularis.*
(3) The part lining the remainder of the uterine cavity—*decidua vera.*

As the ovum grows the decidua capsularis becomes progressively thinned out, and, at the end of the third month, when the ovum fills the uterine cavity, the decidua capsularis blends with the decidua vera, obliterating the decidual space.

Development of Placenta

The plasmodi-trophoblast has the power of eating into the endometrium. In this way small vessels are opened up, and

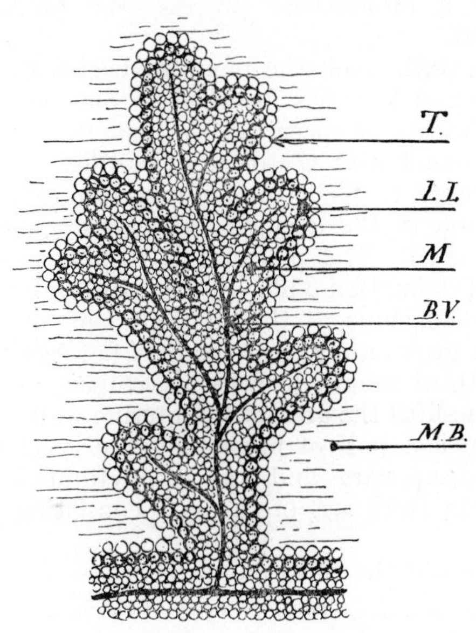

Fig. 4.—Structure of Villus.

M, Mesoderm.
L.L, Langhans' layer } Trophoblast.
T, Syncytium }
B.V, Blood-vessel.
M.B, Maternal blood.

for the first two weeks the ovum derives nourishment by blood flowing through the meshes of the plasmodi-trophoblast. About the third week the trophoblast is replaced by the formation of chorionic villi, which, at first, entirely surround the ovum. These villi consist of (1) an epithelial covering, (2) a connective tissue core, and (3) a blood-vessel system. The epithelial covering is made up of two layers, an outer layer, the syncytium, derived from the plasmodi-trophoblast, and an inner layer, Langhans' layer, which comes from the cyto-trophoblast. The syncytium consists of multi-nucleated protoplasm with no definite cell outline, while Langhans' layer is made up of large well-defined cells with oval nuclei. The blood-vessels are the terminal ramifications of the umbilical arteries and vein. The villi are of two types, the "fixation" villi, which stretch right down to the surface of the decidua, and the "nutritive" villi, which lie free in the chorio-decidual space. The blood flows round these villi and in the spaces between the villi, the intervillous spaces. At this stage the embryonic area is connected with the outer envelope by a mesoblastic process—the precursor of the umbilical cord.

About the sixth week the placenta begins to take on discoidal shape and becomes localised to one part of the periphery. At the site of specialisation, usually that part of the chorion in contact with the decidua basalis, the villi grow in size and number to form the chorion frondosum, while the villi in relation to the decidua capsularis atrophy to form the chorion læve. The placenta is firmly attached to the decidua by (1) fixation villi, and (2) subchorionic decidua, a reflection of decidua at the circumference of the placenta. The placenta grows quickly in the first few weeks and at the end of the third month is fully developed, occupying one-quarter or one-fifth the area of the uterine wall.

During the last half of pregnancy the layer of Langhans completely disappears and the syncytium becomes very thin, the main thickness of the villi consisting of distended capillaries.

The placenta at the third month consists of :—

(1) Decidua basalis, spongy layer of decidua.
(2) Chorio-decidual space.
(3) Chorion frondosum.
 (*a*) Syncytial layer.
 (*b*) Langhans' layer.
 (*c*) Mesoderm with blood-vessels.
(4) Amnion.
 (*a*) Mesoderm.
 (*b*) Ectoderm.

When the placenta separates in the third stage of labour, it does so through the base of the spongy layer of the decidua, which is thinned by the dilated glands. It then consists of :—

(1) Decidua basalis.
 (*a*) Spongy layer nearly to base (fibrotic degeneration).

(2) Blood clots.
(3) Chorion frondosum.
    (*a*) Syncytial layer.
    (*b*) Mesoderm with blood-vessels, many of which are obliterated with endarteritis.
(4) Amnion.
    (*a*) Mesoderm.
    (*b*) Ectoderm.

Placenta

The normal human placenta is usually discoid, measures 6 to 8 in. in diameter, and is $\frac{3}{4}$ to 1 in. in thickness. The placenta weighs 12 to 20 oz., the relative weight to that of the fœtus being about 1 to 6·5. The normal position of the placenta is in the upper segment of the uterus and on the anterior or posterior wall in equal frequency.

The fœtal surface is smooth and covered with amnion, while the maternal surface is rough, divided into cotyledons and covered with a greyish membrane, the decidua basalis. The chorion is thin. From the seventh month onwards the placenta undergoes infarction, and there may be areas of calcareous degeneration present.

Functions of the Placenta.—These are (1) respiratory; (2) nutritive; (3) glycogenic; (4) excretory; (5) barrier; (6) internal secretory.

1. *Respiratory.*—The fœtal blood containing carbonic acid is conveyed to the placenta by the umbilical arteries. Through the placenta an interchange is effected with maternal blood, the fœtal blood ridding itself of carbonic acid, picking up at the same time oxygen, which is conveyed to the fœtus by the umbilical vein.

2. *Nutritive.*—It is difficult to say how food is transferred from the mother to the fœtus. Some believe that a process of diffusion and osmosis, the placenta acting as a semi-permeable membrane, is responsible; others think that the placenta has the power of choosing from the maternal blood those substances which the fœtus needs. In the case of fats there is the idea that these are manufactured by the fœtus from carbohydrates.

3. *Glycogenic.*—Glycogen, absorbed as glucose, is stored by the placenta until the fœtal liver functions.

4. *Excretory.*—Through the medium of the placenta the fœtus throws off any waste products of metabolism.

5. *Barrier.*—This is a protective action which the placenta exhibits, preventing the transference of certain diseases from mother to child. This action, however, is by no means absolute.

6. *Internal Secretory.*—Chorionic gonadotrophic hormone is found in the urine very soon after implantation of the ovum and it is believed that this hormone is formed, almost entirely, by the placenta. Progesterone and œstrogen are also derived from the placenta.

Anomalies of Shape and Size.—May be irregular (*horseshoe*), and sometimes is diffuse, surrounding entire ovum (*P. membranacea*). It may be divided into distinct lobes (*P. bipartite* and *tripartite*), or may have small accessory lobules (*P. succenturiata*).

If situated in the lower uterine segment, it is called placenta prævia.

Diseases of Placenta.—

1. Superficial cysts derived from the chorion—fairly common.

2. Inflammation—associated with inflammation of the decidua.

3. Infarcts (white) occur in over 60 per cent. of placentæ. If very numerous or large they are often associated with albuminuria and eclampsia.

4. Calcification—small calcareous nodules or larger areas of calcification on the maternal surface are fairly common. The area seems to undergo a hyaline change first, followed by calcification.

5. Syphilis—the placenta is large, pale and œdematous. The villi are thickened and show round cell infiltration of the stroma while the vessels are few and the site of endarteritis.

6. Placenta Accreta—absence of the spongy layer of the decidua (see p. 18).

Umbilical Cord

The cord is usually inserted into the placenta eccentrically, and measures from 18 to 24 in. in length, but may vary from 2 to 80 in. It is composed of a mucoid tissue (Wharton's jelly) and contains two arteries and one vein (umbilical vessels). It is usually spirally twisted, in the majority of cases from left to right.

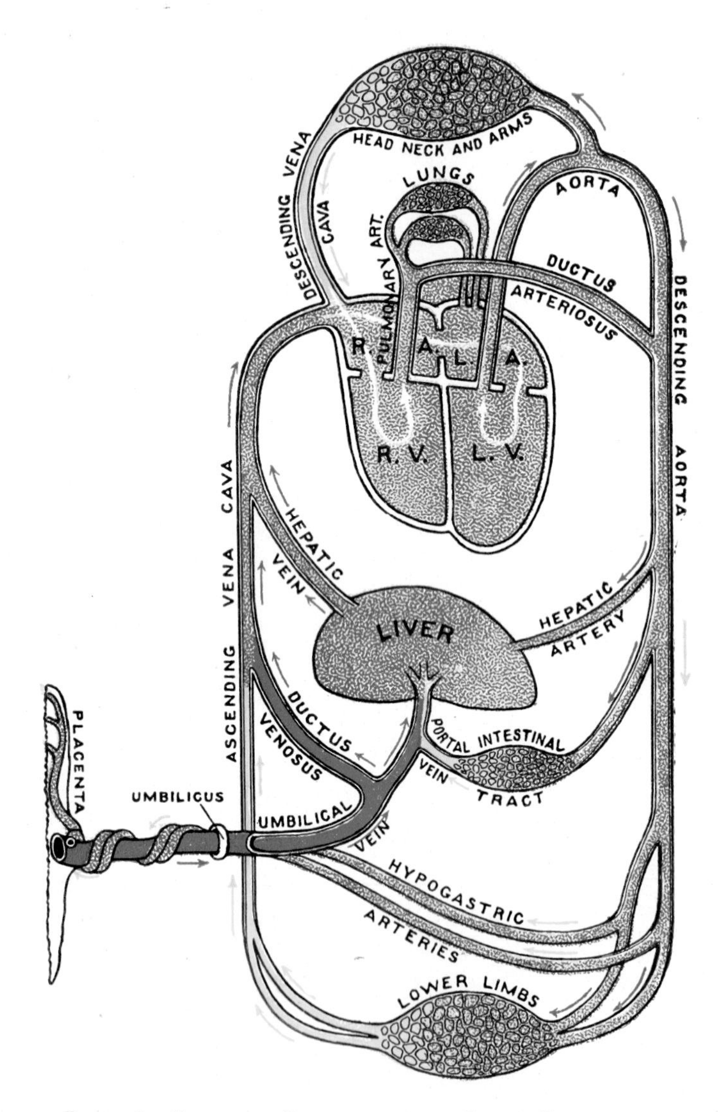

PLATE I.—SCHEMATIC DIAGRAM OF THE FŒTAL CIRCULATION.

ion.

acenta (*battledore*) ; 14 per cent. of

to the amnion and the umbilical
ie membranes before reaching the

.—

cord from fœtal movements ; if
the fœtal circulation, and may

round the limbs or neck of the
re with its growth. From this
so shortened as to impede labour
rd).

pithelium
oneum of
pearance.
ped nuclei,
mediately
the *tunica*
vum. It is
lated to it

CIRCULATION

urified arterial blood passes by way of the umbilical vein to the umbilicus, and then to the liver, to which several branches are given off. The larger stream carries on as the ductus venosus to the inferior vena cava which gathers, from the hepatic veins, blood from the liver and portal circulation. The blood then enters the right atrium, passes through the foramen ovale into the left atrium, and then into the left ventricle. From there it enters the large vessels of the head and neck.

The venous return from the head and neck enters the right atrium and, passing in front of the arterial stream flowing through the foramen ovale from right to left atrium, gains the right ventricle. Thence it enters the pulmonary artery. A little may flow through the lungs, but most goes into the ductus arteriosus, and eventually into the aorta below the arch. From there it passes into the vessels of the abdomen and lower extremities, into the hypogastric arteries, into the umbilical arteries and so back to the placenta.

After Birth.—When the child cries, the lungs are expanded, and once this happens, the blood is diverted into the pulmonary arteries rather than into the ductus arteriosus. The ductus arteriosus shrivels up and loses patency. The pressure rises in the left ventricle and falls in the right ; the foramen ovale closes ; the ductus venosus and hypogastric arteries thrombose and become obliterated.

PHYSIOLOGY

STRUCTURE OF OVARY

The ovary is made up of (*a*) Cortex and (*b*) Medulla
The **Cortex** consists of :—

(1) Germinal Epithelium.
(2) Stroma.
(3) Graafian Follicles.

Germinal Epithelium—a single layer of cuboidal
covering the ovary and continuous with the peri
the broad ligament at the hilum. Bluish-white in a

Stroma.—Connective tissue cells with spindle-sha
blood vessels, lymphatics and nerves. Stroma i
under germinal epithelium is thickened and forms
albuginea.

Graafian Follicles.—Each follicle contains an o
believed that the ovum and cells immediately r
are derived from the germinal epithelium. During the reproductive period, follicles in all stages of development are seen,
but each month, from puberty to the menopause, one follicle
becomes mature, and ruptures—*ovulation.*

Structure of Mature Graafian Follicle.—

From without inwards, the follicle consists of :—

(1) Theca externa—ordinary stroma cells.
(2) Theca interna—polygonal para-lutein cells, with granular brownish protoplasm.
(3) Stratum Granulosum—several layers of cuboidal epithelium.
(4) Cumulus Ovaricus—heaping-up of granulosa cells at one point—contains the ovum.
(5) Liquor Folliculi—fills rest of cavity and is derived from disintegration of cells in the interior of follicle.
(6) Corona Radiata—cells of cumulus ovaricus in immediate contact with ovum.
(7) Ovolemma—a thin layer of structureless material between corona and ovum.

Ovum.—

Protoplasm—(*a*) Outer—clear.
(*b*) Inner—fatty, with albuminous granules : deutoplasm.

Nucleus—lying in deutoplasm, which supplies nourishment.
Nucleolus—inside nucleus.

As the follicle becomes mature, it approaches the surface of the ovary and finally projects at a point called the stigma.

Formation of Corpus Luteum.—

When ovulation occurs, about the fourteenth day before first day of next menstrual period, the walls of the ruptured follicle collapse and there may be some bleeding in the cavity.

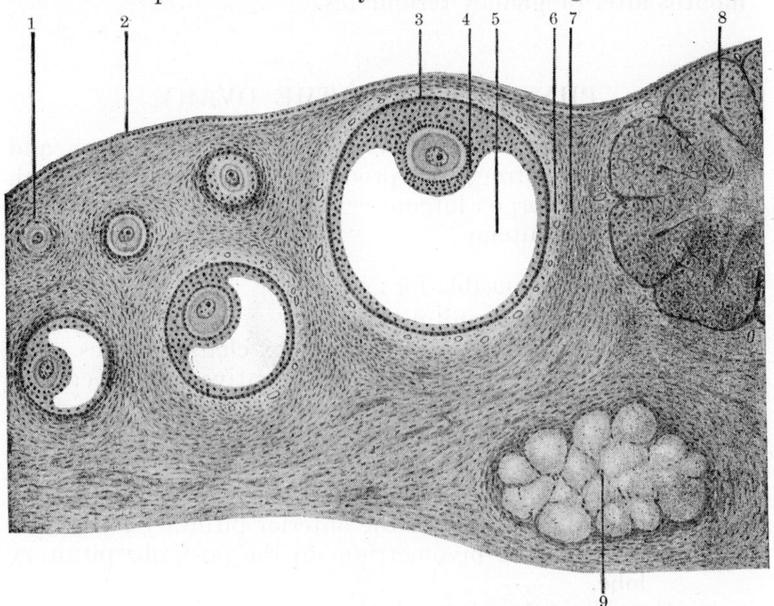

Fig. 5.—Section of Cortex of Ovary, showing Graduated Stages of Maturation of the Graafian Follicle (diagrammatic).

1. Graafian Follicle (primordial).
2. Germinal Epithelium.
3. Membrana Granulosa.
4. Cumulus Ovaricus containing Ovum.
5. Liquor Folliculi.
6. Theca Interna.
7. Theca Externa.
8. Corpus Luteum.
9. Corpus Albicans.

The theca interna becomes hyperæmic. The cells of this layer enlarge and their protoplasm becomes granular and brown—the para-lutein cells. The cells of the stratum granulosum, or as they are now called the lutein cells, multiply, enlarge and swell to fill up the cavity of the follicle. A mature corpus luteum corresponds in size to a cherry.

If conception does not occur the corpus begins to degenerate about two days before the onset of the next period. This takes the form of hyaline change while the lutein cells assume a yellow colour due to the formation of a fatty substance—lutein. The corpus luteum is finally replaced by hyaline tissue—the corpus albicans—the whole process taking some six to eight weeks.

Should the ovum be fertilised the "corpus luteum of pregnancy" is active into the third month and then begins to degenerate so slowly that traces may still be evident two months after pregnancy terminates.

PHYSIOLOGY OF THE OVARY

Two hormones are secreted by the ovary—œstrogen and progesterone. Œstrogen is produced by granulosa, thecal, interstitial and corpus luteum cells; progesterone is derived from the corpus luteum.

Œstrogen is responsible for:—

(1) Growth of the genital tract.
(2) Development of the secondary sex characteristics.
(3) Endometrial changes of proliferative and secretory phases.
(4) Increasing the tone of uterine muscle and inducing frequent contractions of low amplitude.
(5) Stimulating further the luteinising process.
(6) Inhibiting the FSH of the anterior pituitary lobe.
(7) Sensitising the myometrium to the posterior pituitary lobe.
(8) Growth of the uterus during pregnancy.
(9) Development of the duct system and enlargement of the breast.

Progesterone is responsible for:—

(1) Endometrial changes of the secretory phase.
(2) Lowering the tone of uterine muscle and inducing less frequent contractions of greater amplitude.
(3) Desensitising the myometrium to œstrogen and the posterior pituitary lobe.
(4) Inhibition of ovulation.
(5) The "decidual reaction."
(6) Growth of the uterus during pregnancy.
(7) Growth of the mammary acini.

The ovary is directly under the influence of the gonadotrophic hormones produced by the anterior pituitary lobe. Those hormones are thought to be three in number—

Follicle-stimulating hormone—FSH.
Luteinising hormone —LH.
Luteotrophic hormone —Luteotrophin.

They regulate the development of the mature Graafian follicle with the formation of œstrogen and later they control luteinisation of the follicle with the production of progesterone and continued formation of œstrogen.

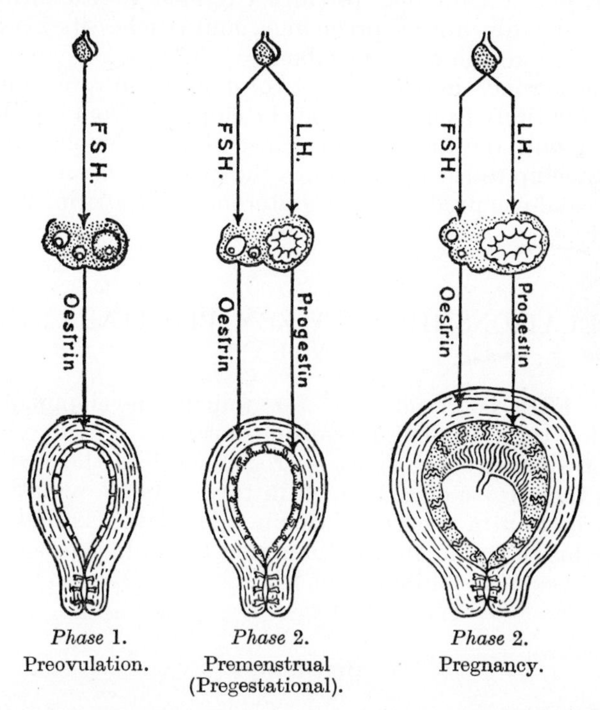

Phase 1. Preovulation. *Phase* 2. Premenstrual (Pregestational). *Phase* 2. Pregnancy.

Fig. 6.—Diagram showing the Sources, Action, and Correlation of the Various Hormones Acting on the Uterus during Three Phases of the Sex Cycle.

The luteotrophic hormone is a progesterone-stimulating agent. In pregnancy, a hormone with an action corresponding to the luteinising hormone of the anterior pituitary is produced by the chorionic villi—chorionic gonadotrophic hormone—and it is thought that this latter has a luteotrophic action. The chorionic gonadotrophic hormone is found in large quantity in the urine reaching its maximum about the sixtieth day and falling to a low level about the hundredth day—this low level is maintained until the end of pregnancy.

Injections into immature female mice of urine from pregnant women which contains much chorionic gonadotrophic hormone, cause luteinisation of the follicles and the appearance of a blood spot. This fact has been used by Aschheim and Zondek in their test for pregnancy, a correct result being obtained in over 98 per cent. of cases after one period has been missed.

Œstrone, a catabolic product excreted in the urine, increases steadily during pregnancy, and reaches its maximum shortly before the onset of labour.

Progesterone, in the first two months of pregnancy, is derived entirely from the corpus luteum, but from the third or fourth month onwards it is produced also by the placenta, and from then up to the ninth month the quantity of pregnanediol —a breakdown product of progesterone—in the urine increases steadily.

RELATIONSHIP BETWEEN PITUITARY AND OVARY

The FSH is responsible for follicle development and, provided there is some luteinising hormone present, the production of œstrogen. This œstrogen inhibits the FSH, promotes the release of LH which in turn induces ovulation and the formation of a corpus luteum. The latter is maintained by the luteotrophin and is stimulated to produce progesterone with subsequent inhibition of LH.

PUBERTY

1. Menstruation occurs.
2. Breasts enlarge and growth of hair takes place on the pubis and axillæ.
3. The mons veneris and labia become fully developed.
4. The body of the uterus enlarges.
5. Ovaries increase in breadth and mature Graafian follicles may be noted.
6. The pelvis assumes the adult female shape.
7. There is a consciousness of sex with increasing reserve and shyness.

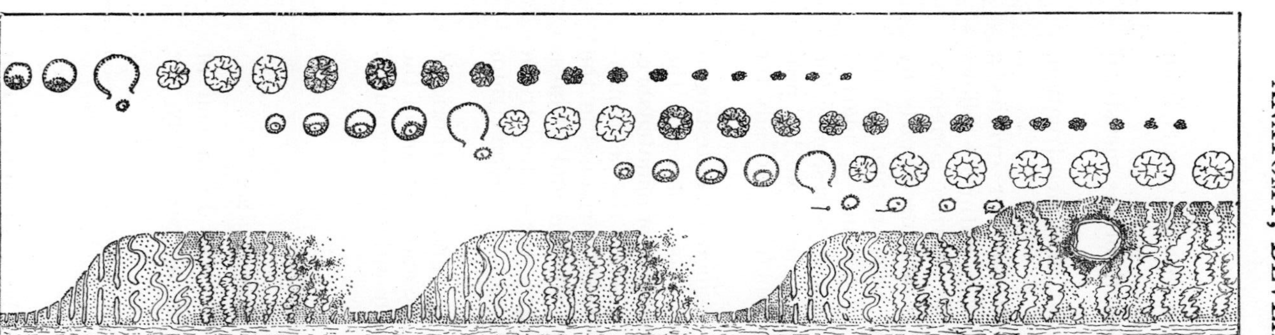

FIG. 7.—SCHEMATIC REPRESENTATION OF THE CORRELATION IN TIME BETWEEN THE STRUCTURAL CHANGES IN THE OVARY AND IN THE UTERUS DURING THE MENSTRUAL CYCLE AND EARLY PREGNANCY. (Modified from Schröder and Graves.)

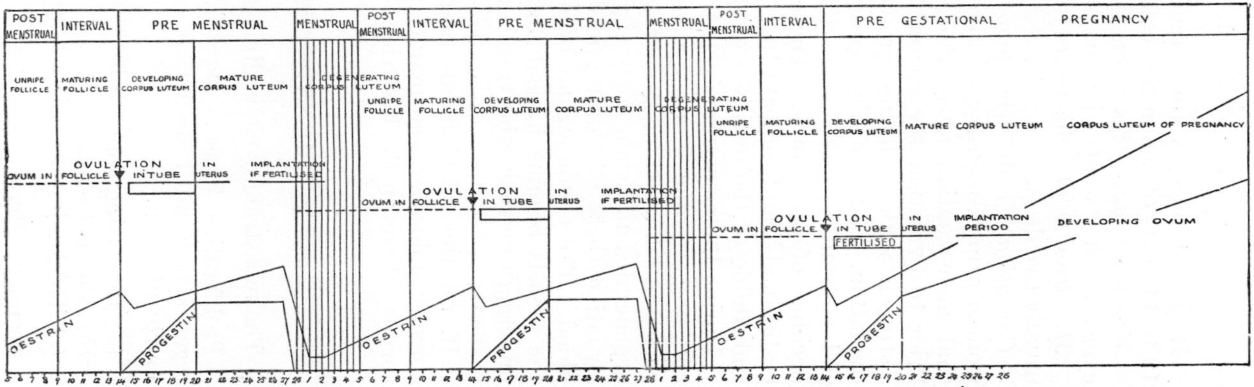

POST MENSTRUAL | INTERVAL | PRE MENSTRUAL | MENSTRUAL | POST MENSTRUAL | INTERVAL | PRE MENSTRUAL | MENSTRUAL | POST MENSTRUAL | INTERVAL | PRE GESTATIONAL | PREGNANCY

UNRIPE FOLLICLE | MATURING FOLLICLE | DEVELOPING CORPUS LUTEUM | MATURE CORPUS LUTEUM | DEGENERATING CORPUS LUTEUM | UNRIPE FOLLICLE | MATURING FOLLICLE | DEVELOPING CORPUS LUTEUM | MATURE CORPUS LUTEUM | DEGENERATING CORPUS LUTEUM | UNRIPE FOLLICLE | MATURING FOLLICLE | DEVELOPING CORPUS LUTEUM | MATURE CORPUS LUTEUM | CORPUS LUTEUM OF PREGNANCY

OVUM IN FOLLICLE | OVULATION | IN TUBE | IN UTERUS | IMPLANTATION IF FERTILISED | OVUM IN FOLLICLE | OVULATION | IN TUBE | IN UTERUS | IMPLANTATION IF FERTILISED | OVUM IN FOLLICLE | OVULATION | IN TUBE | FERTILISED | IN UTERUS | IMPLANTATION PERIOD | DEVELOPING OVUM

OESTRIN | PROGESTIN | OESTRIN | PROGESTIN | OESTRIN | PROGESTIN

5 6 7 8 9 10 11 12 13 14 15 16 17 18 19 20 21 22 23 24 25 26 27 28 1 2 3 4 5 6 7 8 9 10 11 12 13 14 15 16 17 18 19 20 21 22 23 24 25 26 27 28 1 2 3 4 5 6 7 8 9 10 11 12 13 14 15 16 17 18 19 20 21 22 23 24 25 26 27 26

Key Diagram explaining Fig. 7 (modified from Corner), and showing a Diagrammatic Graph of the Hormonal Content of the Blood.

MENSTRUATION

Begins at puberty (menarché), which usually occurs from 12 to 14 years of age in this country.

Menstrual type—this refers to the length of the menstrual cycle, usually twenty-eight days.

Menstrual habit—this refers to the duration of menstruation, usually five days.

Causation.—From the fact that without her ovaries a woman cannot menstruate, the assumption naturally follows that menstruation must depend on the ovarian hormones. Prior to ovulation the endometrium is influenced solely by œstrogen with resulting growth and proliferation. After ovulation, œstrogen and progesterone produce a marked endometrial hyperplasia where the appearances resemble the decidua of pregnancy. Those changes are termed "progestational" and indicate that the endometrium is ready for embedding of the fertilised ovum.

During the menstrual cycle there is an increase in œstrogen and progesterone levels. Should conception not occur the corpus luteum, lacking the necessary stimulus for maintenance, degenerates and some forty-eight hours before the next menstruation there is a dramatic drop of both hormones in the blood. The endometrium becomes dehydrated and shrinks, the vessels become kinked and engorged, the endometrium undergoes necrosis, the vessels rupture and the endometrium is shed.

If, on the other hand, pregnancy occurs, the chorionic gonadotrophic hormone maintains the life and function of the corpus luteum in the first three to four months of pregnancy.

MENSTRUAL PHASES

The menstrual cycle is divided into four phases :—

Proliferative Phase.—Duration eight days. From end of regeneration until ovulation occurs on approximately the fourteenth day.

(*a*) Increasing congestion.
(*b*) Glands tortuous.
(*c*) Thickening of endometrium.

Secretory Phase.—Duration fourteen days. From ovulation until beginning of menstruation.

(*a*) Increasing congestion.
(*b*) Glands enlarged, distended and tortuous.

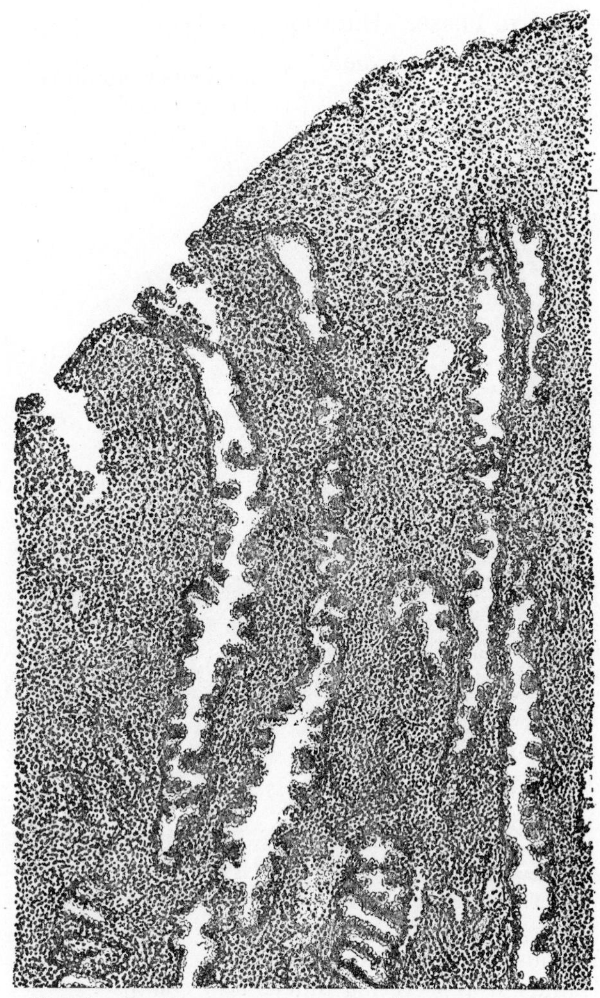

FIG. 8.—THE ENDOMETRIUM IN THE SECRETORY PHASE.

(*c*) Stroma cells enlarge—resemble decidual cells.
(*d*) Stroma becomes œdematous.
(*e*) Marked increase in thickness to as much as $\frac{1}{4}$ in.

Menstruation.—Duration four to five days.

(*a*) Subepithelial hæmatomata are poured out.

(*b*) Surface epithelium gives way.
(*c*) A few surface cells are also extruded.

Regenerative Phase.—Duration two days.

(*a*) Regeneration of stroma
(*b*) Regeneration of surface epithelium.
} From deeper portions of endometrium.

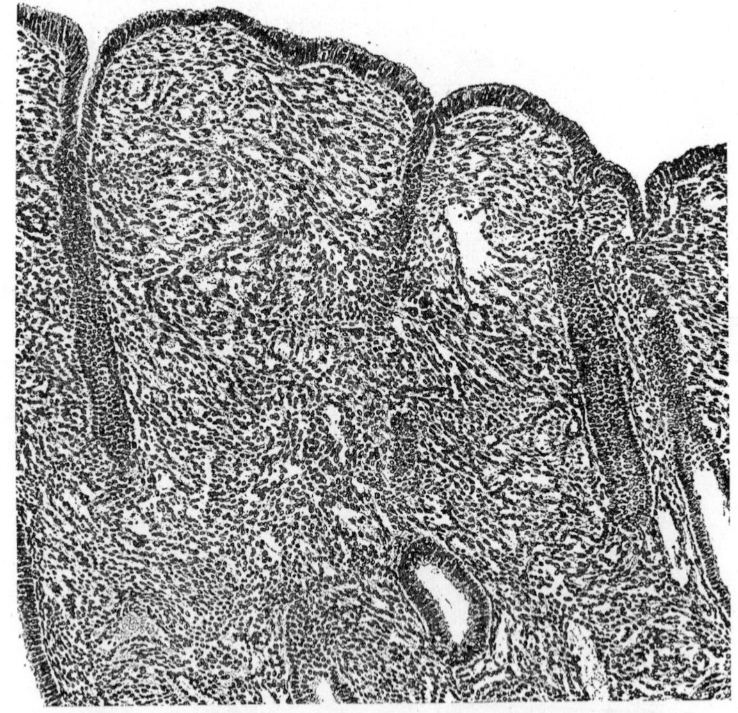

FIG. 9.—THE ENDOMETRIUM IN THE REGENERATIVE PHASE.

(*c*) Mucous membrane shrinks.
(*d*) Glands stop secreting mucus and collapse.

COMPOSITION OF MENSTRUAL FLOW

(1) Blood containing an excess of calcium salts. (2) Mucin (33 per cent.). (3) Lactic acid. (4) Epithelial cells. (5) No fibrinogen or fibrin ferment present.

Menstrual blood normally does not clot.

GENERAL FACTS IN REGARD TO MENSTRUATION

(1) Begins earlier in hot countries.
(2) Enlargement of mammæ, thyroid and parotid may occur.
(3) Most likely time for acne eruptions.
(4) Headaches, lassitude, etc., common.

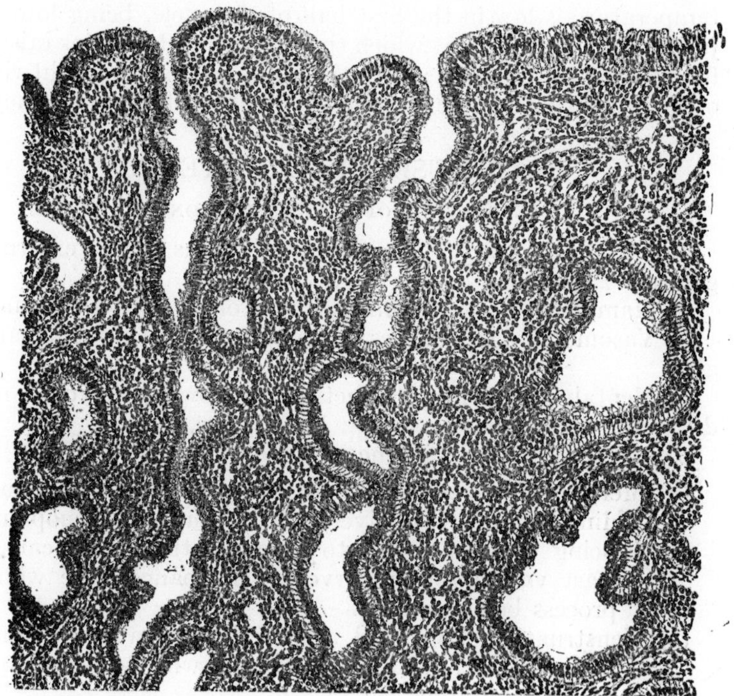

FIG. 10.—THE ENDOMETRIUM IN THE PROLIFERATIVE PHASE.

(5) Pulse slowed, blood pressure raised during secretory phase and lowered after menstruation starts.
(6) Red blood corpuscles are increased before, and decreased after, menstruation begins.
(7) Coagulability of systemic blood is diminished during menstruation.
(8) Diminution of calcium content of blood.
(9) Nervous system more susceptible. Reflex irritability is increased.

OVULATION

Usually occurs fourteen days before next period is due, *i.e.* about twelfth to sixteenth day of menstrual cycle, the exact day depending on menstrual type. If the ovum is fertilised the corpus luteum enlarges, being dependent on the chorionic gonadotrophic hormone from the growing ovum, and materially helps the nidation of the ovum in the uterus; if the ovum is not fertilised the corpus luteum regresses and menstruation occurs. The morning rectal temperature is low in the first half of the cycle, being lowest just before ovulation, at which time it rises and remains raised for the rest of the cycle; if fertilisation occurs this slight rise of temperature continues during the first months of pregnancy.

MENOPAUSE OR CLIMACTERIC

(Cessation of Menstruation)

1. Atrophic changes in ovaries, uterus and external genitals.
2. Mammary tissue atrophies, but is often replaced by fat.
3. Vasomotor disturbances (flushings). Temperament variable.
4. Mental derangement sometimes, following nervous and dyspeptic phenomena.
5. Menopause occurs in one of three ways:—

(*a*) Menstruation becomes less frequent and the loss diminishes progressively, the complete menopause being effected in six to nine months. This causes least vasomotor or nervous disturbances, the whole process being gradual.

(*b*) Menstruation stops and amenorrhœa is at once complete. This is usually associated with severe menopausal symptoms.

(*c*) Periods of amenorrhœa, followed by a severe bleeding in each case, until there is permanent amenorrhœa, usually in six to nine months.

(*N.B.—Such cases should always be curetted for diagnostic purposes, as it is impossible to be certain that carcinoma is not the cause of the bleeding.*)

INTERNAL SECRETORY ORGANS IN WOMEN

(*a*) Thyroid

1. Intimately related to generative organs and function.
2. The thyrotropic function of the pituitary is depressed by a high level of thyroid function and stimulated by a low level.

3. The thyroid hormone may have a specific effect on the gonadotrophic activity of the pituitary or upon the ovary.

4. The ovary is depressed by large doses of thyroid hormone and stimulated by small doses.

5. Enlarges at puberty, during pregnancy and at the menopause.

6. More liable to disease in women. Thyrotoxicosis produces a relative deficiency of œstrogen and is associated with oligomenorrhœa or amenorrhœa while in myxœdema there is hyperœstrinism with menorrhagia and metrorrhagia.

7. Hypofunction in the very young may inhibit full sexual development.

8. In hyper- and hypo-thyroidism there is relative sterility and a tendency to miscarry.

9. The libido is increased in hyperthyroidism and lessened in myxœdema.

10. Aids embedding of the ovum either by an effect on the ovum or by an effect on tissue growth.

11. Is given in sterility and habitual abortion.

12. Accelerates involution and plays a part in the process of lactation.

(*b*) Anterior Pituitary Body

1. The anterior lobe produces: (*a*) gonadotrophic hormones —FSH, LH, Luteotrophin; (*b*) the growth hormone; (*c*) the thyrotrophic hormone; (*d*) the adrenotrophic hormone; (*e*) the lactogenic hormone; (*f*) the mammogenic hormone.
The anterior lobe may also be concerned with the metabolism of carbohydrates, fats and proteins.

2. When removed, the ovaries atrophy and œstrogen is completely suppressed, whereas grafts of anterior pituitary re-establish activity.

3. Castration promotes increase in size and function suggesting that an ovarian hormone has an inhibiting effect. Œstrogen and, to a lesser extent, progesterone have this effect.

4. Hypersecretion causes gigantism and acromegaly; hyposecretion causes dwarfism and hypophyseal cachexia (Simmonds' disease).

(*c*) Posterior Pituitary Body

1. Increases in size during pregnancy and after oophorectomy.

2. Produces oxytocic factor which stimulates myometrial contractions. Those vary in intensity according to the phase of the menstrual cycle and whether the uterus is gravid or not. In pregnancy the maximum effect is produced during labour; in early pregnancy and in the puerperium the response is slight.

3. Produces vasopresser factor which acts on the muscle of the vessels causing blanching of the skin and a rise of pulse rate, oxygen consumption and cardiac output. The respiratory rate is accelerated and the smooth muscle of the small and large intestines is stimulated.

4. Is responsible for an antidiuretic principle which plays an important part in water metabolism.

(*d*) Chorionic Gonadotrophin

1. Produced by placenta and is said to have a luteotrophic action.

2. Presence in the urine is used as a basis for pregnancy tests. A positive result may be obtained within seven days of the first missed period. In hydatidiform mole and chorionepithelioma the titre level is increased.

(*e*) Adrenal Cortex

1. Produces desoxycorticosterone, a hormone essential for life, which leads to the conservation of water, chloride and sodium and excretion of potassium.

2. Produces corticosterone which affects carbohydrate metabolism.

3. Produces an androgenic hormone with masculinising properties; metabolites are excreted in the urine as 17-keto-steroids.

4. Produces an œstrogenic hormone.

5. The adrenal glands may enlarge during pregnancy.

6. Excessive secretion causes sterility, defeminising, and, later, masculinising characteristics.

(*f*) Thymus

The functions of the thymus are not known with certainty. There is the possibility that this gland is concerned with somatic growth and genital development. The gland atrophies at puberty.

CHAPTER II

DIAGNOSIS OF PREGNANCY

TABLE OF SIGNS AND SYMPTOMS IN ORDER OF OCCURRENCE

Months.	1	2	3	4	5	6	7	8	9
Suppression menses	x	x	x	x	x	x	x	x	x
Pulsation in fornices vaginæ	?	x	x	x	x	x	x	x	x
Morning sickness	..	x	x	x	..	..	..	..	..
Softening of cervix and L.U.S.	..	x	x	x	x	x	x	x	x
		P.V.	P.V.		ab	dom	inall	y	
Regular enlargement of uterus	..	?	x	x	x	x	x	x	x
Mammary areola	..	..	x	x	x	x	x	x	x
Dusky hue of vagina and cervix	..	..	?	x	x	x	x	x	x
Uterine souffle	..	..	..	x	x	x	x	x	x
Ballottement	..	..	..	x	x	x	x	..	..
Fœtal heart	..	..	..	?	x	x	x	x	x
Quickening	..	..	..	x	x	x	x	x	x
Uterine contraction	..	..	..	x	x	x	x	x	x
Palpable fœtal parts and movements	..	..	..	..	x	x	x	x	x

The signs and symptoms of pregnancy may be divided into **probable** and **absolute.**

The **probable** are only of value when taken collectively, for independently they may all result from other causes. They are, however, the only guides during the first half of gestation.

The **absolute** are represented by the detection of the fœtal heart and parts, and are not recognisable till the latter half of pregnancy.

PROBABLE SIGNS AND SYMPTOMS

1. Amenorrhœa

Occurs usually immediately after conception and is thus commonly relied on for calculating the probable date of confinement. Alone it is of little value in diagnosing pregnancy or calculating the date of confinement, because—

1. It arises from other causes—

    (*a*) Anæmia (gradual in onset).
    (*b*) Fear of being pregnant.

(*c*) Desire of being pregnant.
(*d*) Menopause and superinvolution.
(*e*) Lactation.

2. Menstruation may continue during pregnancy—
(*a*) In early months before deciduæ capsularis and vera have united.
(*b*) To term, from an empty horn of a double uterus (rarely). Bleeding may be due to cervical polypi, erosions and cancer of cervix.

3. Conception may occur during abeyance of menstruation—
(*a*) During lactation.
(*b*) Before menstruation is established.
(*c*) In anæmia.

2. Pulsation in Anterior Vaginal Fornix
(**Osiander's Sign**)

Of value in early weeks if associated with enlargement and softening of uterus. It is due to the increased vascularity of the uterus following impregnation.

3. Morning Sickness

A reflex symptom, usually represented by a feeling of nausea, occurring any time during the day, but frequently more marked on first rising in the morning, hence name.

It begins, as a rule, after the first menstrual period is missed and ceases during the fourth month, when the uterus rises out of the pelvis. It may, however, be entirely absent or be so severe and prolonged as to form a serious complication. It is thus of little value alone in diagnosing pregnancy.

4. Softness of Uterus, Cervix, and Lower Uterine Segment

In the early weeks the uterus and cervix become softish (**Rasch's sign**), but it is not till the sixth to tenth week that the excessive softness of the lower uterine segment is marked. This is probably due to the increased vascularity of the parts and is a most valuable sign. From the excessive softness of the lower uterine segment it is difficult to follow the continuity of the cervix with the body and they thus appear separate on bimanual examination. This condition is known as **Hegar's sign** of pregnancy; after the tenth week it gradually disappears.

5. Enlargement of the Uterus

This is of a progressive nature and is the most valuable aid to diagnosis before the detection of the fœtal heart. In the early months it is to be recognised by the bimanual method of examination.

For the first three months the size increases chiefly antero-posteriorly and transversely, the uterus becoming globular and remaining in the pelvis. After this time it increases vertically as well and thus the fundus rises into the abdomen.

If it be remembered that at the end of the first month the ovum is the size of a pigeon's egg, at the end of the second month a hen's egg, and the third month a goose's egg, a better idea of the size of the uterus will be gained than by a detailed description and measurements.

The increase in the size of the abdomen becomes apparent during the fourth month, at the end of which period the fundus uteri may be felt three finger breadths above the pubis. As this enlargement closely coincides with the period of pregnancy, the position of the fundus uteri is a valuable guide in estimating the probable date of confinement when other means are absent. This regularity of growth is also of value in determining pregnancy from other abdominal swellings whose growth is irregular.

On account of this rapid enlargement, the abdominal skin stretches, causing *striæ* to form. These are pinkish when recent, and white when due to previous pregnancies.

A dark line (*Linea Nigra*) often appears in the midline between the umbilicus and the symphysis, especially in brunettes.

Average Rate of Increase in Size of Uterus During Pregnancy

In 12 weeks—level with symphysis.
In 16 weeks—two finger-breadths above symphysis.
In 18 to 20 weeks—midway between pubis and umbilicus.
In 24 weeks—immediately below umbilicus.

In 28 weeks—two finger-breadths above umbilicus.

In 32 weeks—midway between umbilicus and xiphisternum.

In 36 weeks—at xiphisternum.

In 40 weeks—in primigravidæ two finger-breadths' descent owing to head entering pelvis.

Too rapid increase may indicate hydatidiform mole, hydramnios or twins.

During the ninth month, in primigravidæ with an average-sized pelvis—

1. The uterine tumour falls slightly.
2. Breathing becomes more easy.
3. Locomotion more difficult.
4. Micturition more frequent.

These symptoms form the so-called *lightening* before labour, and are due to the " taking up " of the cervix from above downwards, which results in the absorption of its canal into the general uterine cavity and thus permits of descent of the head into the pelvis.

6. Mammary Changes

1. Enlargement of glands and distension of superficial veins, associated with a feeling of fullness in the organs, which are frequently painful.

2. After the third month formation of areolæ and turgidity of nipple, with the secretion of serous fluid. The areola of pregnancy is characterised by—

(*a*) A darkening of the normal pink areola, varying from a light brown in blondes to black in brunettes.

(*b*) An enlargement of the sebaceous glands (10 to 20) surrounding the nipple, forming papillæ (*Montgomery's tubercles*).

(*c*) A secondary areola may develop later outside the papillæ.

Value of Sign.—Though characteristic of pregnancy, it is by no means absolute, similar changes occurring in spurious pregnancy, and occasionally with ovarian cysts. In multiparæ the mammary changes are of little value, as the areolæ, once formed, never fade entirely, while fluid may be squeezed out of the breast years after lactation has ceased. Pregnancy may be present with few or no breast changes.

7. Dusky Hue of Vagina and Vulva

(**Jacquemier's Sign**)

A violet discoloration, due to engorgement of the vaginal bulbs and venous plexuses, generally well marked by fourth month, but, being absent in about 17 per cent. and present in some cases of uterine fibroids, is not an absolute sign.

8. Uterine Souffle

A soft, blowing murmur, synchronous with the pulse, heard over the uterus by auscultation, due to blood passing through the tortuous uterine arteries; therefore best heard slightly above the symphysis pubis after the fourth month, when the uterus is abdominal, but later can often be heard anywhere below the umbilicus.

It may be present also in fibroids of the uterus, and is therefore valueless alone as a sign of pregnancy.

This must not be confused with a **funic souffle,** which is due to some pressure on the cord and is synchronous with the fœtal heart, being, of course, diagnostic of pregnancy.

9. Ballottement: (*a*) *Internal*

A passive movement of the fœtus, whereby it can be detected floating in the liquor amnii. It is obtained by pushing sharply per vaginam on the lower pole of the uterus through the anterior fornix and retaining the fingers there in situ; by this means the fœtus is pushed up towards the fundus uteri, but sinking again, will be distinctly felt impinging upon the fingers. It is thus most manifest when the liquor amnii is relatively large in amount compared to the size of the fœtus (fifth to eighth month), and most conveniently performed with the patient in the dorsal position, with the shoulders raised.

(*b*) *External*

A similar process, but obtained with both hands placed externally, one on either side of the abdominal swelling.

It may be simulated by a solid ovarian tumour surrounded by ascitic fluid, a pedunculated fibroid or a stone in the bladder.

10. Uterine Contractions. **(Braxton Hicks' Sign)**

Painless contractions of the uterus occurring at intervals of from five to twenty minutes, and continuing from three to five minutes; these can be felt by laying the hand over the uterus after the third month.

Although a valuable diagnostic sign, it may be simulated by soft uterine myomata and hæmatometra.

ABSOLUTE SIGNS

11. Fœtal Heart

An absolute sign, generally first heard from the eighteenth to twentieth week, and is often as distinct then as in the later months.

It resembles closely the ticking of a watch under a pillow.

Frequency.—Normally varies from 120 to 160 beats per minute.

The frequency is diminished—

(*a*) During uterine contractions.
(*b*) In cases of fœtal suffocation.

The frequency is increased—

(*a*) By high maternal temperature (fever, etc.).
(*b*) In fœtal suffocation.

Position of Greatest Intensity.—In earlier months usually near midline, about 2 in. above the symphysis.

In later months according to presentation and position of fœtus (see Fig. 11).

(*a*) *In Cephalic Presentations with the Occiput Anterior.*—At the junction of upper and middle thirds of a line from umbilicus to middle of Poupart's ligament, to right or left, according to the position of dorsum of fœtus.

(*b*) *In Cephalic Presentations with Occiput Posterior.*—About 2 to 2½ in. out from (*a*) towards flanks to right or left, according to dorsum of fœtus.

(*c*) *In Pelvic Presentations.*—Above the plane of umbilicus to right or left, according to dorsum of fœtus.

In twin pregnancy two areas of greatest intensity are heard, the sound diminishing between them and the two rates differing, being heard by two observers at the same time.

Points of Diagnosis Derived from Fœtal Heart Sounds.—

1. Pregnancy.
2. Life of fœtus.
3. Presentation and position of fœtus.
4. Multiple pregnancy.
5. Threatened asphyxia of fœtus.

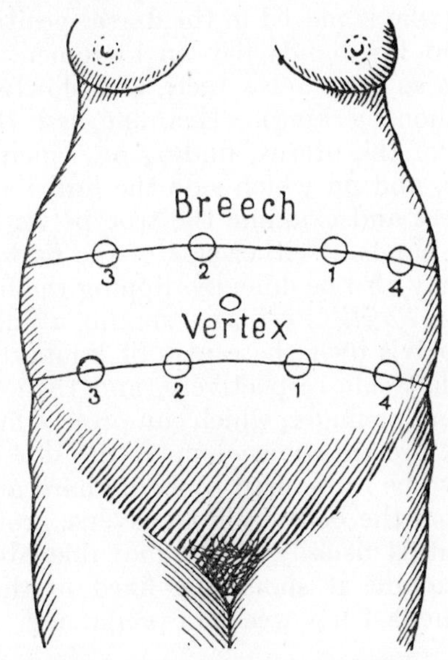

FIG. 11.—POINTS OF MAXIMUM INTENSITY OF FŒTAL HEART-SOUNDS IN VERTEX AND PELVIC PRESENTATIONS.

1. L.O.A. and L.S.A.
2. R.O.A. and R.S.A.
3. R.O.P. and R.S.P.
4. L.O.P. and L.S.P.

12. FŒTAL MOVEMENTS

Usually first felt by the mother about the eighteenth week, but varies from sixteenth to twentieth. This is called **quickening.** The sensation is usually at first of a fluttering or pulsating character and is sometimes associated with faintness. This is almost a positive sign in multiparæ who have felt them before.

In the later months the movements become objective, being recognisable by sight and touch and in some cases they are so severe as to cause the mother much discomfort.

Their prolonged absence, though suspicious, is by no means indicative of death, while their presence is so closely simulated by borborygmi that subjectively they cannot be taken as a guarantee of pregnancy.

13. Fœtal Parts

To be made out in the later months of pregnancy by abdominal palpation.

Palpation: Method of Performance.—Stand at one side of the patient (who is placed in the dorsal position, with knees drawn up), and lay hands flat on abdomen. Keep patient in conversation so as to relax recti, and slowly insinuate tips of fingers (without jerking). Examine first the fundus and then the sides of the uterus, finding on which side the back of the fœtus is, and on which side the limbs are. Then face the patient's feet and examine the true pelvis by passing the fingers of both hands at either side of the part of fœtus lying there. (This may also be done by dipping the fingers in above the pubis, or by *Pawlik's grip*, *i.e.* sinking a finger and thumb into the false pelvis over the centre of Poupart's ligament on the right and left side respectively, and then approximating them.) The hand or finger, which can project farthest into the pelvis in vertex presentations, denotes the side of the occiput.

The head is to be recognised by being hard and smooth and is separated from the body by a transverse groove—the neck. In multiparæ it is usually freely movable above the brim, but in primigravidæ it should be fixed in the brim of the pelvis during the last few weeks of pregnancy.

14. X-rays

The fœtus can be discerned by means of X-rays from the sixteenth to eighteenth week.

15. Biological Tests

By Aschheim-Zondek reaction (see p. 26) and Friedman test (Rabbit). The Xenopus test (spawning of the frog Xenopus on injection of urine) is quicker, giving a result in twelve hours, but recently a more rapid test with the male frog Rana Pipiens has been advocated; 5 c.c. urine are injected into dorso-lateral lymph sac and spermatazoa are found in the urine or cloacal smear four hours later. This test is only accurate during the first three months of pregnancy.

16. Drug Tests

Prostigmin methylsulphate 1 mgm. injected on three successive days will bring on a period if amenorrhœa is not due to a pregnancy.

Differential Diagnosis

The diagnosis of pregnancy should never be communicated unless absolute certainty is entertained. It may most commonly be confounded with—

Ovarian tumours.
Fibroid tumours of uterus.
Ascites.
Pseudocyesis.

Salient Points of Differential Diagnosis.—1. *From Ovarian Tumour*—

(*a*) Regularity of growth of uterine tumour.
(*b*) Amenorrhœa (sudden in onset).
(*c*) Fœtal heart and parts.
(*d*) Uterine contractions.
(*e*) Uterine souffle.
(*f*) Regular outline of tumour.
(*g*) Softness of genital tract.
(*h*) Ballottement.

2. *From Fibroids by*—

(*a*) Amenorrhœa (most important).
(*b*) Softness of uterus.
(*c*) Regular rate of growth.
(*d*) Regular outline of tumour.
(*e*) Fœtal heart.
(*f*) Breast changes.

3. *From Ascites by*—

(*a*) Fœtal heart and parts.
(*b*) Uterine souffle.
(*c*) Softness of cervix.
(*d*) History of growth.
(*e*) Ballottement.
(*f*) Uterine contractions.
(*g*) No dullness in flanks.

4. *From Pseudocyesis by*—

(*a*) Dull note on percussion.
(*b*) Non-disappearance of swelling under anæsthesia.
(*c*) Fœtal heart and parts.

CHAPTER III

ANTENATAL CARE

PREGNANT women require to exercise a certain amount of care at all times, but this varies much in different individuals. Some abort from the least indiscretion, while others can endure much without in the least tending to produce premature expulsion or other untoward symptoms.

Abortion is most liable to occur during the first three months of pregnancy, before the placenta has fully formed, and therefore if special care is to be taken it should be during the early months. Women who have shown a special tendency to abortion should be carefully treated, especially in the early months and at the time a menstrual period would have occurred had the patient not been pregnant.

During pregnancy plenty of fresh air is always beneficial, as there is a normal excess of carbon dioxide in the blood.

Exercise should always be moderate, and specially so in the later months. Fatigue must always be avoided.

Walking is the best form of exercise, but motoring in the country may be encouraged ; long journeys and rough roads are always objectionable.

Crowded entertainments are apt to bring on syncope in some women and are therefore to be avoided.

The method of dress is most important.

Tight corsets are at all times to be condemned, but especially so after the fourth month. When abdominal enlargement manifests itself, elastic-sided corsets or an obstetric belt are to be recommended and are most comfortable ; if these cannot be obtained, a flannel binder forms an excellent substitute.

Garters, if used, should be worn above the knee, and must never be tight ; suspenders are preferable.

Warm under-drawers should always be worn, but especially in later months, when from the prominence of the abdomen the skirts are removed from the legs, and chilling may result.

An ordinary pre-war mixed diet is all that is usually required with perhaps an excess of sugar during the early months. If an ordinary diet is not available, then A, C, and D vitamins should be given. If plenty of milk is drunk, then extra calcium is not usually required unless symptoms of calcium deficiency such as dental caries, etc., show themselves. An excess of calcium would appear to harden the bones of the fœtal skull and retard moulding. Diet should be restricted to ordinary proportions, as an excessive diet may increase size of child.

The bowels during pregnancy have a special tendency towards constipation and should be regulated by light aperients, as cascara, senna, liquorice, etc. Plenty of water should be drunk.

Warm baths should be taken regularly, but cold bathing is contra-indicated.

The breasts, if painful and heavy, should be supported by bandages and the nipples for the last three months of gestation should be bathed daily and if retracted gently drawn out after being anointed with stilbœstrol ointment or lanoline.

Examination of Urine and Blood Pressure

In a normal case the urine should be tested for albumen once a month until the twenty-eighth week, then fortnightly till the thirty-fourth week, and then once a week till delivery. If albumen is found at any time, or if the blood pressure is found to be raised, the urine must be tested more frequently, as occasion demands.

(*N.B.*—If the boiling test is used to detect the presence of albumen, the urine **must be acidified** either before or after boiling, otherwise the presence of even a large quantity of albumen may not be detected.)

(Albumen may be found in the urine owing to contamination with vaginal discharge and, if this is suspected, a catheter specimen is required.)

The urine may also be tested for sugar, but this is not nearly so important as the test for albumen, as 40 per cent. of pregnant women have sugar in their urine at some time during their pregnancy and its presence in the great majority of cases is of no importance.

The blood pressure should be estimated on the occasions when the urine is tested.

The normal blood pressure during pregnancy tends to be low, and the systolic pressure is often 100/60 to 110/70 mm. Hg. A blood pressure of over 135/90 mm. Hg. in a woman under thirty years of age should always be treated with suspicion, especially if associated with a trace of albumen in the urine.

(A high diastolic pressure is of particular importance in diagnosing a toxæmia and its severity.)

Regular weighing will reveal on occasion an occult œdema. Normally a woman increases by about 24 lb. during a pregnancy, gaining about 4 lb. monthly during fourth and fifth months, 5 lb. during sixth and seventh months, but only 3 lb. during last two months. Any monthly increase over 5 lb. should be viewed with suspicion.

The patient should be instructed to report at once if she has (*a*) any swelling of the face, feet or hands ; (*b*) headaches ; (*c*) dimness or abnormality of vision ; (*d*) diminished urine output ; (*e*) any bleeding per vaginam, however slight ; (*f*) pain ; (*g*) constipation ; (*h*) sickness.

Sexual intercourse must be prohibited after the seventh month of pregnancy, as in the later months it is a cause of puerperal sepsis. In the early months it is liable to cause abortion and is therefore absolutely contra-indicated for women who have a tendency to abort.

Pelvic Measurements

The following measurements of the pelvis should be taken in all primigravidæ and in multiparæ, who give the history of a difficult previous labour : (*a*) *External*—(1) Interspinous and (2) Intercristal Diameters, (3) External Conjugate, (4) Intertuberischial, and (5) Posterior Sagittal Diameters ; and (*b*) *Internal*—Diagonal Conjugate.

These diameters are measured as follows :—

1. *Interspinous Diameter.*—By means of a pelvimeter, the tips being held between the first finger and thumb of either hand, one tip being placed on the outer edge of one anterior superior spine and the other on the opposite, the distance between being read off on the scale. This should normally measure 9-10 in.

2. *Intercristal Diameter.*—Slide the tips of the pelvimeter along the outer edges of the crests of the ilia until the farthest points apart are reached and then read the scale. This diameter usually measures 10-11 in.

(*N.B.*—It is the 1 in. of difference between these two readings, which is of importance, for if the interspinous diameter approximates to the intercristal it means that there is a flaring out of the iliac spines, which is commonly associated with rickets and makes one suspect a contracted pelvis due to rickets. Very small measurements, *e.g.* 8 and 9 in., would tend to show a generally contracted pelvis.)

3. *External Conjugate.*—Place one tip of the pelvimeter on the fifth lumbar spine and the other on the anterior surface of the symphysis pubis. This should measure 7½ to 7¾ in. and on subtraction of 3½ in. the true conjugate is estimated. This measurement is apt to be erroneous on account of adiposity over spine.

(*N.B.*—The fifth lumbar spine can always be found by drawing a line between the posterior superior spines of the ilium and taking 1½ in. above its midpoint. In some women it is seen as the top angle of a rhomboid (Michaelis'), which is found on the back, the two lateral angles being the posterior superior spines, and the lower angle being the base of the sacrum.)

4. *Intertuberischial Diameter.*—Best measured with a ruler or tape measure between the inner borders of the ischial tuberosities, the patient lying on her left side with her knees well drawn up. This diameter normally measures 4 in.

5. *Posterior Sagittal Diameter.*—Measured by similar means as (4) from the midpoint of the line joining the ischial tuberosities (middle of anus) to the lower border of the sacrum. This normally measures 2½ in.

Diagonal Conjugate.—Pass two fingers into the vagina, the patient lying on her left side with her head well flexed and the knees drawn up. Locate the promontory of the sacrum with the tip of the second finger and mark off with the other hand where the lower anterior border of the symphysis touches the vaginal hand. Measure the distance between that point and the tip of the second finger. This normally measures at least 4½ to 4¾ in., and on subtraction of ½ in. gives the Conjugata Vera.

(*N.B.*—This is a much more reliable measurement than the external as there is no fat or muscle to cause error. It, however, cannot be made easily till the parts are relaxed and soft, a condition not usually present until six weeks before labour is due.)

Definitions

1. **Attitude** is the relation of fœtal parts to one another in utero. The normal attitude is complete flexion.

2. The **lie** is the relation of the long axis of the child to the long axis of the mother.

3. The **presentation** is the part of the fœtus occupying the

lower uterine segment. The **presenting part** is the part felt on vaginal examination.

4. The **position** is the relation of the presenting part to the pelvis of the mother. The **denominator** is the area of the presenting part which indicates the position, *e.g.* occiput for vertex, sacrum for breech, mentum for face.

EXAMINATIONS DURING PREGNANCY

In a normal case the patient need only be examined three times before her confinement is due, but if any abnormality is found then frequent examination may be required.

First Examination.—As early in pregnancy as possible, preferably as soon as a period has been missed. By this means many abortions due to retroversion can be saved, sickness treated at its earliest appearance and excessive sickness avoided, constipation treated early, which may prevent toxæmia at a later date, and the comparatively rare condition of ectopic gestation diagnosed before acute and dangerous symptoms are caused. At this examination—

1. Medical and obstetric history is taken, patient is physically examined and blood pressure recorded.
2. External pelvic measurements are taken.
3. Vaginal examination to corroborate diagnosis of pregnancy, having special regard to the position and size of the uterus, condition of appendages and presence of constipation or vaginal discharge.

Second Examination.—Five weeks before confinement is due. This examination is especially made at this time: (1) To diagnose presentation of fœtus—if malpresentation is present this is probably the optimum time for correction, as the relative size of fœtus to amount of liq. amnii allows of external version, and when performed the head begins to fix in the pelvis and recurrence of malpresentation is unlikely; (2) to measure diagonal conjugate in primigravidæ or cases with history of difficult labour—the parts being fairly soft at this time; if contraction is found there is time to induce premature labour if considered necessary, as this should never be done before the thirty-sixth week in the interests of the child; and (3) to take the blood pressure and test the urine. At this examination:—

1. Abdominal palpation to diagnose presentation and position.

2. Auscultation of fœtal heart.
3. Blood pressure and urine.
4. Estimation of diagonal conjugate (primigravidæ).

Third Examination.—Two weeks before confinement is due. This examination is especially useful in primigravidæ, and is made especially to find if the head is fixed in the pelvis, as it ought to be, and if not, the reason for the non-fixation along with the estimation of the size of the head with the size of the pelvis. At this examination :—

1. Diagnosis of presentation and position.
2. Fixation of head in pelvis.
3. Auscultation.
4. Blood pressure and urine.

Causes of Non-fixation of Head in Primigravida.—The commonest causes for non-fixation of the head at this time in a primigravida are : (1) Occipito-posterior position ; (2) slight extension of child's head ; (3) contracted pelvis or large head ; (4) constipation with loaded rectum ; and (5) placenta prævia.

Methods of Estimating Size of Head with Size of Pelvis

If the head is not fixed, the question is whether it will enter the pelvis, and this can be estimated by several methods : (1) **Pinard's**—the head being pushed down into the pelvis, estimating with fingers sinking in above symphysis if head enters pelvis or if there is any overlap ; (2) **Fahmy's**—a hand is pressed firmly down upon the fœtal head at the pelvis with the patient lying flat. She is then told to sit up, the hand still being kept on the fœtal head, which will be felt to slide into pelvis if there is no disproportion or one's fingers can be inserted between head and pelvis ; and (3) **Munro Kerr's** (especially useful under anæsthesia in difficult cases)—the head being pushed into the pelvis from above, whilst, with two fingers in the vagina and the thumb over the symphysis, it is felt (1) by the fingers if the head comes down into the pelvis, and (2) by the thumb how much space there is between symphysis and head, or how much overlap of symphysis by head.

CALCULATION OF DATE OF CONFINEMENT

The probable length of gestation is, from the most reliable statistics, 266 days from the date of impregnation, and is usually calculated as the 280th day from the first day of the last menstrual period, but naturally, it is subject to the following fallacies :—

1. Ovulation may occur independent of menstruation.
2. Labour may be premature in women who have a short menstrual cycle or delayed in those who have a longer cycle.

From these causes alone it will be seen that precise calculation is impossible, but as menstruation is usually in abeyance after fertilisation, this method of calculation is nearest and easiest. In general, therefore, the 280 days are calculated as being nine calendar months and a week.

This is obtained practically by adding seven to the first day of the last menstrual period and subtracting three months.

Example :—First day of last period, January 14—

14+7=21—3 months=October 21.

Calculation of the date of confinement, if the menstrual history is unobtainable, is made—

(*a*) From the date of quickening. This must at all times be haphazard, as the period of quickening varies as much as a month, the average being the twentieth week.

(*b*) From the size of the uterine tumour (see p. 37).

CHAPTER IV

NORMAL LABOUR

MAY be called confinement or parturition, and is defined as the expulsion of the uterine contents once the child is viable.

It is naturally a physiological process, but so finely balanced that the least deviation renders it pathological.

It is much more complex and tedious in the human race than in the lower animals, chiefly because—

1. The pelvic axis is curved, that of the outlet and the inlet being at right angles to one another.
2. The diameters of the fœtal head are greater than those of the pelvis through which the head passes.
3. The diameters of the pelvis vary from above downwards; the transverse is greatest at the inlet, while the antero-posterior is greatest at the outlet. To become accommodated to those diameters, the presenting part must rotate.

Nature's proof of the greater difficulty in birth is to be found in the great thickness of the uterine wall.

Labour increases in difficulty and danger—

1. In higher grades of civilisation.
2. In intellectual classes (the higher the mental development, the less the reproductive power).
3. With increased size of child.

THEORIES REGARDING THE ONSET OF LABOUR

It is believed that œstrogen is the main sensitising factor of the human uterus, and when adequate priming has occurred any further stimulus, *e.g.* pressure of the presenting part on the lower segment or some emotional disturbance, may be enough to establish the onset of labour. Some hold that the œstrogenic hormone provokes the onset of expulsive uterine contractions while others say that the growth response is limited by this hormone, and when further uterine enlargement is prevented by increasing œstrogen, labour commences. Kneer suggests that withdrawal of œstrogen, as in menstruation, may be a factor in initiating labour. Hoffman enumerates the views that œstrogen may stimulate the posterior pituitary lobe to secrete its oxytocic principle or may render the uterus sensitive to the posterior pituitary-like hormone. The view that progesterone withdrawal is at least partly responsible for the onset of labour is based on evidence that this hormone may exert an inhibitory effect on uterine muscle. Undue distension of the uterus (premature labour is frequent in hydramnios), excess of CO_2 in the maternal blood stimulating uterine contractions, and increasing infarction of the placenta, have been suggested as possible factors.

GENERAL CONSIDERATION OF LABOUR

Labour is divided into three stages.

The **first stage** begins with onset of true pains and ends with full dilatation of the cervix. It is the stage of dilatation.

The **second stage** begins after full dilatation of the cervix and ends with expulsion of fœtus. It is the stage of expulsion.

The **third stage** begins after the expulsion of the fœtus and ends with the expulsion of the placenta and membranes. It is the stage of detachment and expulsion of the placenta and membranes.

Factors of Labour

Three factors are concerned in each stage of labour. They are (1) powers, (2) passages, (3) passenger.

Powers.—During pregnancy uterine contractions occur from time to time. In labour the " pains " are an exaggeration of the contractions with, in addition, retraction. This latter property enables the uterine muscle fibres, like those of the bladder, to become progressively shorter, so enabling the uterus to expel the fœtus. Retraction does not occur appreciably during the first stage, but is well marked towards the end of the second stage. One part of the uterus just above the internal os, that part called the isthmus, being sparsely supplied with muscle fibres, does not contract at all, but with every contraction it becomes more thinned out. In contrast, the upper segment is rendered progressively shorter and thicker with the formation of *Bandl's ring* or the *retraction ring* at the junction of the active and passive portions of the uterus. This ring becomes very distinct in cases of obstructed labour. The contractile part of the uterus is termed the *upper uterine segment*, the passive part the *lower uterine segment*, and this property of the lower portion relaxing as the upper part contracts and retracts constitutes *uterine polarity*.

During the **first stage,** when the membranes are intact and the child is surrounded with liquor amnii, the pressure is applied equally in all directions. Due to this function of uterine polarity, the lower segment and cervix begin to open up and the force is now transmitted, as a fluid pressure, downwards. As a result, the membranes are separated from the lower uterine pole and, containing a small quantity of liquor amnii, present through the cervix, a fluid wedge being formed which still further dilates the cervix.

A typical uterine contraction begins gradually, reaches its maximum, and finally ceases. Then comes an interval followed by an even stronger contraction. These intervals give rest to the mother, reduce the pressure on the child, and allow the restoration of the placental circulation, which is stopped when the pain is strong. During contractions the arterial pressure is raised, the maternal pulse is quickened, the fœtal heart-rate is slowed, respiration is slowed, the intra-uterine pressure is raised, the cervix dilates, and the uterus becomes elongated and thrown forwards.

In the **second stage** the uterine contractions (*primary powers*) occur more strongly than in the first stage. In addition, the patient uses her abdominal muscles and diaphragm (*secondary powers*); these latter, at first used voluntarily, later become reflex.

The primary and secondary forces are both in action in the **third stage:** the abdominal muscles, however, contract only at the will of the patient for the expulsion of placenta.

The Passages.—In the **first stage,** as we have seen, the uterus is provided with a weak spot by virtue of (1) uterine polarity, and (2) the formation of the lower uterine segment from the isthmus. These two factors, commencing expansion of the lower uterine segment and relaxation of the cervix, allow of the detachment of the membranes to form the "bag of waters."

Differences between Upper and Lower Uterine Segments

Upper.—

1. Peritoneum firmly attached all round.
2. Several layers of muscle, longitudinal fibres in excess.
3. Membranes firmly attached and separate at end of labour.
4. Active during labour.
5. Becomes shorter and thicker.

Lower.—

1. Peritoneum loosely attached in front and absent at sides.
2. Circular fibres chiefly.
3. Membranes loosely attached, and separate at beginning of labour.
4. Passive during labour.
5. Becomes expanded and thinner.

In this stage the bladder is drawn up out of the pelvis by the ascending cervix and lower uterine segment. If the bladder is full, that part below the symphysis may obstruct the descent of the head or the prolonged pressure of the head in such an obstructed labour may cause necrosis of the bladder and vaginal wall and give rise later to a vesico-vaginal fistula.

In the **second stage** the vagina is canalised by the descent of the presenting part. During the latter part of pregnancy the anterior and posterior segments of the pelvic floor sag downwards. During this stage the anterior segment is drawn upwards with the ascending anterior cervical wall, while the posterior segment, being right in line of the descending presenting part, is pushed downwards and backwards. This is obvious externally in a lengthening, thinning and bulging of the perineum. In addition to the soft passages, the fœtus is passing through the hard pelvis.

The passages in the **third stage** are similar to those of the second.

The Passenger.—The " bag of waters " is the passenger in the **first stage.** If the presenting part fits the pelvic brim accurately, this " bag of waters " is saucer-shaped, but in cases of disproportion or malpresentation the membranes are sausage-shaped, have little dilating power and tend to rupture prematurely. The membranes normally rupture at the end of the first stage.

In the **second stage** the passenger is the fœtus with the remainder of the liquor amnii, while in the **third stage** the placenta and membranes are expelled.

Expulsion of Placenta.—After expulsion of the fœtus, the uterus remains retracted from its inherent tonicity, the uterine cavity being filled entirely by placenta. By progressive retraction the placental site is much reduced in size and placental separation begins. This is aided by the formation of retro-placental clot. The placenta is expelled in one of two ways.

In cases where considerable bleeding has occurred behind the placenta, Schultze's method obtains, the fœtal surface coming away first, with the membranes trailing behind—in the form of an inverted umbrella. In other cases the lower edge appears first, the whole placenta, folded longitudinally on itself, coming away after the manner described by Matthews Duncan. The placenta is finally expelled from the vagina by the secondary powers.

As the placenta separates large vessels are torn across, but bleeding is prevented by retraction of the uterine muscle closing the mouths of the vessels, so allowing clotting to occur. If, owing to uterine exhaustion, there is little or no retraction, post-partum hæmorrhage results.

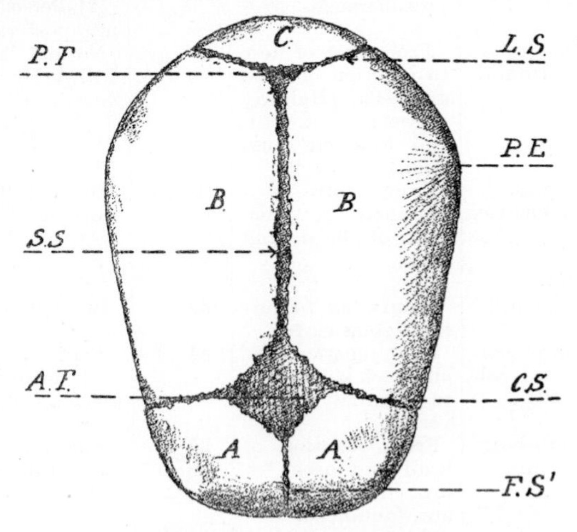

FIG. 12.—FŒTAL SKULL.

A.A, Frontal bones; B.B, Parietal bones; C, Occipital bone; P.F, Post. Fontanelle; A.F, Ant. Fontanelle; L.S, Lambdoidal suture; C.S, Coronal suture; P.E, Parietal eminence; F.S, Frontal suture; S.S, Sagittal suture.

FŒTAL SKULL

This, being the largest and most important obstetrical part of the fœtus, requires a detailed description.

The fœtal skull is divided into the compressible vault and the solid base by a line drawn between the orbital ridges and a point just behind the foramen magnum.

The bones of the vault being small and not apposed, their junction is formed by membranous commissures called *sutures*, which are named—

1. Frontal, between the frontal bones.
2. Coronal, between the frontals and the parietals.
3. Sagittal, between the parietals.
4. Lambdoidal, between the parietals and the occipital.

IMPORTANT DIAMETERS OF THE FŒTAL SKULL

Name.	How Measured.	Measurement.	When Found Engaging.
(*a*) *Antero-posterior.*			
(1) Occipito-mental.	From chin to post-fontanelle.	5 in.	Complete extension of after-coming head.
(2) Occipito-frontal.	From root of nose to external occipital protuberance.	4½ ,,	(1) Incomplete flexion of after-coming head. (2) Persistent occipito-posterior.
(3) Sub-occipito frontal.	From root of nose to junction of head and neck. (Halfway between post.-font. and foramen magnum.)	4 ,,	Normal L.O.A. or R.O.A. Head not fully flexed.
(4) Sub-occipito bregmatic.	From centre ant.-fontanelle to junction of head and neck.	3¾ ,,	Head fully flexed. Normal L.O.A. or R.O.A.
(*b*) *Vertical.*			
(5) Vertico-mental.	From chin to furthest point vertex.	5½ ,,	Brow presentation.
(6) Submento-vertical.	From junction head and neck below chin to furthest point vertex.	4½ ,,	Face presentation with incomplete extension of head.
(7) Submento-bregmatic.	From junction of head and neck below chin to middle ant.-fontanelle.	3¾ ,,	Face presentation with full extension of head.
(8) Mento-nasal.	Chin to orbital plate of frontal bone.	1½ ,,	Smallest diameter produced after complete cranioclasm.
(*c*) *Transverse.*			
(9) Biparietal.	Between points farthest apart on parietal eminences.	3¾ ,,	(1) Largest diameter entering ant.-post. diameter of brim in flattened pelvis. (2) Diameter occupying sacro-cotyloid diameter in occipito-posteriors.
(10) Bitemporal.	Between points farthest apart of coronal sutures.	3¼ ,,	—
(11) Superparieto-subparietal.	From just above one parietal eminence to just below the other.	3½ ,,	Usually replaces biparietal in flat pelvis.

Where more than two sutures meet, membranous spaces are formed called *fontanelles*. Those of obstetrical importance are named anterior and posterior.

Anterior Fontanelle.—Is formed at the junction of the coronal, sagittal, and frontal sutures, thus is the meeting point of four sutures.

It is large and lozenge-shaped.

Is sometimes called the *Bregma.*

Posterior Fontanelle.—Is formed at the junction of the sagittal and lambdoidal sutures, thus is the meeting point of three sutures.

It is small and triangular in shape.

That part of the head situated between the fontanelles and bounded laterally by the parietal eminences is known as the **vertex.**

The measurements of the fœtal head are called diameters.

Clinical Aspects of Labour

Premonitory Symptoms and Signs.—In primigravidæ, where the pelvic measurements are normal, the fœtal head enters the brim of the pelvis and becomes " fixed " about two to three weeks before full time. This allows a slight falling in the level of the fundus with easier respiration, which is described as a feeling of " lightening." At the same time there may be increased bladder irritability and discomfort in walking, the vaginal secretion becomes more copious, and in the last week the vulva gapes.

Normal Labour

The **first stage** begins with the onset of uterine contractions or " pains," and the discharge of some blood and mucus known as the " *show.*" This latter is produced by the membranes being separated from the lower uterine pole with commencing cervical dilatation.

True pains must be diagnosed from false pains.

True.	*False.*
1. Start in back and come to front.	1. Start in front.
2. Occur at definite intervals.	2. Indefinite intervals.
3. Start gradually, become stronger and pass away.	3. Start suddenly (colicky).
4. Uterus felt to contract during pain.	4. No contraction.
5. Cervix drawn up during pain.	5. No drawing up of cervix.
6. Show.	6. No show.

False pains are usually due to constipation, errors of diet or fatigue, and should be treated by rest, enemata and a morphia suppository, $\frac{1}{4}$ gr.

During this stage, if the labour is normal, the patient is able to walk about. The pains, to begin with, occur at half-hourly intervals and last only half a minute, but towards the end of labour they may appear at two-minute intervals and last two minutes. With each pain in the latter part of the first stage, the tendency is to clutch something for support and to cry out. At the end of this stage the membranes rupture. In some cases this may happen before the cervix is dilated, giving rise to a dry labour, while in other cases the membranes, due to abnormal toughness, do not rupture spontaneously, the child being born in a " caul."

The patient should be in bed during the **second stage.** The pains are stronger and more frequent, and now the secondary powers are called into action. During a contraction the patient holds her breath and, with the pains becoming " bearing-down " in character, the fœtal head is driven through the pelvis. The posterior vaginal wall, being right in the line of descent, is pushed downwards and backwards, the rectum is pressed upon and the patient has the desire to defæcate, fæces often being expressed from the rectum. As the head meets the pelvic floor the perineum bulges, is elongated and thinned. The vulva gapes, becomes oval and finally rounded, while the anus becomes D-shaped. Finally, the largest diameter of the fœtal skull engages in the vulva and no further recession takes place between pains, the head is in fact " *crowned*," and, with the next pain, the head is born by a movement of extension. There is now a momentary respite, but with the next pain the head is rotated externally as the shoulders rotate into the antero-posterior diameter of the outlet. The anterior shoulder hitches against the symphysis pubis and the posterior shoulder is born, the trunk and limbs following immediately.

Contractions, which are almost painless in the **third stage,** return after a few minutes' rest. With succeeding pains the placenta is separated gradually from the uterine wall, evident by occasional small gushes of blood. Once the placenta is completely separated it is expelled by a uterine contraction into the vagina, from where it is born by the action of the secondary powers. The fundus uteri, just after the placenta has been expelled, is half-way between the umbilicus and symphysis pubis. The third stage lasts about twenty minutes and may be accompanied by a shivering fit, the " physiological chill " of labour.

The duration of labour in a primigravida is about eighteen hours, the first stage occupying sixteen hours, the second two, and the third half an hour. In a multipara, labour lasts normally about twelve hours, the second stage being often very quick.

MECHANISM OF NORMAL LABOUR

Vertex Presentation

The vertex presents in 96 per cent. of all cases. In these cases the occipito-frontal plane of the head is parallel to the plane of the brim. The vertex is thus in the axis of the brim.

Diagnosis.—

1. By external palpation and auscultation.
2. By vaginal examination.
   (*a*) Before labour, a hard globular mass is felt through the anterior vaginal fornix.
   (*b*) After the cervix is open, the sutures and fontanelles may be felt according to the position.

Positions of the Vertex.—Four, named after the position of the occiput, which is the *denominator*.

1. Occiput anterior and to the left of the symphysis—**left occipito-anterior** (L.O.A.).
2. Occiput anterior and to the right of the symphysis—**right occipito-anterior** (R.O.A.).
3. Occiput posterior opposite the right ilio-sacral synchondrosis—**right occipito-posterior** (R.O.P.).
4. Occiput posterior opposite the left ilio-sacral synchondrosis—**left occipito-posterior** (L.O.P.).

Relative Frequency.—

Usually Quoted.		*One Author's Statistics.* (*From 1,000 cases personally observed.*)
L.O.A.,	65 per cent.	70 per cent.
R.O.P.,	20 ,,	8 ,,
R.O.A.,	10 ,,	20 ,,
L.O.P.,	5 ,,	2 ,,

The L.O.A. position is thus by far the commonest and is called the *normal.* It will be noted that in 78 per cent., at least, the occipito-frontal diameter lies in the right oblique of the pelvis. The pelvic colon encroaches on the left oblique.

(*N.B.*—One of the authors has made an investigation of 1000 cases seen first antenatally and later at labour; the figures so obtained are quoted above. These statistics proved that though the L.O.A. position is the most common, the next most common position is the R.O.A., and the R.O.P. position is not nearly so common as previous figures showed. This fact is corroborated yearly in the various maternity hospital reports when occipito-posterior positions are found usually in 10 per cent. of vertex presentations.)

Diagnosis of Position.—

1. By external palpation and auscultation.
2. By vaginal examination.

In *the occipito-anterior position*, the posterior fontanelle is easily felt to the front, and is to be recognised by three sutures only running from it. The anterior fontanelle is usually inaccessible to the examining finger, being so far up posteriorly to the right or left. If felt, the head is not fully flexed.

In *the occipito-posterior positions*, the head is usually extended to some extent and the anterior fontanelle is commonly felt.

Mechanism of L.O.A. Position

At the beginning of labour the occipito-frontal diameter is in the right oblique of the pelvis, the occiput lying to the left of the symphysis, the sinciput to the right sacro-iliac joint. The movements which constitute the mechanism are (1) Descent, (2) Flexion, (3) Internal Rotation, (4) Extension, (5) Restitution, (6) External Rotation.

1. **Descent** is due to (*a*) intra-uterine fluid pressure, (*b*) direct pressure of the fundus on the breech, and (*c*) uterine contraction and retraction.

2. **Flexion** takes place when the head first meets with resistance, usually at the pelvic brim. Force is exerted through the vertebral column of the child and as the occiput is nearer the fulcrum than the sinciput, according to the two-armed lever principle, it receives more force and sinks further than the sinciput, effecting a substitution of the sub-occipito-bregmatic ($3\frac{3}{4}$ in.) for the occipito-frontal diameter ($4\frac{1}{2}$ in.).

3. **Internal Rotation.**—There are different theories as to why this movement occurs. The old views were that the gutter shape of the pelvic floor sloping down and to the front, the elastic recoil of the pelvic floor and the space available in the sub-pubic angle, all contributed to internal rotation.

The work of Sellheim and Moir is based on "the theory of unequal fœtal flexibilities." If a cylindrical body capable of bending on its long axis unequally in different directions is forced through a curved cylindrical passage, it will rotate in such a way as to adapt itself best to that canal and to allow bending to occur with the maximum ease. Internal rotation results in the long diameters of the skull being brought into the long antero-posterior diameter of the outlet.

4. **Extension** is a movement by which the head is born. This movement occurs at the vulva. The occiput is pressed against the under margin of the symphysis pubis, vertex, brow, face and chin being pushed over the perineum successively. Two factors effect this movment, the uterus acting downwards and the pelvic floor sloping forwards ; also, as the occiput is fixed, all force is exerted on the sinciput (one-armed lever).

5. **Restitution** consists in the rotation of the head through one-eighth of a circle to the left side, the twist on the child's neck resulting from internal rotation being undone.

6. **External Rotation** is a movement of the occiput through a further one-eighth of a circle to the left and is due to the head accompanying the rotation of the shoulders from the left oblique to the antero-posterior of the outlet. This rotation of the anterior shoulder to the front occurs when the shoulder reaches the pelvic floor. The anterior shoulder now becoming fixed beneath the pubic arch, the posterior glides over the perineum and they are born, the rest of the trunk following.

The entire mechanism is thus simply an accommodation of the fœtal head and shoulders to the pelvis.

In R.O.A. positions the mechanism is identical with L.O.A., the occiput rotating forwards from the right to the under margin of the symphysis and then passing to the right again in external rotation.

Changes in the Fœtal Head

During its passage through the pelvis the fœtal head becomes *moulded* in a definite manner, and assumes a characteristic appearance, according to the position it occupied. This is due to changes in the scalp and in the skull.

Changes in the Scalp—Caput succedaneum.—A swelling in the scalp, due to a transudation of serum, forms on the part of the vertex free from pressure and is thus most marked in labours delayed in the second stage. The swelling is not limited by sutures.

In an L.O.A. position this naturally forms on the superior posterior angle of the right parietal bone and the posterior fontanelle.

In an R.O.A. position, on the corresponding part of the left parietal bone and the posterior fontanelle.

In occipito-posterior positions, on the anterior fontanelle and vertex.

Caput succedaneum usually disappears within twenty-four hours of birth.

Changes in the Skull—Head-moulding.—From the mobility of the bones through the sutures, the posterior parietal is pressed beneath the anterior. Thus in an L.O.A. position the left parietal is underneath the right. Later the frontal and occipital bones are overlapped by the parietals, this being more apparent in occipito-posterior positions. The head has a sugar-loaf shape in occipito-posterior positions whereas in occipito-anterior positions it is elongated antero-posteriorly. Thus from the shape of the head the position of the presentation can be told with great certainty.

Cephalhæmatoma.—Is an effusion of blood between the bone and the pericranium. It is usually found on one or both parietal bones and forms a fluid swelling limited to the area of the bone by the sutures. It appears one to two days after birth, increases in size for the next few days and remains thus for some weeks, when it is usually absorbed.

On examination a hard raised edge can be felt, due to irregular ossification, the result of irritation; this causes an apparent depression in the centre, which can easily be mistaken for a pond or depressed fracture.

These swellings should never be interfered with, unless they suppurate, when they require incision and drainage.

It has to be distinguished from a meningocele, which occurs in the line of the sutures or fontanelles and which becomes tense when the child cries.

Occipito-posterior Positions

Diagnosis.—

Abdominal.—The head is in the lower uterine pole and it is suggestive in a primigravida to find the head high and free in the last fortnight of pregnancy. The breech is at the fundus, while the limbs are felt with ease over the front of the mother's abdomen.

Auscultation reveals the fœtal heart sounds farther out in the flank than in anterior positions.

Vaginal examination is helpful only after labour has started. If the head is well flexed the posterior fontanelle is felt behind, with the sagittal suture running forwards to the anterior fontanelle, which is felt in front. Usually the head is not flexed and the anterior fontanelle is very well felt in front with the sagittal suture running back to the posterior fontanelle, which is felt only with difficulty. If the patient is advanced in labour with the fontanelles difficult to feel on account of a caput succedaneum, the whole hand should be inserted into the vagina to feel for an ear, the direction of the pinna indicating where the occiput lies.

Mechanism.—

(*a*) *With the head flexed*—**Descent, flexion, long internal rotation** (the occiput passing through three-eighths of a circle to come to the front). **Extension, restitution** and **external rotation.**

(*b*) *With the head imperfectly flexed or extended*—**Descent, extension, short internal rotation** (the occiput passing through one-eighth of a circle to reach the hollow of the sacrum, the sinciput going to the front). As a rule, in such a position spontaneous delivery is difficult, but if the pelvis be large and the fœtal head small, the subsequent movements of the head are **flexion, restitution** and **external rotation.**

Full flexion of the head is prevented at first by the mother's vertebral column being against the child's back, thus preventing the normal flexed attitude of the back and aiding extension of the head. Extension is increased further by the biparietal diameter of the head ($3\frac{3}{4}$ in.) being held up in the sacro-cotyloid diameter of the pelvis ($3\frac{1}{2}$ in.). Thus the sinciput descends but the occiput is unable to do so until the head is moulded sufficiently to allow the biparietal diameter to pass through. (This accounts for the length of labour in such cases.) If the difference between the diameters is small or the head is easily moulded, the occiput will reach the pelvic floor first and long internal rotation will occur, when labour will end normally. If the sinciput reaches the pelvic floor first, however, it rotates to the front and a *persistent occipito-posterior position* (P.O.P.) occurs. In such cases delivery is very seldom spontaneous and may be effected only with great difficulty by forceps. In some, craniotomy may be required.

Risks to the Mother.—Increased in P.O.P.s because of—

1. The common occurrence of perineal lacerations due to the occipito-frontal diameter engaging the vulva.

2. Prolonged labour and the need for operative interference.

Risks to the Child.—Very much increased in P.O.P.s; difficulty in delivery causing death or injury.

Treatment.—

1. *Preventive.*—Buist's pads, the thicker one being laid on the abdomen on the side of the occiput, kept in place by tight binder. (Can only be successful when the head is not fixed.) Castor oil, to empty the pelvic colon and cause discomfort

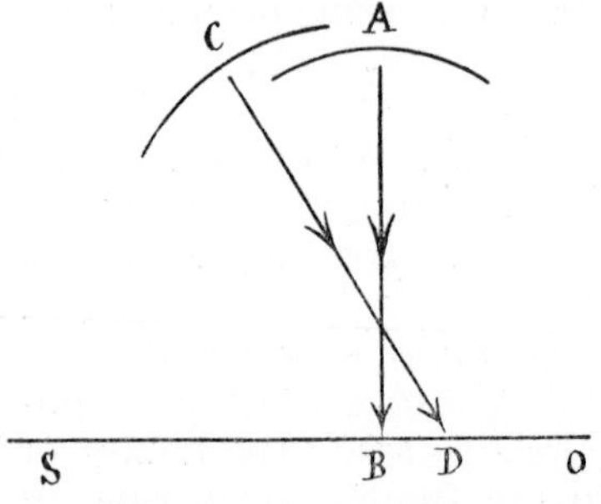

Fig. 13.—Postural Method for Occipito-posterior Positions.

O, Occiput; S, Sinciput; AB, Exertion of uterine force with patient in dorsal position; CD, Exertion of uterine force with patient on side opposite occiput.

to fœtus, should be taken after the application of the pads and the patient advised to stay in bed for twenty-four hours when the pads are removed. If this method is employed, it should be used only in the last two to three weeks of pregnancy and is much more likely to be successful in the occipito-lateral position, where no such treatment is required, than in the true posterior.

2. *During Labour.*—In the first stage the patient should remain in bed to prevent early rupture of the membranes, and it is of advantage that she should lie on the side opposite to that occupied by the back. In the R.O.P. position the patient should lie on the left side; this attitude promotes flexion.

Opinions vary as to when to interfere. In the vast majority of cases (95 per cent.) spontaneous rotation of the occiput to the front occurs. Some teach that interference should be contemplated when the second stage has lasted three hours.

Broadly speaking, this is a satisfactory principle to follow, but it is obvious that should there be maternal exhaustion or fœtal distress, failure of rotation of the head or malrotation, active treatment may have to be carried out earlier. Should the necessity for interference arise, it may take the form of—

(1) Increasing flexion by pressure applied to the sinciput, per vaginam, during pains.

(2) Manual rotation, the head being pushed up out of the pelvis and the occiput rotated to the front, the anterior shoulder being rotated at the same time through the maternal abdominal wall. The vaginal hand may be passed up beyond the head and used to rotate the anterior shoulder if it is impossible to do so through abdominal wall.

(3) Forceps rotation, the head again being pushed out of the pelvis before rotation is attempted. This is often associated with injury to the maternal soft parts and also to the child; it should be practised only by the expert.

(4) Traction by forceps with the object of increasing flexion and so later promoting spontaneous rotation to the front.

(5) Traction by forceps and delivery face to pubis.

(6) If the child is dead and delivery by forceps is difficult, perforation of the skull and craniotomy.

MANAGEMENT OF NORMAL LABOUR

General Rules

Attend at once.

Be above all things cleanly and aseptic. Never introduce anything into the vagina which has not been rendered aseptic.

Arrangements for the attendance of a nurse should have been made.

Contents of Midwifery Bag.—

1. A nail brush and soap. (Brush must always be boiled before use.)

2. A bottle of Dettol for disinfecting the hands and external genitals.

3. Silver nitrate solution, 1 per cent. (to drop in the baby's eyes to prevent ophthalmia), or 10–15 per cent. albucid.

4. Chloroform.
5. A stethoscope.
6. A sterile pair of rubber gloves.
7. A clean gown (sterile if possible).
8. Scissors (for cutting the cord).
9. Thread or tape (for tying the cord).
10. Cotton wool (or tow) to wash the external genitals.
11. Two packets of sterile gauze.
12. A thermometer.
13. A male catheter (rubber) No. 10. (The rubber catheter is used more safely as a glass one is apt to be broken by the pressure of the head in the second stage.)
14. Apparatus for giving a vaginal and intra-uterine douche.
15. Apparatus for giving a subcutaneous or intravenous saline, if required, and normal saline tabloids.
16. A hypodermic syringe with the following drugs: Morphia, $\frac{1}{6}$ to $\frac{1}{4}$ gr.; pethidine 50-100 mgm.,; strychnine, $\frac{1}{60}$ gr.; pituitrin, 5 units; aseptic ergot, 1 c.c. or ergometrine, 0·25–0·5 mgm.; lobeline hydrochloride, $\frac{1}{20}$ gr.; coramine, 0·5–1·0 millilitre of a 25 per cent. solution; methedrine, 20 mgm.
17. Midwifery forceps.
18. Needles, large and small, always lying in lysol or dettol in a needle-case.
19. Sterilised catgut (for vaginal and perineal tears). Some advise silkworm gut for the latter.
20. Dissecting forceps. Two pairs of artery forceps.

It is possible to obtain a sterile drum containing gowns, caps, masks, gloves, squares, cotton wool, gauze, ligatures for cord, vulvar pads, etc.

The obstetrician may also take with him apparatus for giving gas and air or trilene analgesia.

On Arrival

1. Question the patient as to :—
   (*a*) Pains—
   The time of onset.
   The character.
   The site.
   (*b*) The escape of the waters.
   (*c*) The condition of bowels and bladder.

2. Make examination :—
   (*a*) External palpation.
   (*b*) Auscultation—to learn if the child is alive and in good condition.
   (*c*) Vaginal but preferably rectal. Before this the vulva should be shaved and cleansed by washing with soap and water and then swabbing with an antiseptic lotion.

Points to be made out by examination :—
   (*a*) Is she pregnant and what period of gestation ?
   (*b*) Is the child alive ?
   (*c*) Is she in labour ?
   (*d*) What stage and how far advanced ?
   (*e*) The condition of the membranes.
   (*f*) The state of the canals.
   (*g*) The presentation.
   (*h*) The position—may be difficult unless the os is well dilated.

Examine vaginally or rectally between pains.

3. After examination :—
   If all is well, tell patient so.
   If there is any abnormality, do not inform the patient but tell her husband or relatives.
   Do not risk forecast of the duration of labour.
4. See that the nurse has necessaries ready, viz. :—
   (*a*) Plenty of hot water.
   (*b*) Ligatures for cord.
   (*c*) Binder.
   (*d*) Bed—
      (*a*) In proper position.
      (*b*) Mattress covered by mackintosh to prevent soiling.
      (*c*) With no sag in the middle. Boards are of great use.
   (*e*) Cotton-wool swabs in an antiseptic solution.
5. Order enema to be given :—
   Castor oil, ʒss.
   Olive oil, ℥i.
   Hot water, a pint.
6. See that the bladder is emptied.
7. Take the temperature and pulse.

Management of the First Stage

1. If the cervix is less than half dilated, leave the house and if at night, request to be called when the pains are stronger or the membrances rupture; if during the day, call again in a few hours.

2. If the cervix is half to three-quarters dilated in multiparæ, stay in the house but not in the patient's room; make periodic visits. In primigravidæ always stay when the os is fully dilated.

3. Let the patient walk about, but do not allow bearing-down during the pains.

4. See that urine is passed every three hours.

Management of the Second Stage

(*a*) ***When the Head is in the Pelvis.***—

1. May examine vaginally whenever the membranes rupture—
   (*a*) To determine the position more accurately.
   (*b*) To rule out any complication (prolapse of the cord, etc.).

2. Keep the patient in bed lying on the left side or back. If the head is not entering the pelvis well, try Walcher's position. (*Walcher's position* consists of allowing the thighs to hang over the bed, the patient lying on her back. This extends the hip joints and causes the true conjugate to be increased slightly, all other antero-posterior diameters of cavity and outlet being slightly decreased.)

3. Tell the patient to strain during pains and not to cry out.

4. Tie a rope or towel to the left top corner of bed and tell the patient to pull on that during pains. This fixes the pelvis, allows full scope for the abdominal muscles and keeps the patient in proper obstetric position.

(*b*) ***When the Head is at the Vulva.***—

1. Pains are now more severe. Swab the distended perineum thoroughly with an antiseptic solution.

2. Do not support the perineum, but with the left hand between the patient's thighs keep the head flexed by pressing on the sincipital end of the head. After the head has advanced so far that it cannot recede between the pains, lightly anæsthetise the patient with chloroform and by pressing

forwards with a pad placed posterior to the anus, the head should be delivered between pains. In this way the head is born more gently and with more control.

3. In primigravidæ allow the head to distend the perineum for fifteen minutes, pushing it back between the pains and not letting it progress too far during the pains. In this way the perineum is gradually distended and perineal lacerations prevented.

4. Receive the head in the right hand.

5. If the cord is round the neck, slip it over the occiput.

6. Do not hurry the birth of the trunk ; if there is delay, express by fundal pressure, but do not pull on the head.

7. Follow the fundus uteri down with the left hand during the expulsion of the trunk ; thus hæmorrhage is prevented and the presence of twins is diagnosed.

(*c*) *After the Birth of the Child.*—

1. If there is no hæmorrhage, attend to the child and make the nurse grasp the fundus.

2. Wipe out the mouth, eyes, and upper air passages.

3. Wait until pulsation stops before tying the cord (one to two minutes) and during that time attempt to make the child cry.

4. Milk cord to child's abdomen to prevent any loop of bowel being cut across and then tie the cord at two places, 2 and 4 in. from the umbilicus respectively, and cut between.

5. Examine the fœtal end, and if there is no hæmorrhage, hand the child to the nurse and attend to the mother.

Management of the Third Stage

1. The fundus should be controlled with the right hand during this stage and it is a good thing to palpate the uterus occasionally and see how it is behaving.

2. Examine the perineum for laceration ; if any, stitch at once with chromic catgut or silkworm gut. Any vaginal laceration should also be stitched with cargut.

3. Feel the pulse, and treat shock if present. (See p. 197.)

4. If the uterus is flabby at all—knead it gently. Probably in the course of twenty to thirty minutes after the birth of the child it will contract and expel the placenta into the vagina.

5. The expulsion of the placenta from the uterus may be known by—

(*a*) The increased length of the cord visible externally.

(*b*) The increased mobility of the uterus.
(*c*) The higher level of the fundus uteri in the abdomen.
(*d*) The bulging of the abdominal wall above the pubis.

5. After expulsion into the vagina, the placenta is assisted in its birth by the action of the abdominal muscles, or failing that, by firm supra-pubic pressure on the uterus downwards and backwards, the uterus being contracted at the time.

6. After repeated trials, should this be ineffectual, introduce the fingers into the vagina and hook the placenta out.

7. After extrusion from the vulva, rotate the placenta so as to get the membranes away entire; do not pull. Keep pressure on the fundus all the time.

8. Never pull on the cord.

(*a*) The cord breaks.
(*b*) Inversion of the uterus is apt to occur.

9. Grasp the fundus of the uterus for ten minutes after birth of the placenta.

10. Give ext. ergot liq. ʒ1 to ʒ1½ by mouth, pituitrin 5 units or ergometrine 0·5 mgm. intramuscularly or 0·25 intravenously.

After-treatment

(*a*) *Of Mother.*—

1. Make the patient clean and comfortable and apply a sterile pad to the vulva.

2. If the uterus is well contracted apply a binder.

3. See that the binder passes below the trochanters; apply it tightly at this point and over the anterior superior spines, but slackly above.

4. Let the patient now have some light nourishment (a cup of tea) and rest.

5. Wait half an hour longer before leaving the house; see that all is well, taking the pulse and temperature before departure.

6. Return in approximately twelve hours; on return inquire after sleep, pain, micturition and discharge.

Take the pulse and temperature and feel height of fundus.

Tighten the binder and ascertain if the uterus is contracted.

(*b*) *Of the Child.*—

1. Put one drop of 1 per cent. silver nitrate into each eye.

2. Bathe the child in water not hotter than 100° F.

3. Dry the cord thoroughly, dust with boracic powder, and put on a sterile dressing.

4. Sew a binder round the child to keep on the umbilical dressing.

DRUGS IN LABOUR

A. Ecbolics

1. Quinine Bihydrochloride.

Uses.—

(*a*) Ante-natally—for two weeks before date of confinement, gr. ii twice daily—
 (i) tones up uterus ;
 (ii) acts as tonic and increases resistance against sepsis.

(*b*) As an adjuvant for medical induction of labour (see p. 218). (*N.B.*—Large or frequent doses may cause fœtal death, so dosage should be restricted to one dose of gr. x.)

(*c*) During labour for primary inertia. gr. v.

(*d*) In post-partum pill with ergot for sub-involution,
 ℞
 Ergotin.
 Quinine Bihyd. aa. gr. ii.
 Ext. Nux Vomica gr. ¼.

2. Ergot.

Must never be given during labour as it may cause irregular and tetanic contractions and cause rupture of the uterus.

Uses.—

(*a*) After delivery of placenta if uterus is not contracting well.

(*b*) Combined with other methods of treatment for post-partum hæmorrhage.

(*c*) For subinvolution in post-partum pill.

(*d*) Ergometrine 0·5 mgm. intramuscularly or 0·25 mgm. intravenously has lately been widely recommended during birth of anterior shoulder to cause easy delivery of placenta and prevent post-partum hæmorrhage.

Useful Preparations.—

(*a*) Ext. Ergotæ Liquidum ʒi-i½ after labour.

ʒ½ thrice daily in puerperium for sub-involution.

(*b*) Ext. Ergotæ (Ergotin) gr. ii.-gr. iii. thrice daily in post-partum pill.

(*c*) Ergometrine.—

(i) 0·5 mgm. orally thrice daily for sub-involution.

(ii) 0·5 mgm. intramuscularly for flabby uterus after parturition or into uterus in Cæsarean section.

(iii) 0·25 mgm. intravenously for severe post-partum hæmorrhage.

Ergot by the mouth takes 20–30 minutes to act, but its action lasts for about four hours, intramuscularly it acts in about 5 minutes and intravenously almost instantaneously.

3. **Pituitary Extract** (posterior lobe). Consists of Pitocin and Pitressin.

Uses.—

(*a*) Combined with castor oil and quinine for medical induction of labour, 5 units half-hourly for 3–4 doses as required. (See p. 218.)

(*b*) For delay at perineal stage due to inefficient powers, there being no obstruction present. May prevent use of forceps (2–5 units).

(*c*) With delivery of anterior shoulder as stated for Ergometrine, 5 units.

(*d*) After delivery of placenta to ensure contraction of uterus, 5 units.

(*e*) For post-partum hæmorrhage, 5 units, along with ergot preparation. Pituitary acts in about two minutes, but its action only lasts 20–30 minutes.

B. Analgesics

Essentials for an ideal analgesic.—

1. Does not endanger life of mother or have harmful effect upon her.
2. Does not harm the child.
3. Does not diminish uterine contractions and thus delay labour and increase the number of instrumental deliveries.

4. Does not affect the co-operation of the patient in the second stage and thus delay labour.

5. Does not cause prolongation of the third stage or any undue tendency to post-partum hæmorrhage.

6. Easy to administer and fool proof.

7. Always successful in its action.

No such ideal analgesic has yet been found and there is definite evidence to show that the excessive administration of analgesics and anæsthetics during labour raises the maternal mortality and morbidity rates.

Very many methods have been advocated, but the following have been found of most use.

1. **Chloral and Bromide.**—

Very useful in first stage of labour to give patient rest and often helps in cases of spasmodic rigidity of the cervix.

Dosage.—(*a*) Syr. Chloral ♏60–90, or (*b*) Chloral gr. xv. Sod-Bromide gr. xx. to which Tinct. Opii. ♏x. may be added.

2. **Twilight Sleep.**—

(*a*) Morphia $\frac{1}{4}$ gr. and hyoscine $\frac{1}{150}$ gr. are injected as soon as labour has definitely started.

(*b*) Hyoscine $\frac{1}{450}$ gr. is injected every hour after, until labour is completed.

(*c*) The patient lies in a quiet room with the blinds drawn and the ears plugged with cotton wool.

(*d*) See that the bladder is emptied regularly.

(*e*) If the patient appears to be getting away from the influence of the drugs, give chloral gr. xv-xx in first stage or a whiff of chloroform in second stage, and then administer hyoscine $\frac{1}{450}$ gr. hourly as before. **It is never advisable to give a second dose of morphia,** for, should the baby be born within three hours of the administration, it is very apt to be oligopnœic and to give trouble in resuscitation.

3. **Pethidine Hydrochloride.**—

100–150 mgms. injected intramuscularly when os is nearly half dilated, followed by further injection of 100 mgms. if required, in an hour and then four-hourly if necessary. Besides causing analgesia, often helps cervical dilatation. Hyoscine gr. $\frac{1}{150}$ may be combined with first injection and gr. $\frac{1}{450}$ hourly thereafter. If given earlier in labour than indicated above, labour may be stopped temporarily.

4. **Barbiturates.**

All have been recommended by different observers, but

their actions are irregular and may be dangerous for both mother and child even in usual dosage. All are respiratory depressants when given in large doses and have cumulative effects which may cause danger, when followed by inhalation anæsthesia.

5. **Gas and Air** (35 per cent. nitrous oxide).—

Given by means of special apparatus such as Minnitt's. Very useful as patient may regulate dosage herself and can be supervised by duly certificated midwives. Apparatus is cumbersome and it may be difficult to have cylinders always ready.

6. **Trilene** (Trichlorethylene) (0·65 per cent. in air).—

Given by the Freedman inhaler or Trilite pocket inhaler, etc. Use associated with 89·3 per cent. success. May act as anæsthetic and be dangerous, if the fluid in the apparatus is shaken, or if the patient's temperature is raised or she respires too quickly and deeply. When foolproof apparatus is discovered, Trilene will be a most valuable analgesic for use by midwives as well as doctors.

7. **Chloroform.**—

Given à la reine, *i.e.* small whiffs being given, *only* with the pains, on an open mask or through a Junker's or Simpson's vapour apparatus, which patient can regulate herself, under supervision.

Very useful in the second stage of labour as patient's full co-operation is obtained and yet the pains are greatly eased and often amnesia as well as analgesia is produced.

Easy to administer and to carry, speedy and certain in action.

C. Anæsthetics

1. **Chloroform.**—

Best anæsthetic when absolute uterine relaxation is required for difficult rotation or version, but is dangerous if not given by an anæsthetist conversant in its use.

Never to be given more than once in a labour, as delayed chloroform poisoning may occur.

Not to be given in toxæmic cases or for a difficult and traumatising delivery.

Liable to cause post-partum hæmorrhage from uterine relaxation if much given.

2. **Ether.**—

Valuable as a real anæsthetic, but may cause excitability and restlessness if given as analgesic.

Dangerous in pulmonary conditions and in eclampsia, due to risk of pulmonary œdema.

3. **Gas and Oxygen.**—

Best general anæsthesia for labour when apparatus is available, as in hospitals.

Non-toxic and can be used in toxæmic cases or when frequent anæsthetics are required.

Specially trained anæsthetist required so as to obtain satisfactory anæsthesia without causing cyanosis from a deficiency in oxygen; this may endanger child's life as oxygen consumption by the woman in labour is very great. (Just before delivery oxygen 100 per cent. should be given for 30–60 seconds.)

Does not produce sufficient relaxation for difficult intra-uterine manipulations and thus may contribute to a rupture.

4. **Cyclopropane.**—

Powerful and rapid anæsthetic.

Useful in toxæmic and cardiac cases and as an addition to gas and oxygen for the perineal stage.

Requires special apparatus and specialist anæsthetist.

Pituitary extract should not be used, as several cases have been quoted, where severe shock and collapse has followed its injection with patient under cyclopropane.

5. **Low Spinal.**—

Opinions vary greatly as to its uses and its dangers, but it would seem to be of greatest benefit for difficult forceps deliveries, especially when associated with a manual rotation of the occiput.

6. **Caudal.**—

Has been used lately in various clinics in America with excellent results, but it is not free from danger and special technique has to be acquired for its administration.

7. **Pentothal** (intravenous).—

Useful for easy forceps delivery, but is not without danger. Oxygen should always be available in case of spasm.

Useful just for delivery of head in lower uterine segment Cæsarean operation under local anæsthesia.

Should not be used in toxæmic or cardiac cases.

8. Local.—

Can be used for—

(*a*) Infiltration of perineum for suturing tears or episotomy wounds.

(*b*) Infiltration of whole pelvic floor for painless second stage of labour or forceps delivery.

Technique.—1 per cent. procaine hydrochloride can be injected as follows :—

(i) Insert long needle 1 cm. medial to tuber ischii and guide with finger in vagina to a distance of about 4 in. postero-laterally and inject 15 c.c. near ischial spine (pudic nerve).

(ii) Insert needle just inside and posterior to ischial tuberosity and inject 10 c.c. (inferior pudendal nerve).

(iii) Pass needle to subcutaneous tissue of perineum and inject 10 c.c. This is repeated on the opposite side and anæsthesia is complete in from 5–10 minutes and lasts for 1–2 hours. The action is prolonged by the addition of 0·25 c.c. adrenaline (1–1000) to the total amount of procaine.

(*c*) Cæsarean sections especially for toxæmic and cardiac cases.

Technique.—

In classical and lower segment sections only the abdominal wall requires infiltration, but if sterilisation is being carried out then broad ligaments are infiltrated as well.

CHAPTER V

THE PUERPERIUM

THE puerperium is the period following delivery, during which the body is returning to its normal state. It normally lasts from six to twelve weeks.

PHENOMENA

1. The uterus involutes.
2. The decidua is entirely cast off.
3. The mucosa of the uterus is regenerated.
4. The vagina and the supporting ligaments of the pelvic organs contract.
5. The secretion of milk is instituted—lactation.

It is perhaps the most critical period connected with childbirth, as all phenomena, though physiological, easily become pathological.

Involution of the Uterus.—A definite process which takes six weeks to complete.

The uterus diminishes from 32 oz. to 2 oz. in weight. This is effected chiefly by a great reduction of the muscular wall of the uterus, which is achieved by the contractions and retractions of the uterus, cutting off blood supply and making uterus anæmic. This causes autolysis in the muscle, the protoplasm being digested into a soluble peptonoid substance, which is removed by the lymphatics. The vessels diminish in size by new vessels growing inside the dilated vessels of pregnancy. The veins show hyaline change in their walls and the arteries show granular atrophy of muscle fibres.

During the first ten days the process may easily be noted, the fundus uteri normally being felt about the following levels :—

Immediately after labour—below the level of the umbilicus.

The first day after labour—two finger-breadths above the umbilicus. (The rise in the fundus is due to regain of tone of the L.U.S., which collapses after labour.)—5 in. above symphysis.

The second day after labour—one finger-breadth above the umbilicus—4½ in. above symphysis.

The third day after labour—just above the umbilicus—4 in. above symphysis.

The fourth day after labour—just below the umbilicus—$3\frac{1}{2}$ in. above symphysis.

The fifth day after labour—one finger-breadth below the umbilicus—3 in. above symphysis.

The sixth day after labour—two finger-breadths below the umbilicus—$2\frac{1}{2}$ in. above symphysis.

The seventh day after labour—mid-way to the symphysis—2 in. above symphysis.

The eighth day after labour—two finger-breadths above the symphysis—$1\frac{1}{2}$ in. above symphysis.

The ninth day after labour—one finger-breadth above the symphysis—1 in. above symphysis.

The tenth day after labour—level with upper margin of symphysis.

Note.—The umbilicus is not a fixed point, but is useful as an adjacent landmark.

Involution is frequently associated in multiparæ with painful uterine contractions—*after-pains*. Due to excessive uterine contractions to expel blood clot (see p. 224).

Lochia.—During the initial stages of the puerperium, there is a vaginal discharge (lochia). These, for the first five days, are red and hæmorrhagic (lochia rubra), after which they gradually become paler and more serous (lochia alba), till they cease in from ten days to three weeks. This discharge is due in the first instance to the remains of decidua, *i.e.* deep part of spongy layer, being discharged.

They are composed of blood, mucus, and degenerated cells in varying proportions, according to the length of time after delivery. They are alkaline and thus the vaginal bacillus does not thrive until quantity diminishes.

The odour is slightly heavy, but should not be fœtid.

Sudden, early stoppage is indicative of septicæmia, whereas excess is often associated with sub-involution.

The uterine mucosa is fully regenerated after a month, though the placental site can still be discerned.

Secretion of Milk.—Usually commences on the third day, but may be earlier or later. Free lactation is inhibited in the first few days of the puerperium by the large amount of œstrogen and progesterone still circulating in the blood.

Colostrum is secreted for the first two days. It is a viscid fluid, which is colourless at first, but it soon becomes white. It contains fully five times as much protein as mature human milk, but less fat and half as much sugar. It has a purgative action on the child.

Transition milk is secreted from the third day until one month after parturition. Its composition depends on the stage of the puerperium.

Mature milk, having a more constant composition, is secreted after the first month of the puerperium.

General Conditions of Puerperal State.—Pulse slow at first, 60 to 70.

Temperature usually below normal, though there may be a reactionary temperature within twelve hours of delivery; if above 100·4° F. for twelve hours or more, this is suggestive of sepsis. May rise on third day to 100°, due to engorgement of breasts.

Liver and bowels sluggish; other excretory organs active, especially the skin.

The patient should sleep well all the time and feel well by the third day.

MANAGEMENT

Call daily until the tenth day. Post-natal examinations should be made between tenth and fourteenth days and again at fourth to sixth week after delivery (see p. 85).

Inquire as to the lochia, micturition, pain, and sleep.

Diet as usual, with plenty of milk, milk puddings and porridge.

Order an aperient after thirty-six to forty-eight hours (castor oil ℥i) and see that the bowels move daily thereafter, less drastic purgatives being used, such as cascara, vegetable laxative, senna, etc. No drastic purge should be given, but if still constipated with moderate doses, then augment with paraffin, petrolagar or agarol.

(*N.B.*—The anthracene purgatives, such as cascara, may be excreted in the breast-milk and may cause diarrhœa in the infant. Certain fruits and vegetables may have a similar effect.)

Pay special attention to the pulse and temperature (morning and evening readings). The pulse is a most important indicator and if it is maintained above 100 it usually means something pathological is occurring.

The vulval pads must be changed frequently by the nurse, and always after micturition and defæcation. All aseptic precautions must be taken.

Examine abdominally for the fundus uteri daily to see that involution is progressing normally (see p. 77).

It may be advisable to keep the patient in bed till the tenth day, but no bad results have been observed by one of the authors (W. F. T. H.) or his father who have allowed normal cases with no large perineal tears up on the third to fifth days. Such treatment has been adopted for over 2500 cases during the last forty years and no untoward effects have been observed. In fact it has appeared to be entirely beneficial and has been much appreciated by the patients. The time allowed out of bed should be increased daily.

Though the patient is allowed to get up early, if there is no one to help her at home to look after the house and the baby, she should be sent to a convalescent home with her child until at least three weeks have elapsed since her confinement, so as to give her every chance of being fit to tackle her daily routine work. It is the hospital patient who requires most rest and convalescence after her confinement, and, unfortunately, she is usually the patient who is allowed home quickest.

Some patients benefit by massage to legs and abdominal wall, and exercises taught and supervised by a physiotherapist are of great benefit to the hospital patient.

If the patient is confined in her own house and cannot be kept under supervision, then probably it is best for her not to be allowed to rise early as she might be inclined to overdo it, especially if she has several children at home to be looked after. The patient should always be encouraged to rest for at least one hour in the afternoon for a month after delivery.

(*N.B.*—Early rising has been advocated by many authorities especially in the U.S.A. during the past few years, and patients are recommended to get up for a little daily from the twelfth hour after delivery. This has been practised by one of us (W. F. T. H.) both in hospital and private practice for the last three years in over 1,000 cases (Cæsarean sections included) with most satisfactory results for all concerned. Patients with perineal tears are treated similarly, and it has been found that healing is not delayed.)

Benefits of Early Rising.—

1. Secures better drainage of the genital tract.
2. Prevents backward uterine displacements.
3. Promotes free circulation in the lower limbs and pelvis by increasing the muscle tone. Probably helps to prevent embolus and venous thrombosis.
4. Increases intra-abdominal pressure, favouring involution.

5. Prevents muscular weakness and helps the figure.
6. Mitigates constipation.

GENERAL RULES FOR BREAST FEEDING

Breast feeding should always be practised unless there are strong contra-indications.

Benefits.—The natural method of feeding is better for the physical and psychological health of both mother and child than any method of artificial feeding. Suckling is beneficial during the first forty-eight hours, as it :—

(*a*) Teaches child technique of feeding.
(*b*) Helps to draw out nipples and gradually accustoms them to the trauma associated with suckling.
(*c*) Stimulates the secretion of milk.
(*d*) Aids involution of uterus.
(*e*) Provides the child with colostrum.

Supervision.—Each feed should be supervised by the nurse during the first week in the case of a primipara, and for a shorter time as necessary in the case of a multipara. This ensures the establishment of a correct nursing technique and engenders confidence in the inexperienced mother.

It is very important to ensure successful breast feeding of the first child if possible, as the mother's attitude towards breast feeding in all subsequent pregnancies will be determined by her experience with the first child.

Frequency of Feeding.—The first feed should be given 6–12 hours after parturition, depending on the condition of the mother and the baby, and also on the time of birth. Two or three feeds in the first 24 hours are sufficient. Thereafter regular three-hourly feeds should be given as follows—6 A.M., 9 A.M., 12 noon, 3 P.M., 6 P.M., and 10 P.M. Four-hourly feeding should be adopted as soon as the milk supply becomes abundant, except in the case of small babies.

Duration.—Short feeds should be given until the breasts fill with milk about the third day. A few minutes at each breast is long enough to obtain the small amount of colostrum available. More prolonged suckling at this stage may traumatise the nipples.

After the inception of free lactation, twenty minutes should be allowed for each feed.

Method.—One or both breasts may be given at each feed. If the infant obtains insufficient from one breast, as indicated by cry of hunger, infrequent stools and failure to gain in weight, both breasts should be given—ten minutes at each breast.

If the baby is still underfed by this method, continue to give both breasts at each feed and give a complementary feed of cow's milk mixture immediately after each feed except the first (the 6 A.M. feed follows the longest interval and is therefore the largest). Infants do not, as a rule, take more complementary milk mixture than they need. (For composition of mixture, see p. 378.)

Eructation of Air.—Infants always swallow a considerable amount of air during suckling. As much of this as possible must be allowed to escape up the œsophagus by holding the baby upright and gently patting its back (" breaking wind ") once or twice during feed and at end of feed. If baby is laid down without allowing air to escape, distension of stomach may cause vomiting and, later, distension of bowel may cause colic and loose greenish stools. If baby cries soon after being returned to cot, lift again to see if more air can be brought up.

Breast Milk Requirements.—The amount of breast milk suckled per day by average mature babies is as follows :—

½ week	10 oz.
1 ,,	15 ,,
1 month	25 ,,
3 months	30 ,,
6 ,,	35 ,,

These are basic requirements. Much greater amounts are sometimes taken. Wakeful, nervous babies require more.

Test-weighing.—When accurate scales are available, this procedure indicates the amount of breast milk suckled by the baby. The baby is weighed in its clothes after being changed and before going to the breast, and again at the conclusion of the feed in the same clothes and before being changed. The difference between the two weights indicates the amount of breast milk suckled, which, in the first fortnight, should be at least 2½–3 ounces. A single test-feed has little value, as the amount suckled at individual feeds varies greatly. A consecutive series of test-feeds should be carried out, preferably for the whole day.

Pre-requisites of Successful Lactation.—

1. Heredity is an important influence. A family history of successful lactation is desirable.
2. Ante-natal preparation—(*a*) Psychological ; (*b*) of nipples.

3. A nourishing well-balanced diet—(*a*) During pregnancy; (*b*) during lactation.

First-class proteins are more often deficient than any other factor. Deficiency of protein diminishes the quantity of milk secreted but not the quality. Milk, which is an excellent source of protein, should be taken freely in some form.

4. An ample fluid intake. Deficiency of fluid is spontaneously corrected by the development of thirst.
5. Freedom from overwork and fatigue.
6. Freedom from worry. Worry seriously inhibits lactation.

Contra-indications of Breast Feeding.—

1. Chronic ill-health of the mother as follows :—
   (*a*) Pulmonary tuberculosis. Child should be kept apart from mother as danger is from her breath.
   (*b*) Severe heart disease. Breast feeding is practicable in most cases of heart disease.
   (*c*) Severe asthma, chronic bronchitis or bronchiectasis.
   (*d*) Chronic nephritis.
   (*e*) Severe diabetes.
   (*f*) Insanity.
   (*g*) Other conditions according to circumstances.
2. Illegitimacy, sometimes, according to circumstances.
3. Breast abnormalities :—
   (*a*) Retracted nipples which cannot be drawn out.
   (*b*) Hypogalactia, when severe and habitual in all previous pregnancies.

Suppression of Lactation.—If the mother is not to nurse her child or if child be stillborn, milk secretion is suppressed by the administration of an œstrogen in sufficient dosage to inhibit the anterior pituitary. Stilbœstrol, dienœstrol, ovendosyn or hexœstrol, may be given 5 mgm. thrice daily for three days, twice daily for two days and once daily for four days.

POST-NATAL CARE

Two routine examinations necessary, the first twelve to twenty-one days after delivery and the second six weeks later. By such investigation slight local lesions, which would otherwise give rise to chronic disablement, may be treated early. Post-natal care should also cover the general health of the patient as well as the pelvic condition, this being especially necessary in cases which have exhibited toxæmic symptoms during pregnancy.

The chief causes of complaint during this period are: (1) Leucorrhœa; (2) irregular bleeding; (3) pelvic discomfort or pain; (4) backache; and (5) disturbances of micturition. (All these may follow a normal spontaneous delivery.)

1. **Leucorrhœa.**—Usually due to infection of cervix and may be profuse even though no clinical evidence of sepsis was apparent during the puerperium. Delay in treatment may result in chronic cervicitis, chronic infection of pelvic cellular tissue and delay in involution of the uterus. Early erosions should be treated by daily douching with 1–5000 perchloride of mercury, but if they should resist this treatment, the application of silver nitrate or the actual cautery may be required. A purely vaginal leucorrhœa may be present due to organisms growing in a vagina made alkaline by the lochia, in which Döderlein's bacilli have not reappeared. This is a thin white secretion and usually clears up quickly by the administration of lactic acid to the vagina (see p. 265).

2. **Irregular Bleeding.**—Usually due to subinvolution and is often associated with retroversion. Subinvolution should be treated with ergot pills and hot douching. If the uterus is retroverted it should be replaced manually, and the patient be instructed to lie face downwards for ten minutes three times daily. Usually this treatment is sufficient, but if the uterus is still retroverted four weeks later, a pessary must be inserted after reposition of the uterus. The pessary should be worn for three to four months. (A recurrence of red lochia about the twelfth to sixteenth day of the puerperium frequently denotes a retroversion.)

3. **Pelvic Discomfort or Pain.**—Often due to early prolapse of the uterus and vaginal walls, the patient also complaining of the feeling of something coming down. A subinvoluted and retroverted uterus is most likely to give rise to these symptoms. If slight degree of prolapse is present, rest, cold douching and tonic treatment with strychnine is usually efficacious, the ligaments tighten and the condition is cured. If condition is at all severe a pessary may be inserted as well, to keep patient comfortable, but should only be used with discrimination as it retards the toning-up of the musculature in the ligaments.

May also be due to chronic infection of cellular tissue, which is best treated by hot douching, combined at times with vaginal plugging with ichthyol and glycerine (10 per cent.). (The cervix must also be treated, as it is often the initial source of the inflammation.)

4. **Backache.**—May be due to retroversion, early prolapse, utero-sacral cellulitis, chronic pyelitis or excessive strain of sacro-iliac and lumbo-sacral joints. Remedial exercises and the wearing of a good supporting belt are required for the last-named cause. Chronic pyelitis is by no means rare, and should be treated early with urinary antiseptics such as sulphacetamide (albucid), hexamine, pyridium, etc., as it is apt to become very obstinate and may cause acute exacerbations, ureteric spasm, or stenosis.

5. **Disturbances of Micturition.**—May result from bruising or tearing of bladder or urethra during labour, infection of bladder or kidneys, or sagging of the base of the bladder. Patient complains usually of frequency of micturition, with or without pain, or imperfect control on exertion (exertion incontinence). Early tonic treatment, especially with strychnine, increases tone of bladder and sphincter and is especially useful in sagging of the bladder and exertion incontinence, though in the latter the application of the actual cautery to the posterior lip of the urethral meatus, under anæsthesia, may be required in resistant cases.

At Examination, Tenth to Fourteenth Day.—

1. Examine for subinvolution.
2. Examine for retroversion.
3. Examine for presence of red discharge.
4. Examine for tenderness in fornices.
5. See that perineal tear or episiotomy has healed.

At Examination, Fourth to Sixth Week.—

1. Examine for erosion of cervix and leucorrhœa.
2. Examine for degree of prolapse or any gaping of introitus.
3. Examine for exertion incontinence or other urinary symptoms.
4. Examine for retroversion and involution of uterus.
5. Examine for any parametritis, utero-sacral cellulitis or adnexitis.
6. Examine abdominal wall to see if tone has been regained.

Infective Hepatitis
Polio.

CHAPTER VI

PATHOLOGY OF PREGNANCY

THIS may, for practical purposes, be grouped into three distinct classes :—

1. Intercurrent diseases in no way due to pregnancy, but which exercise a distinct influence upon the gravid state, or are themselves reacted upon by this condition, *e.g.* scarlet fever, syphilis, etc.
2. Intercurrent diseases due to pregnancy, *e.g.* eclampsia.
3. Morbid states of the uterus and ovum, which seriously affect the normal relationship between the mother and fœtus and thereby endanger the life of one or other, or both.

(A) INTERCURRENT DISEASES INDEPENDENT OF PREGNANCY

PNEUMONIA

Effect of Pregnancy on.—The pregnant state predisposes to this affection from the now normal excess of fibrin in the blood. It also aggravates the disease in the later months by increasing the dyspnœa, through—

(*a*) Impeding the movements of the diaphragm.
(*b*) The normal deficiency of red blood corpuscles.

Effect of Pneumonia on Pregnancy.—Great tendency to kill ovum from high temperature and thus bring on premature expulsion.

Terminations.—If slight—

(1) May resolve.
(2) May induce expulsion of uterine contents, which usually gives relief.

If severe : Almost always causes abortion, which usually aggravates disease.

Prognosis.—1. Maternal : grave but has improved greatly with chemotherapy. More serious—

(*a*) If it occurs in later months.
(*b*) If uterine contents are expelled.

2. Fœtal: Very grave. Cause of death, high temperature.

Treatment.—As in ordinary non-complicated cases; but—

(*a*) Do not bring on labour.
(*b*) If labour commenced, hasten.
(*c*) Allow free bleeding.

Acute Tuberculosis of Lungs

Effect of Pregnancy on.—Dangerous times are first four months of pregnancy and first four weeks of puerperium due to increased gonadotrophic hormones and decrease of œstrogen. Patient improves greatly after fourth month due to increase of œstrogen. With new forms of treatment for lung tuberculosis, the effect of pregnancy is much less serious. Nursing aggravates disease.

Effect on Pregnancy.—Nil, unless temperature is high, when abortion may occur.

Effect on Child.—1. May be born healthy, but has low powers of resistance against tubercle bacillus.

2. May be born tubercular—very rare.

Treatment.—Tuberculosis should be treated actively by physician and only in cases where active treatment is impossible, due to presence of adhesions, etc., should abortion be induced. This must be done before fourth month otherwise no benefit will occur.

Rules.—Do not allow pregnancy to go beyond term, but rather induce a week before the expected date.

Do not allow mother to nurse her baby or even have it with her until she is cured, or until the baby has been successfully vaccinated with B.C.G. This should be carried out as soon after birth as possible.

Tuberculous women should not marry unless primary lesions have been quiescent for some time; but, if married, should not become pregnant unless the disease is in the first stage and has been inactive for at least two years.

Smallpox

1. *Effect of Pregnancy on.*—Nil.
2. *Effect on Pregnancy.*—
   (*a*) Varioloid. Has little action.
   (*b*) Discrete variola. Tends to cause expulsion of ovum. Prognosis is favourable in early months, but graver in advanced gestation.

(*c*) Confluent variola. Almost always causes expulsion of ovum. Prognosis grave.

3. *Effect on Fœtus.*—

(*a*) Frequently dies from high temperature.
(*b*) May live and be born healthy at full term.
(*c*) May be born with smallpox.
(*d*) May develop smallpox after birth, as late as three months after mother.
(*e*) May be born with smallpox, though mother escapes.
(*f*) In twins, one may suffer and the other escape.
(*g*) Generally resist vaccination if born healthy.

Scarlet Fever

Puerperal women seem to be especially liable, but it is almost impossible to distinguish rash from septicæmic rash. Very dangerous in puerperium. Incubation period seems to be prolonged during pregnancy. Causes premature expulsion, if temperature is high.

Rubella

When contracted in the early months of pregnancy it is liable to cause serious defects and deformities in the fœtus, such as blindness, deafmutism, mongolism, hydrocephalus, or congenital cardiac defects. In the later months of pregnancy, however, this is not the case.

Malaria

1. *Effect on Pregnancy.*—Powerful oxytocic. Causes intra-uterine death of fœtus by—

(1) Massive infection of placenta with parasites.
(2) High temperature.
(3) Direct infection of fœtus by parasites.

Patient more prone to develop—

(1) Toxæmia and precipitate eclampsia.
(2) Sepsis in puerperium.
(3) Pyelitis.

Collapse may follow labour.

2. *Effect of Pregnancy on.*—Aggravates disease and may cause cerebral malaria. Labour may precipitate attack.

3. *Treatment.*—Quinine in usual large dosage. Acts as placebo rather than oxitocic as it prevents high temperature.

Influenza

Pregnant women seem to be specially liable to epidemic influenza. Abortion common, due to high temperature.

Leucorrhœa

Increased by pregnancy and may occur only during pregnancy, due to increased vascularity of parts. Treated as at other times (see p. 265).

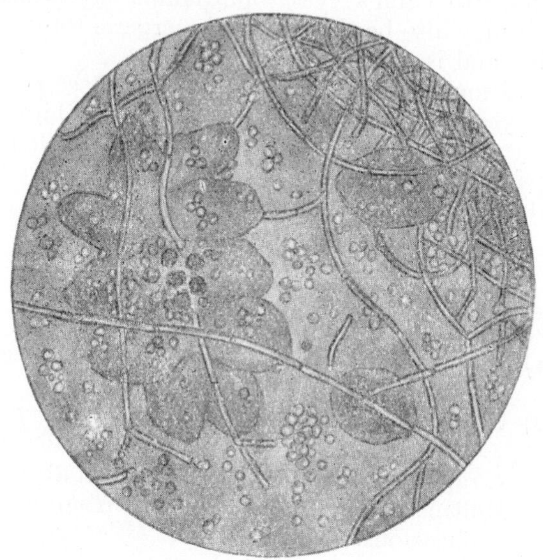

Fig. 14.—Streptothrix—Oidium Albicans.

Monilial Discharge

Due to a streptothrix, *oidium albicans* (see Fig. 14).

Liable to occur with pregnancy especially if there is a tendency to glycosuria.

Discharge is white and lumpy and often very profuse.

Vagina is reddened with small white patches on its surface caused by aggregations of discharge.

Often causes irritation and marked discomfort, but in other cases may not cause any symptoms.

Treated by painting vagina, vulva and surrounding skin, including inside of thighs with gentian violet (2 per cent. aqueous solution), daily for 4 to 5 days and then weekly, if discharge recurs, as it is apt to do, during whole pregnancy.

Always disappears immediately after delivery. Anti-glycosuric diet may be of use.

Gonorrhœa

Vaginal discharge increased by softening of vagina during pregnancy, otherwise not affected by pregnancy; nor is pregnancy affected by it, though sterility may occur, due to salpingitis; tubal gestation may result. Discharge may cause danger to child's eyes (ophthalmia neonatorum) (see p. 388); it may also be the cause of puerperal sepsis—usually salpingitis—and is not fatal.

The condition is treated as at other times (see p. 343).

Child's eyes should be wiped carefully after birth of head with dry cotton wool. Prophylactic drops, which may be irritating in themselves, are not now recommended, as the treatment of ophthalmia is so effective.

Syphilis

1. *Effect of Pregnancy on.*—
   - (1) May not alter the normal sequence of events in acquired syphilis.
   - (2) Usually there is a mitigation of signs, *e.g.* primary sore, if it appears, is often small and heals rapidly. Secondary lesions often absent.
   - (3) Multiparæ are singularly free from grave complications.

2. *Effect on Pregnancy.*—Tendency to miscarry, the fœtus usually dying between the fourth and the seventh months.

Maternal.—(Varies in accordance with age of disease, and if acquired before or after conception.)

(*a*) *Syphilis before Conception.*—Great tendency to premature expulsion. Often the child is carried a month longer each succeeding pregnancy. If gestation is prolonged to term—

- (1) Child may be born apparently healthy, but shows signs of syphilis within three months.
- (2) May show signs of syphilis at birth.
- (3) May die from convulsions in a few days without showing any other sign of syphilis.

(*b*) *Syphilis at Time of Impregnation.*—Conditions same as in (*a*).

(*c*) *Syphilis Acquired after Conception.*—Varies with age of ovum.—

(1) In earlier months child usually shows signs soon after birth as in (*a*).
(2) In later months apparently healthy child often showing signs after three months or in later life.

Successive miscarriages (Habitual) may be the only indication of syphilis.

Paternal.—The ovum may be affected without the mother showing signs of disease. This is very common. Colles' law states that the mother will not be infected by nursing a syphilitic child, but the reason is that she already has the disease, though it is not apparent, *i.e.* " latent syphilis."

Practical Deductions.—

1. Routine blood tests should be taken at all ante-natal clinics. If any deviation from negativity is found, then the patient should be fully investigated—

(*a*) Thorough examination.
(*b*) Blood tests repeated and a provocative injection of arsenic given.
(*c*) Blood tests repeated after five day's interval.
(*d*) If any doubt remains the husband or consort should be asked to report for investigation. The patient may suffer from congenital syphilis herself, in a latent form. It may, therefore, be necessary to examine her parents and siblings.

(*N.B.*—The Wassermann reaction often vacillates during pregnancy and the puerperium.)

2. Forbid marriage until the patient has had at least six months' intensive treatment with penicillin, arsenic and bismuth. The importance of regular attendance for treatment must be stressed as otherwise the patient may later infect her husband should she relapse.

3. Contraception should be maintained preferably until the mother's blood is negative. Ante-natal treatment with penicillin alone is, however, so effective that with due care a healthy infant can be practically guaranteed.

Treatment.—Syphilitic children are treated from birth by intramuscular injections of penicillin, sometimes combined with arsenic and bismuth.

Parents of syphilitic children must be examined and treated.

Mother may nurse a syphilitic baby, but wet nursing of such a child must be forbidden. It must be remembered that the acute syphilitic baby is infectious until treatment has taken effect.

Cardiac Disease

1. *Effect on Pregnancy.*—May cause premature expulsion.
   (*a*) From carbon dioxide poisoning fœtus.
   (*b*) From carbon dioxide causing excessive uterine contractions.
   (*c*) From venous congestion causing hæmorrhage into placenta, etc.

2. *Effect on Fœtus.*—Often small and may be stillborn or die in neo-natal period.

3. *Effect of Pregnancy on Heart Diseases.*—Tends to aggravate all varieties.

The most dangerous period is that following delivery, due to sudden fall in blood pressure.

Three Groups of Cases.—

1. Organic disease present but show no symptoms.
2. (*a*) Can perform usual duties but have slight discomfort and slight limitation of physical activity.
   (*b*) Definite limitation of physical activity.
3. Cardiac reserve at a minimum. No physical activity without discomfort. Heart failure even in bed.

Treatment.—

Group 1.—Pass through pregnancy and labour without any trouble from cardiac condition.

Group 2.—(*a*) Must be watched carefully ante-natally to prevent lapse into 2 (*b*). Normal delivery with no undue prolongation of second stage.

(*b*) Will require frequent periods of rest ante-natally and mild sedative treatment with phenobarbitone and bromide.

Normal delivery in majority of cases, as child is usually small and labour easy.

If any abnormality present, which would make delivery difficult, then Cæsarean section should be done.

Sterilisation will be required in a large percentage of cases which have been persistently in this group during pregnancy and this should be done under local anæsthesia 24 to 72 hours after delivery. (*Cæsarean section is never indicated for sterilisation purposes alone.*)

Group 3.—Absolute rest in bed. Urgent ante-natal treatment with digitalis ♍xxx three to four times daily for three to four days. Mersalyl for œdema. When heart condition is considered satisfactory.

Before the thirty-sixth week Cæsarean section or abdominal hysterotomy should be done without delay under local anæsthesia.

If late in pregnancy and the patient is a multipara, induction of labour should be carried out by rupture of the membranes. If the patient is a primigravidæ, then Cæsarean Section under local anæsthesia will probably be advisable.

Rules for delivery of cardiac cases.

1. Do not allow second stage to be prolonged. Apply forceps if otherwise justified.
2. Allow fairly free bleeding during third stage, as it relieves tension on heart.
3. Keep quiet for at least an hour after expulsion of placenta and be on premises during this time as collapse may occur due to fall of blood pressure by splanchnic congestion.
4. Give twilight sleep or some other analgesia if first stage is delayed and causing patient undue discomfort and worry.
5. Anæsthetist more important than anæsthetic. Best anæsthetics for vaginal delivery are :—
   (1) Gas and plenty of oxygen.
   (2) Chloroform and oxygen.
   (3) Cyclopropane.
   (4) Local.

Each cardiac case must be considered carefully individually so that best form of treatment is carried out.

Diabetes

Effect on Pregnancy.—The untreated patient is usually sterile. When the diabetic condition is controlled by insulin, women frequently become pregnant, and, although specially liable to develop pre-eclamptic toxæmia, the outlook for the mother is good. As regards the child, 40–50 per cent. are stillborn or die in the neo-natal period.

Clinical Features.—Usually none as pregnancy occurs in a woman under treatment. This is not always so, however, and coma, increased adiposity, hydramnios and large child are all possible. Diabetes is frequently preceded by the birth of a very large child several years before.

Diagnosis.—Difficult, as 40 per cent. pregnant women have glycosuria at some time or other during pregnancy. Definitely proved by glycosuria persisting ten days after delivery. Blood sugar high.

Treatment.—Insulin with relatively high carbohydrate diet to avoid acetonuria. Insulin causes decrease of hydramnios.

Labour should be induced at thirty-sixth week, as fœtal mortality after that time is very high. In primigravidæ, Cæsarean Section at thirty-sixth week may be the best treatment. 10 c.c. of 10 per cent. glucose should be injected intramuscularly into baby soon after birth followed by glucose solution orally two-hourly for a month. This is to try to prevent baby dying from hypoglycæmia due to hypertrophy of islets of Langerhans resulting from high blood sugar in fœtus.

If patient develops pre-eclampsia, large doses of œstrogen (150,000–300,000 I.U. œstrodial benzoate daily by injection) may do good as toxæmia may be due to an œstrogen deficiency. (Priscilla White has lowered her fœtal mortality from 30 per cent. to 6 per cent. by such treatment, but others have not been so fortunate.)

Twilight sleep of use during labour, when insulin should be administered. Gas and oxygen best anæsthetic.

Anæmia

May be microcytic, macrocytic, normocytic, hyperchromic, etc.

Continues usually until about 4th to 6th week of puerperium, when condition usually rapidly improves.

Treated with—

(1) Blood transfusions.
(2) Liver injections.
(3) Vitamin C, in large dosage.
(4) Iron.

Chronic Nephritis

Always aggravated by pregnancy.

May only show symptoms during pregnancy (*threshold kidney*), the symptoms becoming more marked and occurring earlier at each successive pregnancy.

Fœtus often dies in utero, but if it survives, is often small and undernourished due to placental infarction.

Diagnosis.—Blood urea high—above 40 mgm. per 100 c.c. Urea clearance of 50 or under.

Urea concentration test low, often below 2 per cent.

Urea range very level with no peak. Albumen and globulin approximate.

Albumen appears early in pregnancy and takes long time to disappear entirely from urine after labour.

Urine output usually increased. Albuminuric retinitis may be present.

Blood pressure remains high for three to four weeks or longer after labour, the diastolic pressure especially being raised.

Treatment.—If blood urea high, above 40 mgm. per 100 c.c. and other signs of chronic nephritis present, pregnancy should be terminated; this should also be considered seriously if symptoms do not respond to treatment, otherwise dangerous kidney damage will result. This is especially necessary if symptoms manifest themselves before the seventh month. Sterilisation required if contraception not practicable.

Essential Hypertension

Pre-existing hypertension associated with generalised arterial spasm.

Familial tendency to disease.

Any blood pressure over 140/90 mm. should come under category. Pressure usually falls during third to sixth month, but increases again during last three months. When the pressure reaches 160 mm. systolic, albuminuria is apt to occur, and this may be followed by œdema, a pre-eclamptic toxæmia being now superimposed.

Prognosis.—

Mother.—

1. Hypertension by itself is not aggravated by pregnancy.

2. If pre-eclampsia is superimposed, then kidneys may suffer damage if pregnancy is allowed to continue.
3. Incidence of pre-eclampsia is seven times more common and eclampsia ten times more common than for women with normal pressure at beginning of pregnancy.
4. Accidental hæmorrhage may occur.

Child.—

1. Fœtus liable to die from concealed accidental hæmorrhage.
2. If blood pressure does not fall in second trimester of pregnancy, prognosis bad ; otherwise good.
3. If blood pressure is over 150/100 mm. at beginning of pregnancy, only one-third give birth to viable infants.

Treatment.—

1. Rest, the amount depending on severity of hypertension.
2. Avoid strong tea, coffee, tobacco, alcohol, spices and red meat.
3. Saline purges.
4. Sedatives such as phenobarbitone gr. ½ and bromide gr. vii twice or thrice daily.
5. If kidney function tests show deficiency or there is marked retinal papillœdema or persistent albuminuria, pregnancy should be terminated; this is especially necessary if persistent albuminuria develops before 20th week.
6. If blood pressure is above 160 mm. the pressure should be taken at least weekly, and if condition deteriorates, patient should be admitted to hospital when daily readings and urinary examinations should be done.
7. It should be endeavoured to keep blood pressure below the danger point of 160 mm. systolic.
8. If albuminuria develops there is great danger of intra-uterine death, so if a child is viable, Cæsarean Section under local anæsthesia or induction of premature labour should be carried out.

(B) DISEASES DUE TO PREGNANCY

Pre-eclamptic Toxæmia

A most anxious condition during pregnancy.

May occur at any time, but it is much more frequent in the later months.

77 per cent. occur in primigravidæ.

Twins and hydramnios seem to predispose.

May be superimposed on an essential hypertension.

Clinical Signs.—

(1) *Œdema*, (2) *hypertension* and (3) *albuminuria*.

All occur in typical case, but in others only one or two of the three signs may be present or pronounced.

Mild or Moderate Cases.—May have no symptoms, but at routine antenatal examination albumen is found in urine and blood pressure is raised.

May have œdema of hands, face, ankles, legs, etc.

Output of urine often diminished.

Increase of weight (over 5 lbs. per month).

Severe Cases.—Increased œdema, often including vulva.

Increased hypertension and albuminuria.

Very much decreased urinary output.

Frontal headaches.

Black specks in front of eyes, amblyopia and possibly blindness.

Buzzing of ears, giddiness and deafness.

Kidney function tests within normal limits.

No albuminuric retinitis.

Results.—

1. Complete recovery (75 per cent.). Albumen disappears from urine and blood pressure becomes normal again, usually within ten to fourteen days after labour.
2. Permanent kidney disease.
3. Convulsions. (Eclampsia.)
4. Fœtus may die in utero if blood pressure is high or albuminuria pronounced.
5. Death of the fœtus in utero is often followed by complete disappearance of symptoms.

Prognosis.—If slight and not increasing, favourable.

Treatment.—

Prophylactic.—Routine antenatal examination of urine and blood pressure.

General.—High protein diet is now recommended—100–120 gm. being given daily.

Salt-free diet (Neo-Selarom or Ruthmol can be used instead).

Saline purges.

Stimulate skin secretion with hot baths, packs, etc.

Blood pressure, amount of albumen and urinary output should be watched daily in moderate and severe cases.

Special.—

(1) For œdema.—Restrict fluid to amount of urine passed, but not less than one and a half pints per diem. Ammonium chloride gr. xxx. thrice daily.

(2) For scanty output urine.—Thyroid gr. v. 4-hourly if output less than ten ounces per diem.

(3) For high blood pressure.—Veratrone $\frac{1}{4}$ to $\frac{1}{2}$ c.c. (over 180 mm. systolic), once or twice daily as required. Venesection.

Obstetric.—

1. Induction of premature labour (*a*) if condition gets worse, despite treatment; (*b*) if condition does not show signs of improvement with three weeks' treatment; (*c*) if early signs of albuminuric retinitis (fluffing of vessels in discs) show themselves.

2. If symptoms suddenly get worse, Cæsarean section is often required to prevent eclampsia occurring. (Sterilisation is never required.)

In all but mild cases constant supervision in hospital is essential.

Prognosis.—10–15 per cent. recurrence in future pregnancies; the cases who suffer longest from the toxæmia are most likely to have a recurrence.

Eclampsia

A convulsive seizure simulating epilepsy, but without any cry. Preceded usually by pre-eclampsia, but in some cases may be fulminating.

Types.—*Tonic and Clonic.*—These usually occur one after the other during the same fit, but may occur independently and alternately with each other.

Description of Fit.—*Tonic:* Fixation of eyes, protrusion of tongue, trismus and distortion of face, often associated with opisthotonus.

Clonic.—Twitching of facial muscles and rolling of the eyes, causing great facial contortion, combined with rapid spasmodic movements of head and extremities, stertorous breathing and marked cyanosis; to these add injection of conjunctivæ, and the horrible picture requires no further description.

Each fit as a rule lasts from thirty to sixty seconds or

longer and leaves the patient in a dazed condition—*coma.* It is usually accompanied by a slightly raised temperature.

The attacks vary in severity and frequency. If fits are numerous, the patient is in a state of complete stupor during intervals and eventually becomes comatose before death, which frequently results from œdema of the brain and lungs, apoplexy or toxic myocarditis.

May develop during pregnancy, labour, or puerperium; less than 25 per cent. developing in puerperium.

Eight times more common in primigravidæ.

Incidence and severity vary in different parts of the world.

Pathology.—

Liver.—Enlarged and mottled by fatty areas, necrosis and hæmorrhages. Degeneration of cells at periphery of lobule. Thromboses and hæmorrhages with necrosis of cells in thrombosed areas, which vary in size.

Kidney.—Enlarged. Degenerative tubular nephritis with degeneration of tubular epithelium. Glomeruli unaffected. Usually no permanent kidney damage, though 20 per cent. develop toxæmia at future pregnancy and 70 per cent. a residual hypertension (Browne).

Heart.—Degenerative myocarditis.

Brain.—Hyperæmia, capillary thromboses and hæmorrhages. Œdema.

Blood.—Increase of fibrinogen content and blood uric acid, but blood urea not increased. Alkalinity diminished. Leucocytosis.

Placenta.—Infarcts, big and small. Hæmorrhages and at times retroplacental clots. Absence of B_1 vitamin.

Lungs.—Marked œdema. Giant cells (? syncytial) may be found in capillaries.

Eye Changes.—Œdema sometimes or detachment of retina may occur. Never albuminuric retinitis unless kidney is becoming damaged, when cotton wool patches and hæmorrhages may occur.

Possible Causes.—

1. Increased intra-abdominal pressure, leading to alteration in circulatory conditions in liver and kidneys and causing degenerative changes (Paramore). This is more common in primigravidæ and stout women of short stature.

2. Hypoxia producing intense injury to trophoblast brings about the liberation of thromboplastin into intervillous sinuses. This in turn is responsible for a deposition of fibrin or a

complete intervillous thrombosis which give rise to infarction. Circulating thromboplastic products may cause liver damage ; according to Young, a toxin may be liberated from the infarcts.

3. Increased intra-uterine tension, *e.g.* hydramnios, twins, etc.

4. Mechanical compression of uterine vessels during labour.

5. Systemic diseases producing effect on arteries of uterus, *e.g.* diabetes, hypertension, nephritis.

6. Œstrogen and progesterone deficiency causing vaso-constriction and ischæmia. The excess of chorionic gonadotrophic hormone in pre-eclampsia may reflect a failing utilisation of this hormone for the production of œstrogen and progesterone (Smith). This results in cerebral œdema, increased intra-cranial tension, hypertension and cerebral anæmia which, according to Browne, are the prelude to convulsions.

Prognosis.

Maternal.—Very grave, but has improved recently, the mortality being now about 10 per cent.

Delivery arrests fits in three out of four cases, but patients may die after arrest of fits.

Slightly more grave in multiparæ.

Intra- and post-partum eclampsia usually give the best prognosis, if the latter is not associated wth cerebral hæmorrhage, when the condition is most fatal.

Fœtal.—Grave. Mortality around 40 per cent.

Fœtal mortality is due—

(*a*) To premature expulsion, 25 per cent.
(*b*) To asphyxia.
(*c*) To toxæmia.

Danger Signs.—The case is reckoned severe if any two of the following danger signs are present :—

(1) Deep coma.
(2) Maximum pulse rate 120 or more.
(3) Maximum temperature 103° or more.
(4) Systolic blood pressure over 200 mm.
(5) Anuria.
(6) Numerous fits.

Treatment.—

1. *The imminence of a fit is recognised by*—

(1) Intense frontal headache ;
(2) Perversions of special senses ;

(3) Great scantiness of urine;
(4) High blood pressure (above 170 mm.);
(5) Vomiting with epigastric pain (almost a sign of eclampsia, as a fit usually follows within thirty minutes).

Treated by induction of labour by rupturing membranes or by Cæsarean section especially if any gross abnormality is present.

2. *If fits develop during pregnancy or labour*—

All cases, whether mild or severe, are best treated with a minimum of obstetric interference, as sepsis is specially liable to occur; low forceps may be required to prevent a prolonged second stage.

Cæsarean section gives high mortality, but may be indicated in fulminating cases or in cases before 34th week of pregnancy.

Stroganoff claims a mortality of only 2·5 per cent., and a fœtal mortality of 12·5 per cent., and therefore one of his methods of treatment is usually adopted.

Stroganoff's Method (Old).—Patient kept in dark room and all possible noise prevented.

All operations, *e.g.* catheterisation, injections, etc., carried out under chloroform. Chloroform should be inhaled in ambulance before admission and on admission.

Morphia gr. ¼ at end of anæsthesia. Colon lavage under chloroform. One hour later, chloral gr. xxx, aq. destillata ℥iss, milk ℥ii, and normal saline ℥iiiss per rectum under chloroform. Two hours later, morphia gr. ¼; two hours later, chloral mixture per rectum under chloroform, and repeat again five hours later.

If no other fits or prodromata have occurred, a rectal injection of chloral mixture is given thirteen hours after admission without chloroform, but if fits or prodromata have occurred, chloroform is again given; this is repeated at twenty-third hour after admission.

If no prodromata, chloral gr. xv t.i.d., orally, till delivery occurs.

Chloral gr. xx to be given after delivery of placenta, as that is a usual time for a fit to develop.

If labour does not start within twenty-four hours of first fit, the membranes should be ruptured.

Venesection of 400–600 c.c. of blood if blood pressure is very high and is not being lowered by the treatment.

Milk is given by mouth if patient conscious; if not, it is given per rectum.

Oxygen after a fit to remove anoxæmia.

Position of patient changed from right to left and vice versa to prevent hypostatic pneumonia developing.

Stroganoff Method (New).—

(1) Morphia gr. $\frac{1}{4}$ after first convulsion at 0·00 hours.

(2) 40 c.c. of a 15 per cent. solution magnesium sulphate, subcutaneously at 0.5 hours.

(3) Morphia gr. $\frac{1}{4}$ to $\frac{1}{6}$ at 2.00 hours.

(4) 20 to 25 c.c. magnesium sulphate solution are injected if no fits have supervened; if further fits then 40 c.c. again at 5.50 hours.

(5) Magnesium sulphate solution as in (4) at 11.50 hours.

(6) Magnesium sulphate solution as before at 19.50 hours, but if eclampsia puerperal and no further fits, 5 to 10 gr. veronal can be given instead.

(7) If patient has had five convulsions before beginning treatment, 400 to 600 c.c. blood should be removed by venesection and the membranes ruptured.

(8) Only minimal amount fluid for forty-eight hours.

(9) Oxygen should be given for four to six minutes after each convulsion.

(10) Amount of urine estimated (best done by indwelling catheter) and tested. (If very scanty, glucose 500–1000 c.c. of a 20 per cent. solution intravenously is often beneficial.)

(11) Patient should be nursed on her right side, but position should be changed to left four or five times during twenty-four hours.

(12) Continuous nursing required until twenty-four hours after last convulsion. Mouth, pharynx and nose should be cleansed frequently and patient must be kept warm.

(13) All interference with patient should be carried out under chloroform.

Rectal Bromethol (Avertin) advocated by Dewar and Morris.

0·075–0·1 ml. of bromethol per kilo of patient's body weight is added to necessary quantity of water to make up a final 3 per cent. solution at 40° C. This is administered by slow rectal injection. If patient is restless three hours or more after the injection, a second similar dose is injected and others may be required at not less than three-hourly intervals. Very rarely are more than three doses required, and patient sleeps for twenty-four hours. (The originators of this treatment claim a 4·3 per cent. maternal mortality in forty-four cases, and it has been used in Edinburgh for the past three years with almost equally satisfactory results.)

Various other forms of treatment have been used, such as that advocated by the Dublin School and the treatment by injections with veratrone (½ to 1 c.c.) after each fit as first advocated in Edinburgh in 1914, and latterly in many U.S.A. obstetric clinics.

3. *Of fit itself*—

(1) Place a gag between teeth—the handle of a spoon wrapped round with gauze or a handkerchief is useful. This prevents biting of the tongue.

(2) Turn head to the side, so that saliva, etc., can escape, otherwise patient may suffocate.

(3) Restrain patient gently so as not to let her injure herself.

4. *After-care*—

The patient must be watched carefully in case puerperal eclampsia should develop and her urine should be measured carefully as bilateral cortical necrosis of the kidneys may follow.

Bilateral Cortical Necrosis of Kidneys

A very dangerous condition, which may be sequela of eclampsia, concealed accidental hæmorrhage or septic abortion; it may, however, occur after a normal labour or a Cæsarean section, but this is very rare. The condition is not confined to obstetric cases.

Clinical Features.—

Patient passes no more than 1 to 2 ounces of urine to begin with and this gets less until anuria occurs.

Patient becomes drowsy about the fifth day and dies of uræmia about the tenth day.

Treatment.—

Must be treated early before the kidneys are irretrievably damaged, otherwise condition is hopeless.

All cases of eclampsia and concealed accidental hæmorrhage should have the amount of urine passed daily carefully checked and if less than ℥10 is passed in thirty-six hours intravenous sodium sulphate (4·285 per cent.), or hypertonic glucose (15 to 25 per cent.) as a continuous drip, or glucose 50 per cent. in 200–400 c.c. water should be given until free kidney secretion is established again. In order to prevent end products of protein catabolism which are believed to be toxic, a high carbohydrate intake is desirable and the following treatment has been advocated by Bull, Jockes and Lowe:

A plastic tube 2–3 mm. in diameter is passed into stomach through nose, and a drip of glucose ℥14, peanut oil ℥$3\frac{1}{4}$, acacia q.s., water ℥31, administered giving steadily 1 litre in twenty-four hours. All vomitus is filtered and returned with drip. This ensures accurate fluid intake, and no loss of food or electrolytes through vomiting. When urine is passed the same quantity of water must be added to the drip.

Hyperemesis Gravidarum—Excessive Sickness

Onset.—Usually insidious.

Generally before fourth month.

If in later months, is generally associated with albuminuria, acute hydramnios or pyelitis.

Most common in primigravidæ.

May be due to vitamins B_1 or C deficiency.

Types.—(*a*) *Reflex* caused by—

(1) Retroversion of uterus.

(2) Too rapid distension due to hydramnios, twins, hydatidiform mole.

(3) Overloaded rectum.

(*b*) *Neurotic*—most common.

(*c*) *Toxic*—a toxæmia of pregnancy.

Symptoms.—

Neurotic Type.—Vicious circle. Vomiting—starvation—acidosis—vomiting.

The patient usually complains that she can keep nothing down and vomits after everything she eats and drinks. (If she can keep down any food at all it is always a good sign.) Pulse and temperature are usually normal. Dehydration occurs as condition progresses. Urine diminished. Urea excretion decreased and high ammonia coefficient (10 to 40 per cent.). Acetone and diacetic acid often present in urine as starvation increases. Dimness of vision may occur followed by optic neuritis and temporary blindness.

Toxic Type.—

(1) Fast pulse over 100 (continued).

(2) Jaundice of face and conjunctivæ.
(3) Rapid emaciation with cachexia and marked dehydration.
(4) Albumen and bile present in urine and output scanty.
(5) Coffee-ground vomit.
(6) Nystagmus.

In Wernicke's Encephalopathy the vomiting suddenly stops after several weeks, but pulse rate remains high. Patient becomes apathetic and drowsy. Sometimes nystagmus, polyneuritis and squint occur followed by mental confusion, coma and death.

Pathology of Toxic Type.—

Kidney.—Glomeruli engorged with blood, and tubal epithelium swollen and necrotic (toxic nephrosis).

Liver.—Resembles acute yellow atrophy. Necrosis of central parts of lobules.

Brain.—Areas of congestion and petechial hæmorrhages in grey matter round third ventricle due to toxin from liver or B_1 deficiency (Wernicke's Encephalopathy).

Treatment.—

Preventive.—1. Examine patient in early pregnancy and correct any error, *e.g.* retroversion, constipation.

2. Treat all cases of slight sickness (morning or otherwise) as early as possible with glucose, bromides, luminal, or vitamin B_1 as necessary.

Actual.—1. If vomiting persists despite preventive treatment, remove patient to nursing home or hospital. This is often sufficient to cure the more moderate cases, and some advise then full diet and removal of all sick basins, etc.

2. Usually, however, starvation is required with nutrient enemata of glucose (10 per cent.) and soda bicarbonate (ʒi to pint) four-hourly. Potassium bromide can be added to these enemata, and in the last enema at night gr. xxx should always be added.

3. After two days' treatment patient is allowed fluids and solids alternately, two-hourly; the solids consisting of toast, biscuits, jam and stewed fruit with plenty sugar; and the fluids of milk, weak tea or cocoa with plenty sugar. Glucose is given freely either in fluid or as barley sugar to suck.

4. If this fails, intravenous glucose (10 per cent.) by a continuous drip.

5. If this fails or if any two clinical features of the toxic type appear, then the case is considered toxic, and abortion

should be induced immediately. (Many patients die because abortion is not induced early or quickly enough once the case is definitely proved to be toxic.)

(*N.B.*—Always consult colleague before induction of abortion is decided upon and performed.)

6. The quickest and easiest method of induction of abortion, which will give rise to least shock, is indicated, and without doubt this is abdominal hysterotomy, provided an operating theatre is available. (This operation is especially useful as the abdomen can be filled with saline before closure, and dehydration is benefited greatly.)

7. If theatre facilities are not available one of the other methods of induction must be tried, but most are slow and uncertain, and dilatation of the cervix with immediate evacuation is associated with shock and hæmorrhage, so that, except in very early cases, this procedure is inadvisable. Vaginal hysterotomy is permissible if done by an expert, but is a difficult operation in a primigravida.

Cramps

Very common in calves of legs, thighs and feet, especially on going to bed. *Treated* by calcium lactate gr. x thrice daily and parathyroid gr. $\frac{1}{12}$ every day. Once relief has been attained treatment can be stopped unless symptoms recur.

Heartburn

Commonest abnormality of pregnancy. May occur early, but not usually until after mid-term. Best treated by attending to diet and giving antacid treatment either with powders (soda bicarbonate, Maclean's powder, etc.) or with lozenges (Antacid (P.D. & Co.) or Jenner's). A frequent change of medicine is required in some cases when the benefit of the initial doses of one prescription is soon lost. Injections on successive days (three) of prostigmin 1 c.c. may cure intractable cases.

Chorea

Rare, but important from its gravity.

Causes.—Primiparity.

Previous attacks.

Rheumatic diathesis.

Period of Development.—At any time during pregnancy. More frequent in early months.

Symptoms and Course.—Those of ordinary chorea often exaggerated.

Usually commences gradually, but may be sudden.

May cease, but usually persists till expulsion of uterine contents.

Generally continues into puerperium in a milder degree, and may even appear to develop at this time.

Does not always recur in future pregnancies, although liable to, if attack severe.

Results.—May cause abortion.

Mortality, 17 per cent. ; more dangerous in multiparæ.

Exhaustion is the usual cause of death.

May cause mania by preventing sleep.

Treatment.—As in ordinary cases.

Bring on premature expulsion if severe, especially if movements persist during sleep.

Pruritus

Irritation usually of vulva. Worst at night. Most often occurs during second half of pregnancy. May be due to vaginal discharge, which must be treated. In the majority of cases of true pruritus no discharge is present and many of these clear up on milk diet for several days. Local anæsthetic ointments such as anethaine, nestosyl, etc., may be tried, or a fluid such as liq carbonis detergens ; if these are unavailing, painting with iodine (1 per cent.) daily or injection of proctocaine into vulva may be required (see p. 334).

Varicose Veins

Due usually to increased abdominal tension and pressure of uterus on iliac veins. In early months may be due to dilatation of unstriate muscle generally, *e.g.* the ureter and is probably caused by progesterone.

Chiefly affects veins of inferior extremities and pelvic plexuses. Worst in multiparæ.

Treatment.—*In lower extremities* as in non-pregnant cases. As much rest as possible is important.

If *vulvar* or *vaginal*, there is a great tendency to hæmatoma formation during labour ; treat, therefore, rigidly before expected confinement by recumbent position of patient and pressure on the vulva with a pad of cotton wool.

If varicosities are severe and causing marked discomfort

either in legs or vulva, the veins should be injected with sodium morrhuate.

Hæmorrhoids

A common complaint in last three months often continuing into first week of puerperium. Treat with cold compresses, analgesic ointments such as storaxol, anusol, nestosyl, kamillosan, etc., or suppositories of anusol or nestosyl.

Jaundice

1. **Simple.**—Rare, but important, as it may be a precursor of malignant type (acute yellow atrophy), to which there is a special liability during pregnancy.

2. **Malignant (Acute Yellow Atrophy of Liver).**—Very grave.

Pathology.—Liver greatly decreased in size. Capsule wrinkled. Petechial hæmorrhages. Necrosis of centre of lobule with degeneration around. May be due to infective hepatitis.

Signs and Symptoms.—Intense jaundice.

Scanty urine, often hæmaturia.

Continuous vomiting.

Delirium, diarrhœa and coma, often with convulsions.

Frequently commences during puerperium.

Duration.—May kill in twelve hours or last six days ; ends almost always in death.

Treatment.—*Simple :* Medicinal, as uncomplicated case.

Malignant : Empty uterus as soon as possible.

Pyelitis

Ætiology.—May occur at any time during pregnancy, but is most common from the fifth to seventh month.

B. coli is the common causative organism and the right kidney is usually affected.

Probably a blood infection.

Both ureters become dilated during pregnancy probably owing to action of progesterone and the maximum dilatation is reached about the fifth month. The right ureter shows a kink at the pelvic brim with a constriction above the kink and an atony of upper two-thirds of ureter. This causes a stasis and pyelitis occurs when the stagnant urine in the pelvis of the kidney becomes infected, during a period of lowered resistance, from a focus of infection elsewhere, *e.g.* constipation. May be precipitated frequently by insufficient protection by warm underclothing.

Types.—

1. *Acute*—

High temperature, sometimes rigors.
Fast pulse.
Pain in lumbar region (usually right).
Tenderness in iliac area (usually right).
Rigidity over tender area.
Albumen and pus in urine.
Frequency of micturition.
Vomiting and nausea (often).
Constipation.
Headache and malaise.

These cases are often diagnosed as appendicitis, influenza, etc., as urinary symptoms are not prominent.

2. *Chronic.*—Clinical features—

May be preceded by headache and malaise.
Backache.
Slight frequency of micturition.
No albumen in urine, but coliform organisms are present.

Acute—

Diagnosis is only made by the presence of pus in a single drop of uncentrifuged urine, but a tentative bedside diagnosis can usually be made by palpating loin and iliac fossa between two hands with equal pressure. In pyelitis the maximum tenderness is elicited by the hand palpating the loin.

Prognosis.—Good. Nearly all go to full term with medical treatment only.

Treatment.—Rest in bed and lie on affected side, light diet with plenty of water to drink. Hot packs to loin.

Sulphathiazole, or sulphamezathine, 1 grm. four-hourly with sod. bicarb. and pot. cit. āā gr. xx. for two days, six-hourly for two days, and eight-hourly for two days.

In persistent cases, 0·5 grm. twice daily may be required for long periods unless toxic effects are produced.

(*N.B.*—When giving sulphathiazole, the urinary output must always be measured and must be of good amount, otherwise crystals may form in the kidney and give rise to hæmaturia and anuria.)

Five c.c. of 40 per cent. hexamine or cylotropine (Schering) can be given intravenously on four successive days in obstinate cases.

If these measures fail, catheterisation of ureters followed by irrigation of the pelvis of the kidney and drainage may be required.

In very toxic cases induction of labour or abortion may be required rarely and is usually followed by a rapid cure. This treatment may be especially necessary if associated with hyperemesis.

ABNORMAL PREGNANCY

Spurious Pregnancy or Pseudocyesis

Simulation of the pregnant state by the non-pregnant and is occasionally well marked.

There may be present—

Amenorrhœa.
Sickness.
Enlargement of abdomen.
Mammary changes with milk secretion.
Quickening.
False labour pains.

Causes.—Psychological.

From mental perversion met with in—

(1) Sterile women at menopause.
(2) Newly married, who are desirous of offspring, or think it the natural result of matrimony.
(3) Unmarried, who have had illicit intercourse.

Diagnosis.—

(*a*) *History.*—Symptoms of pregnancy usually not in the normal routine.

(*b*) *Signs*—

(1) Percussion of abdomen tympanitic.
(2) Auscultation negative.
(3) Vaginal examination gives negative signs; no softness.
(4) Abdominal tumour disappears when patient is anæsthetised.

Treatment.—Proof to the patient or husband that abdomen becomes flat under anæsthesia.

Ante-flexion of Gravid Uterus

In Early Months.—Normal.

If aggravated, causes frequent micturition and excessive sickness.

In Late Months.—Forms pendulous belly and may project through separated recti.

Cervix is high up and points backwards.

Causes difficult locomotion and dysuria.

Is cause of malpresentations and malpositions from changing axis of uterus.

Met with chiefly in multiparæ, when it is of less importance; but in primigravidæ it is a sign of a contracted pelvis and is of grave import.

Treat by binder or obstetric belt applied with patient in dorsal position.

Deliver in dorsal position, otherwise the head has difficulty in engaging.

Prolapse of Gravid Uterus

Rare, as usually prolapse disappears during latter months of pregnancy.

Partial.—Os externum at vulva.

Tends to right itself as uterus grows.

Complete.—Procidentia.

Uterus entirely outside vulva.

Abortion always occurs if not replaced.

Symptoms.—Bearing-down feeling.

Difficulty in defæcation and micturition.

Treatment.—Replace prolapse and keep in position by ring pessary.

Retroversion of Gravid Uterus

Causes.—

1. Impregnation in an already retroposed uterus.
2. Acquired during pregnancy.
    - (*a*) By a strain or fall.
    - (*b*) By over-distension of bladder.

Course.—

1. Usually rights itself.
2. Abortion may take place.
3. May become completely incarcerated in pelvis.
4. Part may remain in pelvis and part grow into abdominal cavity (sacculation), being due to adhesions or tumour of posterior wall of the uterus. (Very rare.)

Symptoms and Signs.—

(*a*) In early months often absent. May have—

(1) Bearing-down pains.

(2) Vesical and rectal symptoms from pressure.
(3) Excessive sickness.

(*b*) After fourth month (incarceration).

(1) Aggravation of rectal troubles.
(2) Difficulty in micturition followed by retention of urine, with dribbling (sometimes); by far the most important symptom.
(3) Abdominal tumour (distended bladder).
(4) Abdominal pain.
(5) Pain in back and legs.
(6) Sickness.

Diagnosis from—

(1) Ovarian cyst.
(2) Fibroid.
(3) Hæmatocele.
(4) Extra-uterine gestation.

1. History of pregnancy—

Amenorrhœa, etc.

2. Abdominal tumour, with difficulty in micturition, retention or dribbling.

3. Vaginal examination—

Shows softness of parts.

Large swelling posteriorly, which changes in consistency.

Cervix usually inaccessible, being very high up under symphysis.

4. Catheterisation dissipates abdominal tumour.

Prognosis.—In early months favourable.

In later months grave—

(*a*) From disease of bladder (necrosis) or rupture.
(*b*) From sloughing of pelvic organs.
(*c*) From renal congestion and uræmia occurring.
(*d*) Cystitis, pyelitis and pyonephrosis may occur.

Treatment.—

(*a*) Replace and keep in position by a pessary until the fifteenth week.

(*b*) Method of reposition if incarcerated :—

(1) Empty the bladder and keep the patient in bed, when it often rights itself.
(2) If not, put the patient in genu-pectoral position, and, with fingers in vagina or rectum, push steadily on incarcerated uterus upwards, and,

as far as possible, to one or other side of the sacral promontory. Apt to aid abortion if not done very gently and thus extreme Trendelenberg position alone is recommended by some for fifteen minutes at a time.

(3) If previous efforts unavailing, place the patient in Sims' position (abdomino-lateral) and anæsthetise; now repeat previous efforts.

(4) If still unavailing, grasp anterior cervical lip, if accessible, with volsella and drag it downwards steadily, while at the same time push steadily, as before, on the fundus through the rectum.

(5) Laparotomy and reposition of the uterus from above may be required, accompanied by pressure on the fundus, per vaginam, by an assistant.

(6) If reposition and operation are impossible, procure abortion by passing a sound and rupturing the membranes; if the cervix is inaccessible, aspirate liquor amnii through the posterior fornix, after which leave the patient for a few hours before attempting reposition; abortion always takes place after drawing off the liquor amnii.

(7) With sacculation—
  (i) May right itself during labour.
  (ii) Reposition.
    (*a*) Vaginal.
    (*b*) Abdominal.
      If impossible,
  (iii) Cæsarean section with removal of tumour (if present) or uterus (if necessary).

Fibromyomata of Uterus

1. *Effect on Pregnancy.*—

(*a*) Tend to prevent conception by causing uterine congestion and thickened endometrium.

(*b*) If conception occurs, they tend to cause abortion. This specially applies to interstitial and submucous varieties.

(*c*) Cause malpresentation from destroying normal ovoid shape of uterine cavity.

2. *Effect on Parturition.*—Often none, but

(*a*) May impede the passage of the child if low in the uterus.

(*b*) May cause serious hæmorrhage by impeding uterine contraction.

(*c*) May give rise to irregular uterine contractions.

(*d*) May cause uterine inertia.

3. *Effect on Puerperium if Submucous.*—

(*a*) May be the origin of puerperal fever from tendency to necrose after labour.

(*b*) Often give rise to secondary hæmorrhage, perhaps weeks after labour, from pedunculation and extrusion.

4. *Effect of Pregnancy on Fibromyoma.*—

(*a*) Causes great enlargement of the muscular fibres of the tumour, which thus increases in size, and also becomes softer from increased vascularity; may undergo red degeneration (see p. 297), which is usually associated with pain, tenderness and rise of temperature.

Treatment of Red Degeneration.—

(1) Rest in bed, morphia in frequently repeated doses, ice-bags or hot fomentations. If not availing—
(2) Myomectomy, if possible; if not,
(3) Hysterectomy.

(*b*) After labour the uterus, from contracting on a submucous tumour, tends to expel it as a polypus and in some cases so interferes with its circulation that it suppurates or necroses.

(*c*) In some instances interstitial and subperitoneal tumours have been known to atrophy and disappear after the puerperium. Usually, however, they involute with the uterus, though in rare cases they may increase in size, becoming sarcomatous.

Treatment.—Never drag the child past the tumour, as necrosis will be almost inevitable, followed often by septicæmia. *If impeding delivery*—

1. If in parturient canal, remove if possible by torsion of the pedicle after clamping or enucleation.

2. If subperitoneal try to push it out of the pelvis. Genu-pectoral position may help.

3. If diagnosed early in pregnancy as a probable source of impediment to labour, perform myomectomy.

4. If only diagnosed during labour, and cannot be moved, Cæsarean section, with hysterectomy or myomectomy (as required), offers the best chance to both mother and child.

Ovarian and Broad Ligament Tumours

Affect labour differently, according to size.

If large and abdominal—

1. Prevent secondary powers acting.
2. Change axis of the uterus.

If small and pelvic—

May prolapse before head and block passages.

(*N.B.*—Dermoids are most frequently found in this situation.)

Diagnosis.—

1. If large—

Double abdominal tumour. X-ray examination of great use.

2. If small and pelvic—

Soft mass bulging the vaginal wall in front of the presenting part.

Prognosis.—If large and abdominal—favourable.

If small—grave, from—

1. Torsion of the pedicle, which may occur during pregnancy or in the puerperium.
2. Rupture of the tumour.
3. Rupture of the uterus by tumour causing obstruction to labour.
4. Exhaustion from delay.

Treatment.—*During pregnancy*—remove owing to risk of torsion of pedicle, especially in smaller cysts.

During labour.—If large and abdominal—forceps delivery.

If small and pelvic—

1. Try to push it out of the pelvis between pains, with the patient in the genu-pectoral position. If irreducible—

2. Deliver by Cæsarean section and remove tumour. (See that pedicle is tied securely as the ligature is liable to slip.)

3. If discovered in puerperium or post-natal period, removal is indicated.

Diseases of Amnion

1. Defective Secretion of Liquor Amnii—Oligohydramnios. In early months causes—

(*a*) Adhesion of the embryo to the amnion.

(*b*) Intra-uterine amputation of the limbs by amniotic bands causing compression.
(*c*) Impediment to fœtal growth.

In later months causes—
(*a*) Undue sensation of fœtal movements.
(*b*) Delay in labour from absence of forewaters.

2. **Hydramnios.**—Usually chronic, but may be acute, especially in early months.

Definition.—When the amount of liquor amnii is so great that it produces morbid symptoms by its distension of the uterus, causing pressure on the abdominal or thoracic viscera, and the fœtus. It cannot, therefore, be gauged by a given amount. (Normal amount, 1000 to 2500 c.c. In hydramnios may be from 10 to 25 litres.)

More frequently seen in multiparæ.

Most frequently commences in the later months (after the sixth), but may develop in the early months, causing vomiting from excessive uterine distension and frequently ending in premature expulsion.

Possible Cause.—

Fœtal—

(1) Often associated with fœtal deformities, *e.g.* anencephaly, hydrocephaly, spina bifida, club foot, etc., and may be due in anencephaly, hydrocephaly, and spina bifida to pressure on cerebral centres, causing excessive secretion of urine.
(2) May be due to obstruction in umbilical vein due to stenosis or thrombosis or excessive tension of cord, which causes exudate from surface of cord.
(3) Persistence of vasa propria which spring from fœtal end of cord between chorion and amnion. These vessels usually atrophy at sixth month.
(4) Cirrhosis of liver and cardiac abnormalities in fœtus. Thus in uniovular twins, fœtus in hydramniotic sac may be found to have enlarged heart and kidneys.

Maternal—

(1) May be associated with cardiac or renal disease, causing œdema of placenta with excessive exudation.
(2) Diabetics often have hydramnios. May be associated with albuminuria.

(3) Chronic infection of amnion from focal infection elsewhere.

(4) Acute hydramnios may follow trauma.

Symptoms in Later Months.—Undue size of the uterine tumour, giving rise to pressure symptoms, such as œdema of the legs and vulva and sometimes ascites.

If acute, vomiting from rapid distension of the uterus.

Scanty urine and albuminuria in many cases.

Difficult locomotion.

Dyspnœa from pressure on the diaphragm.

Signs.—

1. Large smooth abdominal tumour, which does not correspond with the normal growth of the pregnant uterus.
2. Thrill and succussion wave.
3. Fœtal heart and parts difficult to make out.
4. Internal ballottement well marked.

Effect on Pregnancy and Parturition.—

1. Frequently premature expulsion.
2. Malpresentations common.
3. Prolapse of the cord may occur, especially after sudden rupture of the membranes in the upright position.
4. First stage of labour is unduly prolonged from inability of the uterus to contract.
5. Undue prolongation of the second stage from uterine inertia following over-distension.
6. Post-partum hæmorrhage from uterine inertia.
7. Involution of the uterus apt to be slow.
8. May be associated with albuminuria.

Effect on Fœtus.—

1. Frequently expelled prematurely.
2. Frequently deformed, anencephalic, etc.
3. May die from pressure.

Prognosis.—To mother—favourable as a rule.

To child—unfavourable; 30 per cent. dead born; many who are born alive subsequently die during the first week.

Hydramnios may occur in subsequent pregnancies.

Diagnosis.—May be mistaken for ovarian or parovarian tumour alone or complicating pregnancy. Hydatid mole resembles it.

Ballottement helps, but X-ray most satisfactory.

Treatment.—

1. Rest, if not causing too severe symptoms.

2. Paracentesis of liquor amnii through abdominal wall, removing 1 to 1½ pints at one time. (This may have to be done more than once and usually can be performed without inducing labour.)

(*N.B.*—Always take X-ray first so as to be sure fœtus is not a monster, for if so, there is no point in prolonging the pregnancy.)

3. If near full term or monster present, induce labour by rupture of membranes as far up as possible.

CHAPTER VII

HÆMORRHAGES DURING PREGNANCY

(*a*) IN EARLY MONTHS

In the first half of pregnancy, vaginal bleeding may be due to :—

1. Continued menstruation—decidual bleeding.
2. Erosion of the cervix.
3. Cervical polypi.
4. Carcinoma of the cervix.
5. Abortion.
6. Hydatidiform mole.
7. Extra-uterine pregnancy.

1. ABORTION

If the contents are expelled before the viability of the fœtus (before the twenty-eighth week), this is called abortion or miscarriage.

Premature labour is the term applied to expulsion after the twenty-eighth week.

Frequency.—About one in five pregnancies.

Thirty-seven per cent. of child-bearing women miscarry before thirty years of age.

Multiparæ are more liable than primigravidæ.

More common before the fourth month :—

(*a*) From greater vascularity of the decidua predisposing to hæmorrhage.

(*b*) Attachment of the ovum is less secure before placental fixation.

Most apt to occur at the time corresponding to a menstrual period.

Most Frequent Causes.—*Paternal :—*

1. Constitutional diseases, specially syphilis.
2. Extremes of age.

Maternal.—

1. Toxins—
   (*a*) Syphilis.
   (*b*) Zymotic fevers.
   (*c*) Jaundice.
   (*d*) Excess of carbon dioxide in cardiac and lung affections.
   (*e*) Lead poisoning.
   (*f*) From septic foci, *e.g.* tonsils, pyorrhœa, etc.

2. Impoverished state of the blood from—
   (*a*) Vomiting.
   (*b*) Suckling (prolonged).
   (*c*) Famine, etc.
   (*d*) Too frequent pregnancies.
   (*e*) Deficient vitamins, especially vitamins A, D and E.

3. High temperatures—
   In pneumonia, rheumatism, etc.

4. Nervous—
   (*a*) Mental shock, fear, worry, excitement.
   (*b*) Direct reflex, suckling.

5. Local uterine disease—
   (*a*) Diseases of the decidua.
   (*b*) Diseases of the placenta.
   (*c*) Fibromyomata.
   (*d*) Displacements, especially retroversion.
   (*e*) Congestion from—
   Plethora.
   Cardiac and hepatic disease.
   Excessive coitus.
   (*f*) Chronic endometritis.

6. Direct violence—
   Riding, dancing, etc.
   Jolting from rough driving.

7. Rhesus incompatibility.
8. Drugs, *e.g.* ergot, aloes, phosphorus, etc.
9. Criminal abortion.
10. Endocrine influence—progestin and thyroid deficiency, particularly important in habitual abortion and thyrotoxicosis.

Fœtal.—

1. Death of the ovum.
2. Hydramnios.

3. Myxoma of the chorion.
4. Rupture of the membranes.
5. Anomalies in development.

Mechanism.—During first two months the ovum is usually expelled entire.

During third month the decidua capsularis ruptures and ovum is expelled either entire or after rupture of membranes.

After third month rupture of the membranes is usual—fœtus is expelled first and followed later by placenta and membranes.

Between third and sixth months placenta is often retained through firm attachment to the uterus at that time.

Symptoms.—

1. Hæmorrhage.
2. Pains—uterine contractions, with usually some dilatation of cervix. These may occur independently or together.

1. *Hæmorrhage* is a sign of separation of the ovum and varies in quantity, sometimes being but slight, at other times so excessive as to endanger the life of the mother. The blood is often expelled in clots.

Hæmorrhage at all times tends to cause the death of the ovum from separation and pressure, and this is, in many cases, the direct cause of uterine contractions and expulsion.

2. *Uterine Contractions.*—Pains are always intermittent, and vary much in intensity.

They cause further separation of the ovum and dilatation of the cervix.

Diagnosis.—

1. History of pregnancy, amenorrhœa, etc.
2. Signs of pregnancy, specially enlargement and softness of the uterus.
3. Hæmorrhage and pains, independently or associated.
4. There may be dilatation of the os.

Varieties of Abortion.—

1. Threatened.
2. Inevitable—
    (*a*) Complete.
    (*b*) Incomplete.
3. Missed.
4. Habitual.

An **abortion** is said to be **threatened** when there is some bleeding, but contractions or pains, if present at all, are only very slight. The os is closed or practically so. The amount of bleeding is significant, but even if profuse or constant it is not impossible for the ovum to survive, provided contractions are not occurring.

It is essential to differentiate uterine abortion from tubal pregnancy and there is this difference in symptomatology. In uterine abortion, hæmorrhage is profuse and is the first symptom; this is followed by pain, which often is not severe. In tubal pregnancy, on the other hand, pain is the first symptom and may be severe; vaginal bleeding follows and is usually scanty.

An **abortion** is said to be **inevitable** (1) when uterine contractions are so severe as to cause dilatation of the cervix, (2) when the uterine contents protrude through the cervix, (3) when there has been an escape of liquor amnii and (4) usually when there is profuse bleeding.

(*a*) **Complete abortion** means that the uterine contents have been expelled in their entirety.

(*b*) **Incomplete abortion** means the retention in utero of some portion of the ovum after abortion. This may be—

(*a*) Decidua.
(*b*) Placenta (entire or part).
(*c*) Membranes.

Diagnosis of Incomplete Abortion.—

1. Within twenty-four hours after the supposed abortion—
   (*a*) History of pregnancy, amenorrhœa, etc.
   (*b*) History of expulsion of a mass.
   (*c*) Continuance of pains and hæmorrhage.
   (*d*) Dilatation of the os internum and the cervical canal.
   (*e*) Enlargement and softness of the uterus.

2. After a week or more—
   (*a*) History of amenorrhœa and subsequent history of profuse bleeding with pain, and perhaps expulsion of clots, fleshy lumps, etc.
   (*b*) Persistence of the bleeding.
   (*c*) Enlargement of the uterus.
   (*d*) Occasionally, fœtid discharge and high temperature—**Septic Abortion.**

The above symptoms of hæmorrhage and pains are sometimes closely simulated by a uterine polypus, but the previous amenorrhœa is in these cases always absent. If the pre-existing amenorrhœa be of short duration, the case may be viewed as a delayed menstrual period and the possibility of abortion overlooked.

A **missed abortion** is the term applied to those cases in which the death of the ovum takes place, but expulsion is delayed often for several months. This is due to lack of irritability of the uterus. When cast off, the ovum appears shrivelled and of a brown colour—*Carneous Mole.*

Pathology of Carneous Mole.—Hæmorrhage occurs into decidua and if profuse, the decidua capsularis ruptures. The chorion is destroyed and the amnion is caused to bulge towards the fœtus by effused blood. If the mole is not discharged at once the clot consolidates and the wall of the ovum becomes firm and fleshy. The fœtus and liquor amnii may be absorbed.

Clinical Features.—History of pregnancy and of a threatened abortion, all the symptoms of pregnancy except amenorrhœa passing off; thus the breasts, previously big, become small, and the abdominal enlargement, if present, decreases.

There is a feeling of weight and coldness in the hypogastrium.

The uterus, enlarged and doughy, does not grow, but instead becomes slightly smaller and harder.

Negative A.Z.R. (Aschheim-Zondek Reaction).

X-ray may fail to show normal fœtal shadow.

Treatment.—

Threatened abortion—

(*a*) Absolute rest for at least one week after all bleeding has stopped.
(*b*) Sedatives—morphia gr. $\frac{1}{4}$.
(*c*) Progesterone 10–20 units may be given daily until the bleeding has been stopped for several days. Ethisterone 30 mg. in association with œstrogen—ethinyl œstradiol 0·05 mg. or stilbœstrol 5 mg. daily—is an alternative.
(*d*) Vitamin E—viteolin, six capsules daily or ephynal 25 mgm. twice or thrice daily.
(*e*) Thyroid, gr. 1 daily.
(*f*) Light, easily digested diet.
(*g*) Avoid constipation by mild laxatives or oil enema.
(*h*) Correct any retrodisplacement. This may further detach ovum, but abortion will result if not done.

(*i*) Avoid strenuous exercise, sexual intercourse, etc., after bleeding has been stopped.

Inevitable abortion—

Leave alone unless bleeding is severe, and then—

(*a*) If the os internum is open—

(i) Pituitary 5 units.

(ii) Digital removal of ovum from uterus under anæsthesia.

(iii) Removal of ovum from uterus by ovum forceps or flushing curette, using a douche at a temperature of 118° F.

(*b*) If the os internum is closed—

Pack cervix and vagina for eight hours. This controls the hæmorrhage, excites uterine contractions and dilates the cervix.

Abortion often comes away when pack is removed or soon after.

If it does not, os is now open and treat as described above.

Complete Abortion—

Treated as above.

Incomplete Abortion—

(*a*) Examine all discharge.

(*b*) Under anæsthesia evacuate retained products digitally, by ovum forceps or by flushing curette with hot douche of 118° F.

Septic Abortion—

If the temperature is raised and interference is required owing to bleeding, it is essential that the retained products be evacuated with the minimum amount of interference, after which a glycerine pack may be left in the uterus for several hours.

If there is no bleeding, manipulation is better postponed until the temperature has settled. Antibiotics and/or sulphonamides should be given meanwhile. This therapy may be continued for several days after evacuation.

Missed Abortion—

The uterus should be emptied as soon as possible. (The teaching that a missed abortion should be allowed to come away spontaneously in days or weeks, or even months, is to be deprecated.) This can be effected by œstrogenic therapy and pituitary, by the insertion of tents into cervix or by the intra-uterine injection of utus.

Habitual Abortion.—

This is defined as three or more consecutive miscarriages.

Possible causes—

(*a*) General—

1. General systemic disease—nephritis.
2. Specific infection.
3. Blood dyscrasias.
4. Rhesus incompatibility. (Despite opinions to the contrary, we believe that there is not yet sufficient knowledge to exclude this as a possible factor.)
5. Thyrotoxicosis.
6. Hormone deficiency, particularly lack of progesterone and thyroid.
7. Vitamin deficiency, particularly A, D and E.

(*b*) Local—

1. Congenital maldevelopment of the uterus.
2. Retroversion of the uterus.
3. Uterine fibroids.
4. Deep cervical lacerations which involve the circular fibres at the internal os and so interfere with uterine polarity.
5. Endocervicitis and endometritis.

Investigation—

This should include a thorough medical overhaul and pelvic examination between pregnancies. The Rhesus factor and Wassermann reaction must be determined. Any systemic lesion or local abnormality should be treated. If the patient has had two or more miscarriages the uterus should be curetted.

As soon as the next pregnancy begins a hormone assay may be carried out with advantage. The gonadotrophic, œstrogen and pregnanediol levels should be ascertained. (Pregnanediol is a break-down product of progesterone.) The B.M.R. may, too, be estimated.

Treatment—

If no obvious cause be found it has been our custom either to give such patients, as soon as pregnancy begins : (1) progesterone 20 mg. daily for four days, and thereafter ethisterone 30 mg. and ethinyl œstradiol 0·05 mg. daily ; (2) vitamen E—

ephynal acetate 25 mg. twice or thrice daily ; (3) thyroid 1 gr. thrice daily if the B.M.R. is under -10, thyroid $\frac{1}{2}$ gr. thrice daily if the B.M.R. is under $+10$, or to rely on chorionic gonadotrophic hormone 200 units twice weekly in association with thyroid $\frac{1}{2}$ gr. daily (see p. 358).

Such a course of therapy may be continued throughout the first four months and tapered off in the fifth month. In addition, the patient must be advised regarding a well-balanced diet, limitation of activity and abstinence from coitus. Rest should be enforced at the times of the suppressed periods and indeed the patient may benefit, in some cases, from continued absolute rest in bed throughout the earlier months of pregnancy.

2. HYDATIDIFORM MOLE

Also called *Vesicular Mole* ; is essentially a disease of the chorionic villi, consisting in their enormous development in number and size.

Morbid Anatomy.—Hypertrophy and mucoid degeneration of the connective tissue of the villi, with increase of both layers of epithelium, particularly the plasmodial layer of syncytium, which is irregularly developed and contains large and vesicular nuclei. Langhans' layer is greatly proliferated in patches. The blood-vessels are practically obliterated and the mole is probably nourished by maternal tissues. To the naked eye the hypertrophied villi look like white currants or grapes.

The villi tend to grow into the uterine wall, thus thinning and even perforating it.

Period of Occurrence.—Generally in the first weeks of gestation, when the villi are diffuse over the entire ovum.

If the disease be now general the ovum dies and is absorbed, no trace being found on expulsion of the mass.

If the disease appears later and thus becomes localised, the ovum may continue to grow till full time, the placenta being enlarged and myxomatous.

The growth of the diseased villi is extremely rapid, and distends the uterus to a size quite out of proportion to the period of gestation, thus in four months the uterus may be the size of a full-time pregnancy.

Malignancy is probably due to deep penetration of the uterine walls, so that removal of mole is apt to be incomplete.

Causes.—Doubtful.

Said to be maternal, because—

It is often associated with diseased decidua.

Said to be fœtal, because—

1. In twins, one may be a mole, the other healthy.
2. It is never found without impregnation.

Symptoms and Signs.—Enlargement of the uterus quite out of proportion to the period of the pregnancy.

Pain in the back and loins.

Vomiting from over-distension of the uterus (occasionally absent).

Ballottement absent.

Lower uterine segment tense.

May have discharge of cysts per vaginam.

Hæmorrhage, often severe.

Both ovaries usually cystic (lutein cysts).

A.Z.R. markedly positive. Positive result obtained with urine diluted 1/100.

Treatment.—

Evacuation of uterus per vaginam by cervical dilatation, and removal of the mole by ovum forceps.

When the uterine mass is so large that the fundus is at, or above, the level of the umbilicus, it may be safer to remove the mole by abdominal hysterotomy.

The patient should be kept under observation for one year, and the A.Z.R. done frequently. In this way the early development of chorionepithelioma is recognised. The patient should be instructed to report at once if abnormal vaginal bleeding occurs and a fuller investigation may then be carried out by curettage.

Dangers.—

1. Hæmorrhage.
2. Uterine rupture from thinned or perforated walls.
3. Septicæmia from retained portions which are too adherent to be removed.
4. Chorionepithelioma. Nearly 60 per cent. of all cases of this interesting new growth follow hydatidiform mole.

Chorionepithelioma

(*a*) *Ætiology.*—

1. Arises from the connective tissue and the epithelium of the chorion.

2. Usually starts in the uterus, but may begin in the broad ligament, ovary, vagina or vulva.

3. Only occurs in women who have been pregnant.

4. Usually follows a hydatidiform mole or abortion, but may follow a normal pregnancy.

(*b*) *Pathology.*—

1. *Naked Eye*—

(*a*) A purple-coloured nodular growth containing chiefly blood-clot, intersected by strands of fibrin, necrotic uterine tissue or tumour tissue; arising over an old placental site, *i.e.*, usually near the fundus.

(*b*) Begins in the muscle and then usually invades the endometrium or, more rarely, the peritoneal coat.

(*c*) Very friable and bleeds on touch.

(*d*) Has no blood-vessels of its own and no proper connective tissue stroma.

(*e*) Surface may be covered by a membrane-like decidua and at the base, near the uterine muscle, is a patchy, red and white, narrow area, which consists of actively growing tumour and areas of small blood sinuses.

2. *Microscopically*—

(*a*) Masses of undefined protoplasm with many nuclei (derived from syncytium).

(*b*) Small polyhedral cells with large nuclei found in clumps (derived from Langhans' layer).

(*c*) Mono- and multi-nuclear giant cells form the greater part of the cell masses and are also found destroying and infiltrating the adjacent tissues after the manner of a sarcoma. (Probably syncytial cells.)

(*d*) Chorionic villi.

(*e*) Lutein cysts common in both ovaries.

(*c*) *Dissemination.*—

1. By the blood-vessels—the cells surrounding, destroying, and then growing into the uterine veins.

2. Metastases are common in the vagina, lung, broad ligament and brain, and are similar in character to the original tumour.

3. Malignancy is very variable, but the prognosis is usually bad.

(*d*) *Signs and Symptoms.*—Bleeding—severe and irregular, causing anæmia.

Discharge—offensive, containing shreds of tissue.

Pyrexia—usually slight, but sometimes rigors, probably due to extensive metastases and not to septic infection.

Enlargement of uterus to about the size of a three-months' pregnancy.

Hæmoptysis in late or rapid cases, due to lung metastases.

Cervix often patulous and the growth may be felt.

Secondary nodules in the vagina common.

A.Z.R. strongly positive.

(*e*) *Diagnosis.*—

1. By examination of curette scrapings microscopically, but the clinical features should be taken into account as well.

2. Should be suspected if after curettage for retained products, bleeding and offensive discharge recurs after a short period (two to four weeks).

3. Should also be suspected if any interference with the growth gives rise to a large or uncontrollable bleeding.

(*N.B.*—As little interference as possible should be made, as it is liable to give rise to metastases and sometimes sudden death.)

4. A positive A.Z.R. after hydatidiform mole has been evacuated (see p. 127). (A new pregnancy must, of course, be excluded.)

(*f*) *Treatment.*—Immediate pan-hysterectomy with removal of the appendages, controlling veins wherever possible to start with, so as to prevent metastases due to interference.

(*N.B.*—Operation is not contra-indicated by the presence of metastases, as often they disappear after removal of primary growth.)

(*g*) *Prognosis.*—

1. Malignancy varies greatly, death occurring in a few days after the onset of symptoms in some cases, whilst in others, operation fifteen months after the onset of the symptoms has resulted in cure.

2. Those following hydatid mole seem least malignant. This may be due to thorough removal of the growth; it is in these cases where villi are found, which also seem to denote low malignancy.

3. Those following a full-time pregnancy seem most malignant, due probably to increased width of the vessels, and thus rapid occurrence of metastases is favoured. May

also be due to disease in placenta not being noted; also, there is a longer period for growth compared with those following abortion and hydatid mole and thus the muscle may be more thoroughly invaded. The shorter the interval after pregnancy, the more malignant the tumour; thus, those occurring early in the puerperium are the most deadly.

4. Death may occur by perforation of the uterine wall.

5. Secondary nodules may be partially destroyed by hæmorrhage and thrombosis cutting off the blood supply to the tumour, the surrounding tissue being provoked to tissue reaction. Seldom is the whole nodule destroyed by such means unless after the primary growth is removed, when it commonly occurs.

6. If no recurrence takes place in six months, the chances are good; if none in a year, they are very good; whereas after two years the case may be said to have recovered absolutely. The percentage of recovery in the cases following hydatid mole was 78, which shows the lower malignancy of these tumours (Teacher).

3. CARCINOMA OF THE CERVIX

Pregnancies in quick succession may help the development of cancer at a subsequent pregnancy.

Effect of Pregnancy on.—May tend to hasten disease by increasing the vascularity of the organ.

Effect on Pregnancy.—Pregnancy may occur at all stages and is seldom affected unless disease advanced, when abortion may occur.

The usual symptom of amenorrhœa is generally masked by the discharge, which may be taken for a period.

Some authors state that there is a tendency to abortion or high fœtal mortality, due to bacteria from the cancer acting on the fœtal membranes and endometrium (advanced cases).

Effect on Parturition.—If slight, disease has little effect.

If disease advanced—cervix is undilatable, and therefore tears, with copious accompanying hæmorrhage, which may be fatal.

Septicæmia and rupture of uterus may occur.

Clinical Features.—

1. Loss of weight (very suspicious symptom during pregnancy).

2. Bleeding—usually slight in amount.
3. Hardness of cervix.

Prognosis.—Grave; from rapidity of growth during pregnancy and from risks of parturition, *e.g.*, hæmorrhage and sepsis.

Treatment.—

If the disease is operable, Wertheim hysterectomy, preceded by Cæsarean section if the child is viable, may be done. If inoperable treat with radium and deep X-ray therapy; in such cases the pregnancy is removed in the first place.

4. EXTRA-UTERINE GESTATION

Synonym.—Ectopic Gestation.

Definition.—The fixation and development of an impregnated ovum outside the lining membrane of the uterus. The common situation is the ampullary portion of tube, but it may occur in any situation in the tube or even in the ovary.

Tubal Pregnancy

Types.—Ampullary, interstitial, infundibular and isthmic.

Cause.—Some obstruction in the Fallopian tube insufficient to prevent ingress of the spermatozoa, but enough to prevent egress of the ovum—

(*a*) Tubal abnormalities such as diverticula, accessory ostia, or an infantile condition.
(*b*) Tubal inflammation—salpingitis—resulting in a partial occlusion of the tubal lumen or denudation of mucosa and cilia.
(*c*) Premature activity of the trophoblast.
(*d*) External migration of the ovum.

Symptoms and Signs.—

(*a*) May have none.

(*b*) May have symptoms of a normal pregnancy, the most important being amenorrhœa.

(*c*) Most frequently—

1. Pain in the side.
2. Slight irregular hæmorrhages from the uterus.
3. Occasional feelings of nausea and faintness.

Signs.—

(*a*) Soft pulsating and **very tender** mass at the side of or behind the uterus.

(*b*) Uterus enlarged and soft.

(*c*) Localised rigidity over the affected area.

(*d*) Accelerated sedimentation rate of red blood corpuscles.

Symptoms of Rupture.—Rupture most frequently occurs between the fourth and twelfth week, except in interstitial cases, when it occurs between the fourteenth and the sixteenth week. In isthmic cases it may occur earlier than the fourth week.

Terminations.—

1. **Intra-peritoneal Rupture.**—*Clinical Features.*—

(*a*) Sudden and intense abdominal pain.

(*b*) Shock and collapse; intense and increasing pallor; sighing respiration; small fast pulse and restlessness.

(*c*) Vaginal bleeding (not too excessive).

(*d*) Shedding of the uterine decidua.

(*e*) Pain over shoulder-blades (often).

Signs of Intra-peritoneal Bleeding (only occurring in some cases).—

(*a*) Cullen's sign—blue-green shimmer around umbilicus, especially if associated with hernia (hæmatomphalos).

(*b*) Dewe's sign—pain produced over both shoulder-blades by placing the patient on her back and applying pressure to hypogastrium—due to irritation of phrenic nerve by blood between the liver and the diaphragm. (Only if large effusion.)

(*c*) If long after rupture, post-hæmorrhagic leucocytosis.

(*d*) A diffuse abdominal distension and, vaginally, an indistinct fullness in fornices from blood effusion, which, if left for a day or so, changes in consistency (pelvic hæmatocele).

2. **Extra-peritoneal Rupture.**—*Clinical Features.*—

(*a*) Sudden pain in the abdomen, as if something had ruptured.

(*b*) Shock.

(*c*) Signs of hæmorrhage not so exaggerated as in intra-peritoneal rupture.

The signs are definite :—

Usually, distinct abdominal swelling and, vaginally, a tumour which tilts the uterus to one or other side of pelvis.

3. **Tubal Abortion** (incomplete) through the abdominal

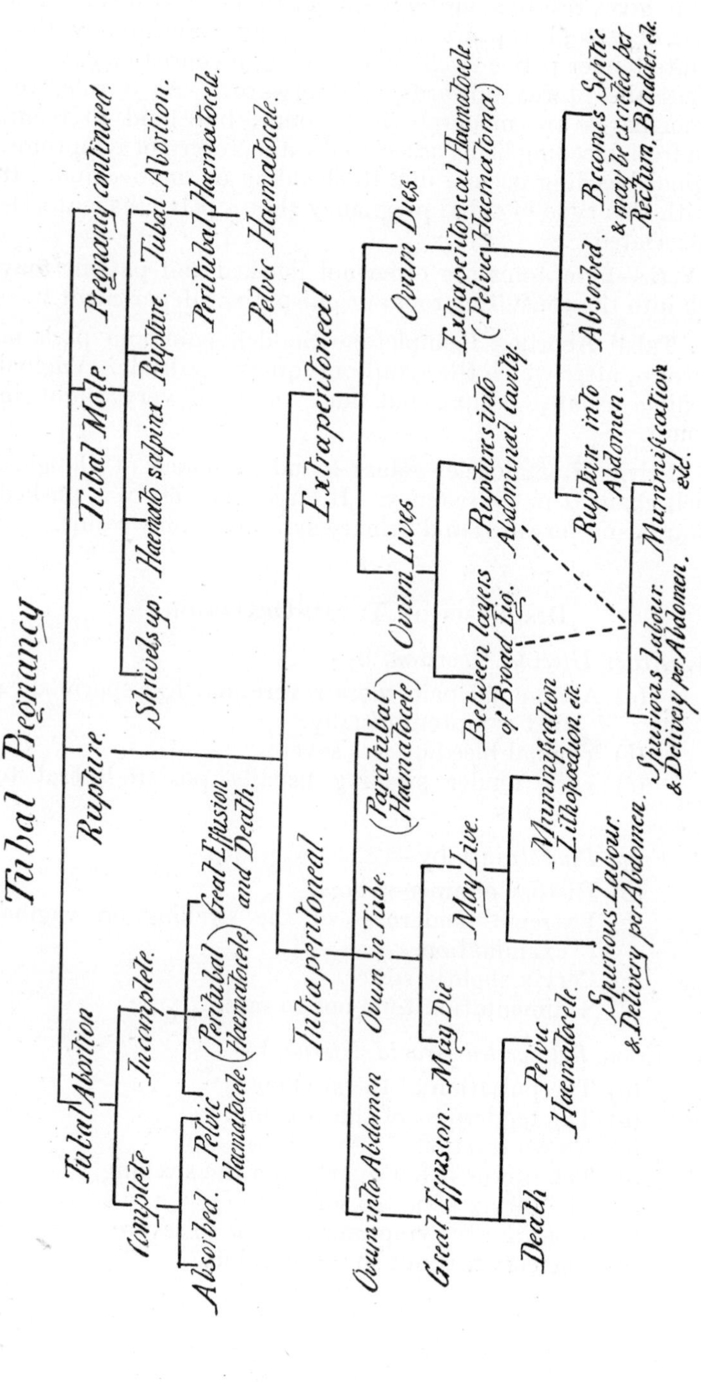

Tubal Pregnancy

Tubal Abortion
Complete
Absorbed.
Pelvic Haematocele.
Incomplete.
(Peritubal Haematocele)
Great Effusion and Death.

Rupture.
Intraperitoneal.
Ovum into Abdomen
Great Effusion.
Death
Pelvic Haematocele.
Ovum in Tube.
May Die
May Live.
Spurious Labour. & Delivery per Abdomen.
Mummification Lithopædion. etc.
(Paratubal Haematocele)
Extraperitoneal
Ovum Lives
Between layers of Broad Lig.
Ruptures into Abdominal Cavity.
Spurious Labour. & Delivery per Abdomen.
Mummification etc.
Ovum Dies.
Extraperitoneal Haematocele. (Pelvic Haematoma.)
Rupture into Abdomen.
Absorbed.
Becomes Septic & may be excreted per Rectum, Bladder. etc.

Tubal Mole.
Shrivels up.
Haemato salpinx.
Rupture.
Tubal Abortion.
Peritubal Haematocele.
Pelvic Haematocele.

Pregnancy continued.

Fig. 15.

ostium gives rise to symptoms similar to, but less severe than, those of actual rupture and is usually associated with a definite tender pelvic swelling, changing in consistency, which pushes the uterus upwards and forwards. As a rule, the hæmorrhages are moderate in amount, but tend to recur, each fresh bleeding being associated with a return of symptoms. Vaginal bleeding occurs, due to shedding of the decidua. It is with this type of tubal pregnancy that a pelvic hæmatocele is associated.

(*N.B.*—Symptoms are often not marked and patient may walk into the consulting room or out-patient department.)

4. **Tubal Abortion** (complete).—Sudden pain and perhaps faintness, after which the symptoms quickly subside. Vaginal bleeding usually occurs, but may only be very slight in amount.

5. **Pelvic Hæmatocele.**—Mass found in pouch of Douglas, which changes in consistency. If large, the cervix is pushed upwards and forwards and urinary symptoms may result.

Diagnosis of Tubal Gestation

1. *From Uterine Abortion*, by—
   - (*a*) Abdominal pain more severe and less spasmodic; first symptom usually.
   - (*b*) Vaginal bleeding less severe.
   - (*c*) Very tender swelling usually postero-lateral to uterus.

2. *From Pyosalpinx*, by—
   - (*a*) History of amenorrhœa.
   - (*b*) Extreme tenderness of the swelling on vaginal examination.
   - (*c*) Cervix slightly softer.
   - (*d*) Sedimentation time not so rapid.

3. *From Retroverted Gravid Uterus*, by—
   - (*a*) The pulsation of the swelling.
   - (*b*) The tenderness of the swelling.
   - (*c*) No contractions.
   - (*d*) The uterus is felt apart from the swelling.
   - (*e*) The cervix is not so soft.
   - (*f*) The urinary symptoms are not so severe.
   - (*g*) The cervix is not so inaccessible.

4. *From Fibroid*, by—
   (*a*) The history—amenorrhœa especially.
   (*b*) Not so hard in consistence.
   (*c*) The pulsation of the swelling on vaginal examination.
   (*d*) The tenderness of the swelling.

5. *From Fibroid and Pregnancy* (very difficult), by—
   (*a*) The pulsation and tenderness.

Extra-uterine Gestation at or Near Term

Diagnosis.—

1. Difficult, as the pregnancy has apparently progressed normally.

2. Fœtal heart and parts may be more easily felt and heard, and the child may lie more to one or other side of abdomen.

3. Cervix harder than normal.

4. Uterus felt as a hard mass to the side of the sac, and is usually mistaken for a fibroid.

5. Symptoms of obstruction may occur, due to sac adhesions.

Intra-peritoneal Rupture

Diagnosis

From Ruptured Ulcer of the Stomach or Duodenum.—

1. The collapse is more marked owing to the hæmorrhage.
2. History of pregnancy.
3. The abdomen is most tender in the hypogastrium and iliac regions.
4. There is no period of apparent well-being, as is often the case in ruptured gastric ulcer.
5. Fullness in the fornices.
6. The vomiting is less prominent.
7. No history of digestive trouble.

From Twisted Ovarian Cyst.—

1. The collapse is much more marked, and the patient is obviously extremely ill.
2. No tender mass on abdominal palpation.
3. By the history in most cases, but pregnancy may be present with a cyst.

4. The patient becomes rapidly worse, whereas with a twisted ovarian cyst the condition usually improves after a time.
5. Fullness in the fornices and slowly shifting dullness may be present.

From Acute Fulminating Appendicitis.—

1. By the history.
2. The pain and rigidity are not most marked over M'Burney's point, as in appendicitis.
3. No vomiting usually.

(*N.B.*—The insertion of a needle into the posterior fornix and withdrawal of blood into a syringe will make diagnosis certain in cases of tubal gestation, when blood has been effused.)

Clinical Course after Rupture.—

1. Intra-peritoneal. The patient nearly always dies from bleeding in a few hours if not treated.

2. Extra-peritoneal. The bleeding usually stops, but may be so severe as to rupture secondarily into the peritoneum, and become intra-peritoneal.

3. Tubal abortion (incomplete). There is usually temporary recovery, but a return of the hæmorrhage occurs and this may prove fatal.

Tubal abortion (complete) is usually followed by complete recovery with little disturbance.

Prognosis.—Very grave; 70 per cent. die if they are untreated.

Treatment.—

1. If diagnosed early before rupture—removal of the tube and sac by laparotomy.

2. If intra-peritoneal rupture—laparotomy; clamp and remove ruptured tube and sac.

3. If tubal abortion (incomplete)—remove the tube and its contents.

4. If extra-peritoneal—remove the tube and sac, clearing out the clot.

5. If recognised late in pregnancy—perform laparotomy; open the sac, remove the fœtus.

(*a*) Understitch and remove the placenta.
(*b*) It may be safer to leave the placenta for ten to fourteen days to die in the sac, which is stitched to abdominal parietes (marsupialisation) and

then remove; attempts at immediate removal may prove fatal from bleeding.

(c) Some advise leaving the placenta in the abdomen to be absorbed or become calcareous.

It is best not to wait until spurious labour occurs, unless the patient can be kept under strict observation, and even then expectant treatment is not advisable.

6. Hæmatocele. Laparotomy—evacuate blood clot. Uterus may be ventro-suspended to avoid retroversion due to adhesions forming in the Pouch of Douglas.

(*b*) HÆMORRHAGE IN LATER MONTHS

ANTE-PARTUM HÆMORRHAGE

Ante-partum hæmorrhage is bleeding from the placental site after the child has become viable, namely, after the twenty-eighth week and prior to the birth of the child. There are two types :—

1. Placenta prævia or unavoidable hæmorrhage.
2. Accidental hæmorrhage (Ablatio Placentæ).

PLACENTA PRÆVIA

This means that the placenta is situated in whole or in part in the lower uterine segment. The condition occurs in 1 in 1000 cases and is more frequently met with in multiparæ.

Causes.—

1. The villi in contact with the decidua capsularis of the lower uterine pole take part in the development of the placenta. When the decidua capsularis fuses with the decidua vera this portion of the placenta must of necessity be placed in the lower uterine segment.

2. Defective vascularisation, due to inflammation or atrophy, necessitating placental spread to gain sufficient nourishment. This spread may encroach on the lower uterine segment.

3. Pre-existing endometritis which may act in much the same way as in 2.

Varieties.—

1*st Degree*—where the placenta encroaches on the lower uterine segment, the greater part occupying the upper segment.

2nd Degree—where the edge of the placenta overlaps, but does not cover, the internal os—partial placenta prævia.

3rd Degree—where the placenta completely covers the internal os—central placenta prævia.

In defining those different types, the internal os must admit at least one finger.

Clinical Features.—

The one sign is hæmorrhage. This bleeding appears after the twenty-eighth week but may sometimes occur only when labour commences. The onset is sudden, the loss is at first moderate but may be profuse, there is a complete absence of pain and there is a definite tendency for the hæmorrhage to recur, maybe on several occasions. It is quite possible that a placenta prævia is the cause of bleeding and abortion in the earlier months, but in many cases it is naturally difficult, and indeed often impossible, to say so with certainty.

Cause of Bleeding.—The painless uterine contractions of later pregnancy promote stretching of the lower uterine segment and a partial detachment of the placenta ; such a separation is bound to occur during the first stage of labour, and the hæmorrhage is therefore termed inevitable or unavoidable.

Source of Bleeding.—(*a*) Principally from the sinuses in the lower uterine segment, (*b*) to a very small degree from partially separated cotyledons of the placenta.

Effect of Placenta Prævia on Pregnancy.—The placenta prevents the head entering the lower segment and so there is a tendency to malpresentations. The onset of labour is frequently premature.

Effect of Placenta Prævia on Labour.—Malpresentations are more common. The first stage is delayed because the head is prevented from engaging and the attached placenta may hinder the " drawing-up " of the lower segment. The position of the placenta may lead to an absence of the bag of waters. There is an increased risk of cervical and lower segment laceration and a predisposition to post-partum hæmorrhage—the passive lower segment may experience difficulty in controlling the sinuses.

Diagnosis.—The bleeding associated with placenta prævia must be differentiated from that of external accidental bleeding. A provisional differentiation can be made by (*a*) history and (*b*) abdominal palpation.

Placenta Prævia.	*External Accidental Hæmorrhage.*
(*a*) *History*—	
Quiet onset.	Stormy onset.
No pain.	Abdominal pain is first symptom.
Hæmorrhage first and only sign. May-be small repeated bleeding.	Hæmorrhage follows pain. Usually prolonged and profuse single bleeding.
Condition of patient varies directly with blood loss.	Condition of patient may be worse than can be accounted for by blood loss.
Intra-uterine death not so common.	Fœtus may die in utero.
Bleeding aggravated during uterine contraction.	Bleeding lessens during uterine contraction.
Bleeding lessened by rupture of membranes.	Bleeding may be unaffected by rupture of membranes.
No toxic symptoms.	May be hypertension, œdema and albuminuria.
(*b*) *Abdominal Palpation.*	
Presenting part high.	Head engaged or can be pushed into pelvis.
May be malpresentation.	No tendency to malpresentation.
Presentation may be difficult to determine.	Not so.
Ballottement is obscure.	Not so.
No tenderness.	Area of tenderness present.

In hospital, if there is no urgency, X-ray examination may show the exact position of the placenta.

(*a*) Inject into the bladder 2 oz. of a 10 per cent. solution of sodium iodide or air. A space of more than 1 cm. between the bladder shadow and the presenting part suggests a placenta prævia.

(*b*) Soft tissue X-ray. If the placental shadow is not seen in the upper uterine segment with a lateral exposure, the placenta is probably in the lower segment.

Vaginal examination is the only sure way of diagnosing placenta prævia. With a finger inserted through the cervix the presence of the placenta in the lower segment can be confirmed or eliminated. Such an examination may still further separate the placenta and induce alarming hæmorrhage. For that reason, **vaginal examination in such cases should be made only in hospital and with everything ready to go ahead immediately, if necessary, with Cæsarean section.** In doubtful cases, when the os is closed, it is best to dilate the cervix sufficiently with Hegar's dilators to admit a finger (the rough granular feel of the placenta and its adhesion to the uterine wall ought at once to distinguish it from blood clot which is so easily broken up).

Prognosis.—

Maternal.—Varies according to the degree of placenta prævia, the 3rd degree or central placenta prævia giving the worst prognosis. Death rarely occurs from hæmorrhage during pregnancy but, results rather from—(1) lacerations of cervix and lower segment at labour, (2) hæmorrhage from such lacerations, (3) hæmorrhage during 3rd stage from atonic lower segment, (4) shock following delivery, (5) infection—predisposed to by manipulation required.

Fœtal.—Bad and varies with the degree of placenta prævia, being worst in the central type. Influenced, too, by the method of treatment employed.

It should be said, however, that with a more radical outlook and a simpler scheme of treatment, the mortality, both maternal and fœtal, has been greatly reduced.

Treatment.—It is important to remember that vaginal bleeding in the last three months of pregnancy may be due either to placenta prævia or to external accidental hæmorrhage. **At the home of the patient no attempt should be made by vaginal examination to differentiate one condition from the other.** The patient should be given morphia $\frac{1}{4}$ gr., a large vulvar pad and T bandage should be applied and the patient transferred to hospital. There her blood is grouped, the Rhesus factor determined, a red count done and the blood pressure taken. As a general rule, should the red count be less than 3,000,000 or the blood pressure below 90/60, the patient is transfused.

In hospital, active treatment may be necessary at once if the hæmorrhage is severe. More frequently, however, the hæmorrhage has been moderate and the " expectant treatment" of placenta prævia is carried out. Complete rest in bed is essential, sedatives may be administered and the patient is dealt with in a way very similar to the case of threatened abortion. X-ray examination may meantime confirm the presence of a placenta prævia. The immediate object is to carry the patient successfully into the last month of pregnancy, and then a vaginal examination is made for the first time. Treatment will depend on the findings at that examination.

1. *Central Placenta Prævia.*—Cæsarean section.

2. *Partial Placenta Prævia*—(*a*) if a primigravidæ—Cæsarean section, (*b*) if a multipara—(1) rupture of membranes, (2) application to scalp of Willett's forceps, with 2 lb. weight (3) if breech presents, a leg may be brought down through the cervix and gentle weight traction applied. Allow spontaneous delivery and *never pull on leg to effect delivery.*

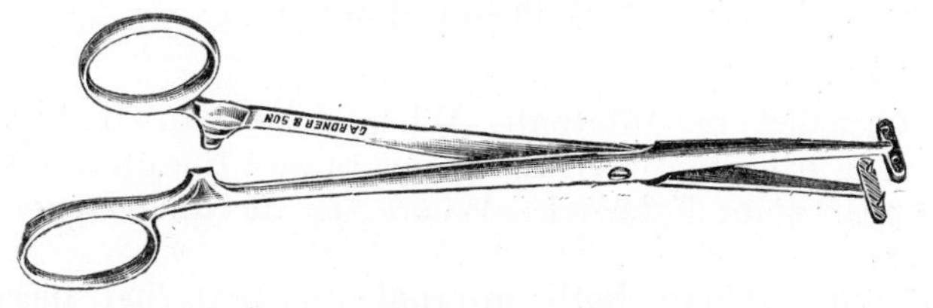

FIG. 16.—WILLETT'S FORCEPS.

3. *First Degree*—rupture of membranes if vertex presents and the application of a tight abdominal binder; if bleeding recurs Willett's forceps may be applied. In a breech presentation a leg may be pulled down if the degree of cervical dilatation is sufficient and light weight traction applied.

Packing the vagina tightly with gauze is required only rarely, *e.g.* severe bleeding before the patient is sent to hospital, especially if the journey is considerable, or profuse hæmorrhage excited in hospital by vaginal examination. Vaginal packing is an emergency measure only and not a standard method of treatment.

There is practically no place for bipolar podalic version and the pulling down of a leg in the treatment of placenta prævia. This method is not radical enough for the more severe degrees of placenta prævia and too radical for the first degree. Version may be indicated—

As a means of promoting uterine contractions where placenta prævia has been diagnosed before the twenty-eighth week of pregnancy.

The possibility of bleeding during and after the third stage should always be remembered. Such bleeding may affect seriously the prognosis. Should it occur, the placenta may have to be removed manually, and if it continues thereafter, despite uterine stimulation, the uterus may have to be compressed, a hot intra-uterine douche given or, if persistent, the uterus and vagina packed.

(*N.B.*—Blood transfusion is required in cases where the blood loss is at all excessive.)

ACCIDENTAL HÆMORRHAGE

This means bleeding from a normally situated placental site after the twenty-eighth week and before the birth of the child.

Occurs more frequently in multiparæ.

Varieties.—

1. **Concealed or Internal.**—Where the effused blood is retained in utero between the placenta and the uterine wall.
2. **Apparent or External.**—Where the bleeding escapes per vaginam.
3. **Mixed.**—Where both internal and external bleedings occur.

Causes.—*Before Labour.*—

1. Associated with toxæmia of pregnancy.
2. External violence.
3. Undue exertion.
4. Emotional stress.
5. Placental disease.
6. Inflammation of decidua.
7. Hypertension.

When Labour has set in.—

1. Abnormally short cord.
2. Sudden diminution of the uterine contents after the escape of liquor amnii in hydramnios.

Symptoms.—

(*a*) *Of Internal.*—

1. Collapse usually, but if not, pulse rate steadily increases.
2. Distension of the uterus, which may sometimes be irregular in outline.

3. Severe steady pain in abdomen.
4. Uterus feels hard and is tender to touch.

(*b*) *Of External.*—Bleeding often associated with abdominal pain.

(*c*) *Of Mixed.*—Symptoms of both (*a*) and (*b*).

Toxæmic symptoms such as a raised blood pressure, albuminuria or œdema may be present in all varieties.

Diagnosis.—Easy if bleeding external.

(**Placenta prævia must always be excluded.**)

Difficult if internal and may be mistaken for a rupture of the uterus, tonic contraction of uterus or even eclampsia with coma.

Differential Diagnosis of Concealed Hæmorrhage from Uterine Rupture and Tonic Contraction.

Concealed Hæmorrhage.—

1. Generally occurs before the membranes rupture.
2. Uterus is increased in size, hard and tender.
3. Presenting part remains in *statu quo.*
4. Steady pain over the distended uterus.
5. No severe intermittent pains.
6. Fœtal parts are felt with difficulty.
7. Cervix often closed.

Rupture.—

1. Generally after the membranes rupture.
2. Uterus is diminished in size.
3. Presenting part recedes or changes.
4. Occurs after uterine contractions.
5. Fœtal parts are usually easily felt.

Tonic Contraction.—

1. Uterus smaller.
2. Obstetric exhaustion.
3. Cervix dilated.
4. Presenting part impacted.

Prognosis.—Very grave in concealed hæmorrhage as the patient is often in an advanced stage of collapse before the danger is recognised. Not grave for mother in external and mixed types but fœtal mortality is apt to be high.

Treatment: External and Mixed Types.—In certain cases where the bleeding is slight, where the patient can be kept under constant supervision, and where the child, through prematurity, is unlikely to survive, palliative treatment as for threatened abortion may be adopted.

Where active treatment is necessary—

1. Rupture membranes and apply a firm abdominal binder.
2. Bipolar or internal version depending on the degree of cervical dilatation, and bring down a foot. This is very rarely required.
3. Treat any shock and collapse.

Concealed Type—

1. Morphia, gr. $\frac{1}{4}$.
2. Treat shock and collapse.
3. Absolute rest.

Watch carefully (*a*) general condition.
(*b*) pulse.
(*c*) size of uterus.

When uterine contractions start, as they usually do in two to three hours or when vaginal bleeding occurs indicating an improvement in uterine tone and contractility, the membranes should be ruptured and the subsequent labour is usually uneventful.

If contractions do not start after the patient has been rested, pituitary extract, 2·5 units, may be given. Should contractions fail to appear, the uterus enlarge, the pulse quicken or the general condition deteriorate, Cæsarean section should be carried out. After the uterus has been evacuated by Cæsarean section, hysterectomy may be required in a few cases, if the uterus fails to contract.

Blood transfusion as soon as all internal hæmorrhage has ceased.

The urinary output must be measured for the following 48 hours in case bilateral cortical necrosis is developing.

CHAPTER VIII

ABNORMAL PRESENTATIONS IN LABOUR AND MULTIPLE PREGNANCY

FACE PRESENTATIONS

Occur 1 in 250 labours.

May be primary or secondary.

Primary—before labour commences—rare.

Secondary—after labour commences.

From marked extension of the head, instead of flexion, in a vertex presentation.

Causes.—

1. Prevention of approximation of chin to sternum, from—

    (*a*) Coils of cord round neck.
    (*b*) Cystic tumour of neck.
    (*c*) Intervention of arms between chin and sternum.
    (*d*) Spasm of muscles in back of neck.

2. Excess of liquor amnii.

This causes extreme mobility of the head above the brim from the globular shape of the lower uterine segment. The occiput may thus impinge on the pelvis and be prevented from descending.

3. Contracted pelvis or large child.
4. Obliquity of uterus.
5. Dolicocephalic head.
    Is more probably the result than the cause.
6. Favoured by low placental implantation.
7. Anencephaly.

Positions.—These are named according to the position of chin (mentum), which is the denominator.

Being due, in the large majority of cases, to extension of vertex presentations, they are named first, second, third and fourth, according to the vertex presentation from which they are derived.

Thus, if in a vertex L.O.A. the head extends and the face presents, the chin will be posterior and opposite to the right sacro-iliac joint, and the position will be named *right mento-posterior* or first face position. In like manner, we get from—

R.O.A.—*Left mento-posterior*, second position.
R.O.P.—*Left mento-anterior*, third position.
L.O.P.—*Right mento-anterior*, fourth position.

In all the above positions the fronto-mental diameter occupies the same position as the occipito-frontal in vertex cases.

Mechanism.—

1. Extension and descent of chin, enabling submento-bregmatic diameter to engage.

2. Internal rotation forwards of chin to back of symphysis; in abnormal mechanism, backwards into hollow of sacrum.

3. Flexion. The chin becomes fixed beneath the pubic arch and the face, sinciput, vertex and occiput pass successively over the perineum and the head is born.

4. Restitution.

5. External rotation as in vertex cases.

Diagnosis.—

On Abdominal Palpation.—

1. A large groove is felt between the back and the occiput and the presenting part is high.

2. Heart sounds are heard below umbilicus and if on the same side as the fœtal limbs, are usually diagnostic of a face presentation.

On Vaginal Examination.—

1. If seen early, easy. The characteristic landmarks are—
   (*a*) The orbits.
   (*b*) Mouth with gums (distinguished from anus by not gripping inserted finger).
   (*c*) Nostrils.

2. If seen late, after the membranes have been ruptured for some hours, the large caput succedaneum so modifies the face that it may be mistaken for the breech, but the mouth should give the diagnosis.

Effect on Labour.—

1. *Causes of Delay in First Stage.*—
   (*a*) From face forming an inefficient plug to liquor amnii and thus membranes present frequently in sausage-shaped form and rupture early.

(b) If membranes rupture early the flat face forms but a feeble dilator of cervix.
(c) Face bones do not mould.
(d) Uterine force transmitted to head at disadvantage because of angle between head and neck.
(e) Unless there is full extension, large diameters engage.

2. *Causes of Delay in Second Stage.*—
(a) The flat face forms an inefficient dilator of passages.
(b) Mento-posterior cases being most common, there is a long internal rotation.
(c) The chin in mento-posterior cases may rotate backwards into the hollow of the sacrum (persistent mento-posterior position), and if this occurs, spontaneous delivery is almost impossible except with a small child or a large pelvis.

Management.—

General Rules.—

1. Be careful, in examining vaginally, not to injure the child's eyes.

2. Preserve membranes if possible till full dilatation of cervix; therefore attempt to make diagnosis vaginally only between pains.

3. Make the patient lie on the side the occiput is on. This favours extension of the head.

Special Rules.—In multiparæ, leave alone and, if there is much delay in the second stage, assist with forceps.

In primigravidæ, and mento-anterior position, treat as above. If mento-posterior, correct the lordosis of the child by fixing shoulder, pressing back the chest and pushing the buttocks in the opposite direction by abdominal manipulation. At the same time push up the face and forehead per vaginam, thus substituting an occipito-anterior position of the vertex, and deliver with forceps (*Thorn's manœuvre*). Should this manœuvre prove impossible, promote extension by pulling down the chin or pushing up the sinciput during pains. As in occipito-posterior cases, the chin may be brought to the front by manual rotation. If such manœuvres are unsuccessful, delivery by forceps traction or version may be attempted. If the child is dead—craniotomy.

Broadly speaking, interference should be carried out when

the second stage has lasted two to three hours and no progress is being made.

Prognosis.—

To Mother.—Slightly less favourable than in vertex, due to—

(*a*) Perineal tears.
(*b*) Manipulations being more often required.

To Child.—Grave. Ten per cent. are born dead—

1. From delayed labour.
2. From compression of head.

In addition, the eyes may be injured by careless vaginal examination.

The child when born usually presents an unsightly appearance from the swelling of the face and the elongation of its head; this disappears in a few days. It should therefore be kept from maternal inspection for 24 hours at least.

BROW PRESENTATIONS

Occur 1 in 2000.

Intermediate between vertex and face presentations.

Causes.—Same as face.

Diagnosis.—The prominence of the forehead, with the orbital ridges on one side of it and the large anterior fontanelle on the other.

Mechanism.—

1. May flex and form a vertex presentation.
2. May extend and form a face. (Most common.)
3. May be born as a brow; if so, the forehead rotates to the front, and, with the superior maxilla resting behind the symphysis, the cranial vault passes over the perineum by flexion; this is followed by extension, whereby the upper jaw, mouth, and chin successively glide beneath the pubic arch. This must always be very rare, as it can only occur in a very large pelvis or with a small head.
4. If the forehead rotates backwards, spontaneous delivery is impossible.

Prognosis.—

To Mother.—Mortality is increased from labour delayed by the longest diameter (vertico-mental) engaging and passing through the pelvis; injuries are common to the perineum, vagina, bowel and bladder. Rupture of the uterus may occur.

To Child.—Grave. Mortality, 18 per cent.

Management.—

1. If met with early, version. If later, try to convert into a vertex presentation as in face presentations ; if this be of no avail and the position is mento-anterior, try to convert into a face presentation by pushing up sinciput.

2. If labour is far advanced and the brow is irreducible, delivery should be attempted by forceps traction ; if mento-posterior, rotation of the chin forwards must be first accomplished before delivery by forceps can be completed. The result is usually unsatisfactory.

3. Cæsarean section, especially if the pelvis is contracted.

4. If the chin has rotated backwards, craniotomy is almost a *sine qua non*.

PELVIC PRESENTATIONS

Include breech, footling, and knee presentations.

Frequency.—Most frequently occur in multiparæ.
Breech, 1 in 40.

(*a*) Complete—with thighs and knees flexed.
(*b*) Frank—with thighs flexed and knees extended.

Footling, 1 in 74.
Knee, extremely rare.
Gross, 1 in 33.

Causes.—

1. Hydramnios and twins.
2. Contracted pelvis.
3. Tumours of uterine wall.
4. Placenta prævia.
5. Hydrocephalus.
6. Monsters.
7. Premature or dead fœtus, due to change of centre of gravity.

Positions.—According to position of sacrum, which is the denominator.

They are numbered as in vertex cases, the sacrum being the denominator.

They are named :—

1. *Left sacro-anterior*, L.S.A., first position.

2. *Right sacro-anterior*, R.S.A., second position.
3. *Right sacro-posterior*, R.S.P., third position.
4. *Left sacro-posterior*, L.S.P., fourth position.

Diagnosis.—

1. By external palpation.

The hard head can be felt at the upper pole of the uterus and *is easily ballotable.* Irregular mass felt over pelvis.

2. By auscultation.

Fœtal heart heard with greatest intensity to one or other side *above* umbilicus unless breech is low down in pelvis, which is rare.

3. Per vaginam—during labour.

(*a*) Soft presenting part, usually high up.
(*b*) Spinous processes of sacrum and ischial tuberosities.
(*c*) Fold of groin and scrotum (if male).

This may be distinguished from the axillary fold by the absence of ribs.

(*d*) Anus.—Meconium frequently found on the examining finger.
Sphincter ani grips finger.
No gums felt.

Diagnosis of Foot from Hand: Foot.—

1. Toes of equal length.
2. Prominence of heel at angle to limb.
3. Big toe not opposable.

Hand.—

1. Fingers vary greatly in length.
2. No prominence of heel.
3. Thumb bends over palm.

The knee may be differentiated from the elbow by offering a depression with prominences at either side, the elbow having a prominence flanked by depressions.

Mechanism.—

Sacro-anterior.—

1. Compaction.

Movement equivalent to flexion, the breech becoming engaged in pelvis, the bitrochanteric diameter being found in one or other oblique.

2. Internal rotation.

The *anterior hip* rotates forward behind the symphysis

(the denominator does *not* rotate forwards as in vertex cases. In L.S.A., therefore, the left hip comes forward).

3. Lateral flexion.

The anterior hip catches under the pubic arch, and the posterior passes over the perineum and is born.

4. The body follows, the shoulders lying in the conjugate.

5. After the birth of the trunk, the occipito-frontal diameter engages with the occiput just in front of the transverse diameter of the pelvis.

6. The occiput now rotates forward behind the symphysis.

7. The nape of the neck catches under the pubic arch, and the head becoming flexed on the trunk, the chin, face, forehead, and cranial vault pass successively over the perineum, and the head is born.

Sacro-posterior.—

1 to 4 as in sacro-anterior positions, but head may come into pelvis with the occiput just posterior to the transverse, and when this occurs the occiput may rotate backwards into hollow of sacrum, when delivery is very difficult; usually, however, the occiput rotates to the front, and the mechanism is similar to sacro-anterior cases.

Management of Normal Breech Case.—

During pregnancy in a primigravida, external version should be attempted at the thirty-fourth to thirty-sixth week (see p. 202).

In labour leave alone so as to preserve the membranes intact till full dilatation if possible. (The bag of forewaters tends to present in a sausage-shaped form and is thus liable to early rupture.)

If membranes rupture, let the breech dilate cervix.

When membranes rupture, examine for prolapse of cord, then leave to nature if possible and protect perineum as in vertex cases.

The vagina, however, may be ironed out manually, the hand being smeared with antiseptic soap: this softens the vagina and allows easier distension.

In a primigravida, episiotomy should be done so as to permit easier delivery of the head, more room for manipulations, if required, and prevention of a severe perineal tear.

When buttocks and thighs are born, cover with a warm towel to prevent premature inspiration due to the effect of cold air.

Pull down loop of cord and, if pulsating normally, leave

delivery to nature. If pulsation feeble, very quick, or absent, delivery must be completed as quickly as possible by supra-fundal pressure and traction. Otherwise *traction must never be used*, as it causes the arms to extend above the head.

When umbilicus is born, feel for arms in front of chest. If present, then leave to nature, if not, they are extended and must be brought down as quickly as possible (see p. 153).

After shoulders and arms are born, catch child with fingers round back of shoulders and flex head with knuckles. Exert supra-fundal pressure as well, and draw child gently downwards and backwards, and then, when nape of neck appears under symphysis, bring body of child over mother's abdomen when head is born easily.

Once the shoulders have been born, it is the custom of some to deliver the head after the manner described by Burns. The body of the child is allowed to hang over the end of the bed, with the object of (*a*) increasing flexion of the head, and (*b*) gradually drawing the head down through the pelvis. When the nape of the neck appears under symphysis, the head is delivered as described above.

(*N.B.*—Never hurry a breech delivery, especially in a primigravida, unless complications are present. A quick delivery is usually detrimental to the child, and tentorial tears and intra-cranial hæmorrhage are common causes of still-birth or neo-natal death.)

Causes of Delay in Breech Cases

1. Impaction of breech in pelvis.
2. Extension of arms at side of head or in nuchal position.
3. Extension of after-coming head.
4. Rotation backward of occiput.
5. Contraction of cervix round neck.

1. **Impaction of Breech in Pelvis.**—Generally due to contraction of pelvis, large fœtus, rigid canals or frank breech.

Management.—

(*a*) *If Knees are Flexed.*—Pull down the anterior foot. This reduces the size of breech, and subsequent delivery is easy. (If the posterior foot is brought down, the anterior buttock may catch on the symphysis.)

(*b*) *If the Knees are Extended.*—

(1) Push up the breech out of the pelvis if possible and then pass one hand inside the uterus, pressing the thigh of

the child against its abdomen and at the same time flexing the head and the back of the child with the other hand through the abdomen. This bends the knees and a foot will be easily reached (*Pinard's manœuvre*).

(2) If it is impossible to push the breech out of the pelvis—

(*a*) Put first finger into the groin and pull the breech down, always exerting traction towards the trunk and *not* the thigh.

(*b*) A blunt hook round the groin, though decried by some authorities, if used carefully, may be efficacious. Traction must always be towards the trunk else the thigh will be fractured and the hook must pass right round the thigh.

(3) Apply forceps to breech. Try a tentative pull; if forceps slip, remove, as further traction is useless. If they hold, however, delivery is usually easily effected.

(4) In very rare cases it may be necessary to comminute breech with the three-bladed carnioclast, as a last resort—this is done by putting the middle blade into the rectum, and the other blades outside the fœtal pelvis; if this is done the head must always be perforated before delivery is completed.

1. **Delay of Breech at Outlet.**—Breech may often be expelled by grasping each side of the fundus with either hand and exerting strong pressure during a contraction (Kristellar's manœuvre).

2. **Extension of Arms above Head.**—May be due to pulling on legs.

Management.—(1) *Lovset's Manœuvre.—When inferior angle of anterior scapula is visible* grasp *pelvis* of child with hands and gently rotate through 180°, the back of the child passing anteriorly; this brings the posterior shoulder to the front, and it appears under the pubis where arm either delivers itself spontaneously or can be lifted out by finger in elbow. The child is then rotated in the opposite direction for 180° and the other arm is similarly delivered. This method avoids any internal manipulations.

(2) Free the posterior arm first as there is more room in the hollow of the sacrum; swing the trunk of fœtus well forward, pass a hand over the back of the fœtal shoulder, pass two fingers along the humerus to the elbow and push the forearm over the face.

To free the anterior arm, swing the trunk of the fœtus well backward, and repeat the previous manipulation; if this is not possible turn the body of child by grasping the trunk with the thumbs posteriorly and the fingers anteriorly and then turning gently by a rotatory movement, pushing the trunk slightly upwards as well, until the anterior arm has become posterior; then deliver the arm as before. (Rotation should be carried out in the direction which turns face to the extended arm and often arm comes down without any further manipulation being required; if turned in opposite direction a nuchal displacement will result.)

The freeing of the arms must always be done with great care to prevent injury to the delicate bones, and tugging on the shoulder or humerus must be avoided as a fracture will occur. Sometimes an arm is displaced behind the head—*nuchal displacement.* This can be freed by rotating body so as to rotate face away from displaced arm.

3. **Rotation Backwards of Occiput.**—This should never occur if the doctor is in attendance during the delivery. In spontaneous delivery with the occiput in the sacral cavity, the nape of the neck catches on the perineum, and by a movement of flexion, the chin, face, forehead, and cranial vault pass successively from beneath the pubic arch, and the head is born.

It is of great value to remember the method of spontaneous delivery, so that it may be followed closely when assistance is necessary. Artificial rotation of the occiput is, however, usually easily accomplished.

If impossible to rotate, try to deliver by the *Prague seizure,* putting the fingers of one hand over the shoulders and raising the feet over the abdomen of the mother with the other hand.

4. **Extension of After-coming Head.**—The commonest cause of delay; frequently caused by injudicious traction on the trunk and want of fundal pressure.

Management.—Compression of the cord is now almost certain; therefore, for the safety of the child, delivery should be completed gently and quietly in at most ten minutes.

It is essential, therefore, to keep in view the two factors required, viz.:—

(*a*) Promote flexion.

(*b*) Assist the secondary powers to expel the head (the uterus has little power to expel the after-coming head through the pelvis).

(1) Make out the position of occiput, whether forwards or backwards.

(2) By supra-pubic pressure try to flex the head, as well as to assist the expulsive force.

(3) If unavailing and the occiput anterior, put the child astride the left arm and place the fingers of the left hand on its upper jaw or in its mouth to cause flexion of the head. With the fingers of the right hand on each shoulder, apply traction first downwards and backwards till the nape of neck is seen, then bring the body over the mother's abdomen and the head will be delivered. An assistant should exert

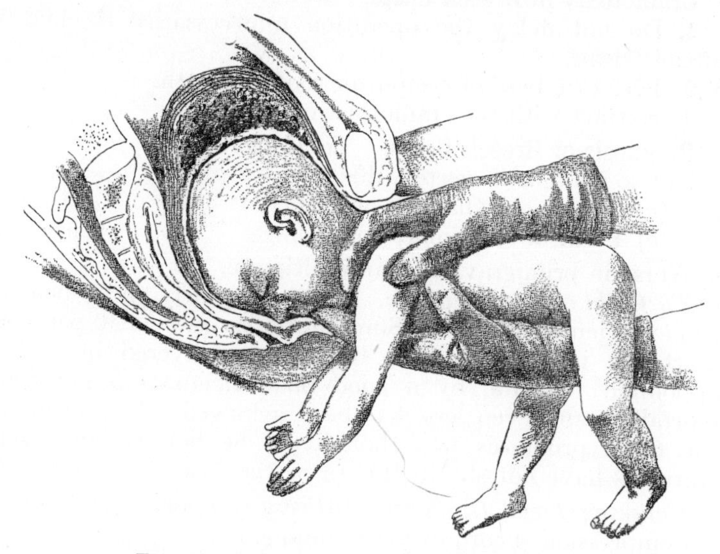

FIG. 17.—MAURICEAU-SMELLIE-VEIT MANŒUVRE.

fundal pressure during the first stage of the manœuvre (*Mauriceau-Smellie-Veit manœuvre*). By this combined movement the chin is made to pass over the perineum in the usual manner. (Fig. 17.)

It is useful to remember that in head-last deliveries the chin must always be born before the occiput.

(4) Forceps. The application of forceps to the after-coming head is most satisfactory and it is well always to have them ready in case of delay.

In occipito-anterior positions they are especially efficacious, and should be applied under the abdomen of the child, its trunk being thrown well forward under the pubic arch during the application.

From the grip of the head now obtained, traction causes well-marked flexion, and birth is frequently surprisingly easy.

5. Contraction of Cervix Round the Neck of the Child.—Undoubtedly the most difficult complication to deal with, and frequently requiring craniotomy.

If met with, anæsthetise and try—

Fundal pressure ; if unavailing—

(*a*) Child in good condition : dilate or incise cervix.

(*b*) Child dead or dying : craniotomy.

Craniotomy in Breech Cases.—*Rules.*—

1. Do not delay the operation unnecessarily if child is already dead.
2. Perforate base of occiput or roof of mouth.
3. Extract with the cranioclast or crotchet.

Prognosis of Breech Cases.—*To Mother.*—

Not so good as in vertex, due to—

(*a*) More manipulations necessary.

(*b*) Perineal tears more common.

Worse in primigravidæ than multiparæ.

To Child.—May be grave. Depends greatly on proficiency and experience of doctor. Some statistics quote a 40 per cent. mortality in primigravidæ, but when delivered in a well-appointed hospital, by a good obstetrician, a 5 per cent. mortality, and even less, has been achieved. In multiparæ, the fœtal prognosis was thought to be better, but recent statistics have not shown this to be the case.

Causes of Fœtal Death after Delivery of Body.—

Compression of cord by after-coming head.

Asphyxia due to premature inspiration.

Delay due to complications.

Intra-cranial hæmorrhage and tears due to rapid delivery of head through partially dilated vagina, there being no time for gradual moulding.

Broken neck through excessive forward leverage of body.

In an elderly primipara Cæsarean Section should be seriously considered owing to the probable difficulty in delivery and risk to the child.

SHOULDER PRESENTATION (TRANSVERSE LIE)

Also called *cross birth.* The lie may be oblique.

Frequency.—1 in 250 cases.

Presentation.—Shoulder, hand, elbow or ribs.

Causes.—

1. Absence of normal ovoid shape of uterine cavity from excess of liquor amnii.
2. Contracted pelvis (especially flat).
3. Obliquity of uterus.
4. Twins, especially second twin.
5. Placenta prævia.
6. Premature labour.
7. Dead fœtus.
8. Multiparity with flabby uterus and pendulous abdomen.
9. Uterine malformations, *e.g.*, arcuatus or subseptus.

Positions.—According to position of acromion, which is the denominator.

First, *Left acromio-anterior*, L.A.A.
Second, *Right acromio-anterior*, R.A.A.
Third, *Right acromio-posterior*, R.A.P.
Fourth, *Left acromio-posterior*, L.A.P.

The positions can thus be dorso-anterior or dorso-posterior. The most frequent position is left acromio-anterior.

Diagnosis.—Most important, as artificial delivery is always called for, and the earlier the diagnosis is made the easier and less dangerous is the treatment.

1. Inspection shows transverse elongation of uterine mass and the fundus lower than normal.
2. External palpation reveals breech and head at different sides, the breech occupying a higher level.
3. *Vaginally.*—The os uteri is high up and the presenting part is difficult to reach.

Presentation of membranes in sausage shape.

The shoulder offers a bony prominence with three radiating ridges—the clavicle, spine of scapula and humerus radiating from acromion.

Higher up, the cleft of axilla with the ribs may be felt.

The elbow offers a bony prominence with a depression on either side.

Diagnosis of a hand from a foot is already given (p. 150).

The right or left hand may be recognised easily from the manner in which the operator may " shake hands " with the fœtus, right to right and left to left. The thumb points to the fœtal head.

Diagnosis of Position.—Is most easily made by external palpation and must be ascertained before treatment is adopted.

Prognosis.—*To Mother.*—Varies according to stage of labour.

If advanced, grave.

Spontaneous delivery is almost impossible.

If diagnosed before the membranes have ruptured—good.

If diagnosed long after the membranes have ruptured—unfavourable.

To Child.—Very grave. Almost 45 per cent. die.

Mechanism of Spontaneous Delivery.—

(*a*) *Spontaneous Version.*—Not rare, and consists in the spontaneous substitution of the breech or head for the shoulder (when the head is substituted it is sometimes called *spontaneous rectification*). This generally occurs before, but has been known to occur immediately after, rupture of the membranes.

(*b*) *Spontaneous Evolution,* which consists of four movements :—

(1) Impaction of shoulder and chest in the oblique diameter of pelvis.

(2) Rotation forwards of shoulder behind the symphysis.

(3) Depression of chest and breech along hollow of sacrum till thorax reaches vulva.

(4) Expulsion of breech and legs followed by head.

(*c*) *Spontaneous Expulsion.*—The presenting part descends, the body doubles up, and the two parts, head and chest, escape together from the vulva. Very rare.

(*N.B.*—The two latter mechanisms can only occur with a small, premature, flexible or macerated fœtus in an enlarged pelvis.)

In the majority of cases untreated, impaction results. Then the uterus may rupture or may pass into a state of secondary inertia or uterine exhaustion. Later there may be sloughing of the soft parts from sustained pressure during labour.

Treatment.—

1. *Diagnosis Made in Last Month of Pregnancy.*—

(*a*) Pelvis normal—Cephalic version (external), and keep in place with a binder (see p. 202).

(*b*) Pelvis contracted—Cæsarean section at term.

2. *During Labour.*—

(*a*) Membranes intact—

(1) Cephalic version, if possible.

(2) Bipolar podalic version ; or

(3) If cervix is nearly fully dilated, rupture membranes and do internal podalic version.

(*b*) Membranes ruptured—
(1) If cervix is slightly dilated—bipolar version, if possible (see p. 202).
(2) If cervix is nearly fully dilated—internal podalic version (see p. 203).

(*c*) Shoulder impacted—
(1) If the fœtal heart is good and the lower uterine segment not too thinned out, anæsthetise patient deeply and perform internal version.
(2) If the child is markedly distressed or dead—decapitation.
(3) If the uterus is tightly contracted on the child or the lower uterine segment markedly thinned out—decapitation (see p. 214).

MULTIPLE PREGNANCY

By *super-fecundation* is meant the fertilisation of more than one ovum at the same inter-menstrual period, but at different times. Proved by a mother being delivered of twins—one mulatto and the other white.

By *super-fœtation* is meant the fertilisation of another ovum after the uterus is already gravid. It thus implies ovulation during pregnancy, which probably does not take place.

Examples of twins of very different size being born are probably due to unequal development although of the same age.

Development.—

If Distinct Ova (Binovular).—Two deciduæ capsulares.

Two chorions and amniotic sacs.

Two placentæ, which may unite at the edges, but the circulation of each is quite distinct.

May be of same or different sex.

Abnormalities.—Decidua capsularis may be common to both.

Chorionic division may be absorbed, giving the appearance of only one chorion.

If from One Ovum (Uniovular).—One decidua capsularis.
One common chorion.

May have one or two amniotic sacs.
One placenta.
Always of same sex.

Abnormalities.—

1. Amniotic division may be absorbed, the two original amniotic cavities being fused.
2. Formation of an acardiac fœtus.
3. Double monsters and teratoma may be found from incomplete fission.
4. Hydramnios is common.

Acardiac Fœtus.—This is the result of the heart and circulation in one twin being stronger than that of the other. By the intimate anastomoses in the placenta of the two circulations, the force of the blood current in the stronger twin causes a regurgitation through the umbilical arteries of the weaker twin, whose cardiac circulation is thus entirely destroyed. The heart, head and upper part of the body are therefore entirely undeveloped, although the lower limbs, etc., continue to grow from the nourishment they receive through the regurgitated circulation.

Size and Weight of Twins.—Each as a rule under the average weight ; combined they average about 9½ lb.
One twin is usually larger than the other.

Sex.—Sixty-four per cent. of same sex. If of same sex, male and female occur in equal proportion.

Course.—

1. Are usually expelled prematurely, 66 per cent.
2. One may be expelled prematurely and the other carried to full time.
3. One may die and be expelled alone.
4. One may die, and, being retained in utero, become shrivelled and flattened (*fœtus papyraceous*).
5. One may develop as a myxomatous mole, or one sac may develop hydramnios. The latter is common.
6. Have a marked tendency to be associated with albuminuria and eclampsia.

Presentation.—Both heads, 40 per cent.
Head and breech, 35 per cent.
Both breech, 10 per cent.
Head and shoulder, 9 per cent.
Breech and shoulder, 5 per cent.
Both shoulder, 1 per cent.

Diagnosis.—Often not made until after the birth of first twin. They may, however, be diagnosed during pregnancy by the excessive size of the uterine mass associated with numerous fœtal parts and two fœtal heads.

Occasionally two hearts may be heard beating at different rates and in different areas, the beats not being heard (or only slightly) in the intervening area. For a positive diagnosis to be made by auscultation, it is essential that the two hearts be heard simultaneously by two observers and that there should be a difference in rate of at least ten to the minute.

X-rays give definite diagnosis.

Prognosis.—*To Mother*, more unfavourable than normal.

1. From the large placental site predisposing to—
   (*a*) Hæmorrhage—post-partum.
   (*b*) Septic absorption.

2. From complications on the part of twins—malpresentations, etc.

3. From the frequency of maternal complications—pre-eclampsia, hydramnios, etc.

4. Some teach that over-distension of the uterus causes inertia. One of us (C. K.) does not believe this as the premature and rapid labours which characterise a twin delivery signify anything but lack of tone.

To Children.—Unfavourable.—
(1) From prematurity.
(2) Frequency of malpresentations.
(3) Small size and malformations.

Labour.—This is usually easy as the children are small.

After the birth of the first twin, the second is usually born spontaneously within an hour.

A protracted interval between the births may be due to inertia or to malpresentation of second twin. The third stage may be delayed.
   (*a*) From the large size of the placenta.
   (*b*) From inertia.

Placentæ.—

1. Nearly always born after the birth of the second child.
2. The placenta of first may be born before the birth of the second child.
3. Both may be born before the birth of second child.

Rules for Management of Normal Twin Labour.—

1. After the birth of the first child, tie the end of the

cord attached to the placenta in case of free communication between the circulations of uniovular twins causing hæmorrhage or asphyxia of second twin. Examine vaginally to determine presentation of second twin. If normal (head or breech), rupture membranes.

2. If the head or breech of the second child presents, wait half an hour for the pains returning spontaneously ; if they do not return, stimulate contractions by kneading the fundus. Pituitary extract 2–5 units may be given.

3. If the second child is lying transversely, rupture the membranes and carry out an internal version, bringing down a leg. Wait for pains to complete delivery.

4. If the pains do not return within an hour, hasten delivery artificially as the os is apt to close ; in cephalic presentation delivery may be effected by forceps or version.

5. Express the placenta soon, as from its size it is apt to be retained in the uterus after its separation and, by preventing complete contraction, may give rise to hæmorrhage.

6. Be alert always for hæmorrhage in the third stage.

Management of Complex Twin Labours.—If the membranes present together and both are cephalic presentations, rupture the lower sac ; if one is a breech and the other a cephalic presentation, rupture the membranes of the cephalic.

If the membranes are ruptured and both heads tend to enter the brim simultaneously, disengage the uppermost and, if accessible, apply forceps to the lower ; if a head and breech present, push up the breech to prevent the chins locking.

Chin Locking in Head and Breech Presentations.—Extremely rare.

If after the birth of the breech of the first child the head of the second enters the pelvis before the head of the first—

1. Push up the second and try to unlock the chins.

2. If this is impossible, decapitate the first child as it is usually born dead, apply forceps to the head of the second and deliver, then deliver the head of the first by fundal pressure, with crotchet or with forceps.

CHAPTER IX

DELAYED LABOUR

WHEN labour is not completed within twenty-four hours.

Assistance is frequently called for before this, thus the classification is arbitrary.

Delay may be due to faults in the powers, passages, or passenger, and may occur in any stage.

DUE TO POWERS

Ineffective Uterus.—

(*a*) Inertia (hypotonic).

(*b*) Inco-ordinate uterine action.

(1) Hypertonic lower uterine segment.
(2) Colicky uterus.
(3) False labour.
(4) Contraction ring.

(*a*) *Inertia*—(i) *Primary.*—

Causes.—

(1) Malpositions and malpresentations.
(2) Over-distended bladder.
(3) Over-distension of uterus, *e.g.* twins or hydramnios.
(4) Elderly primiparity.

Clinical Features.—Little or no progress from beginning of labour. Pains weak and intervals long. No caput on head, which is often high. Cervix is rather persistent and not fully drawn up. No disturbance of pulse or temperature and patient is more wearied than distressed.

Treatment.—If membranes intact no harm results.

Empty bladder and bowels.

Quinnie gr. v-x. Massage uterus. Hot douches.

Chloral gr. x-xx. may help to soften cervix and give patient a rest. Morphia ¼ gr. may also be used.

Posterior pituitary extract, two units if presentaion and position normal and no contraction of pelvis. Thymophysin 0·25 to 0·5 c.c. also useful in such a case. Probably safest method of giving pituitary is intravenously. 1 min. to 100 c.c. 5 per cent. glucose running at 50 c.c. for first half-hour and then 100 c.c. per half-hour later (Hellman), or 10–15 min. in 500 c.c. 5 per cent. glucose dropping 30 times a minute.

(Stone). If severe contractions occur they will cease almost at once if injection is stopped. Keep up strength with light diet and glucose drinks.

In second stage more danger due to exhaustion and more liability to infection. Prognosis for child not so good.

Forceps usually required when head in cavity or at outlet.

(ii) *Secondary.*—When labour is obstructed, the uterus either becomes over-stimulated and tonic uterine contractions and retractions occur (see p. 192 " Premonitory signs of labour ") or the uterus becomes exhausted (secondary inertia).

Clinical Features.—Pains good to begin with, but become progressively weaker until they may cease entirely. Always in second stage.

Dangers.—Little if child undelivered ; but if delivered during inertia, severe atonic P.P.H. may occur.

Treatment.—Any obvious cause should be dealt with. Empty bladder and bowels. Morphia $\frac{1}{4}$ gr. to ensure rest. After a sleep of two to three hours pains will start again and, if not strong enough to deliver child naturally, forceps should be applied whilst uterus is contracting strongly.

(*b*) *Inco-ordinate Uterine Action.*—

Causes.—

(1) Elderly primiparity.
(2) Familial.
(3) Suppressed fear or nervous tension causing contraction of lower segment by stimulation of sympathetic.
(4) Malformation of uterus where fusion is incomplete, *e.g.* U. bicornis-unicollis or subseptus.
(5) Malpositions and malpresentations especially occipito-posterior positions and transverse arrest of head ; high presenting part associated with absence of pressure on cervical ganglia.
(6) *Dystrophia Dystocia Syndrome.*—
 (i) Late primiparity ; frequently only daughter.
 (ii) Familial history of dystocia.
 (iii) Male type of pelvis or slightly justo-minor ; small cervix and rigid vagina ; stout with short extremities ; hyperpituitary type with male characteristics.
 (iv) Often associated with post-maturity and occipito-posterior position ; tendency to pre-eclampsia.

(1) *Hypertonic Lower Segment.*—Feeble action of upper segment (reversed polarity, see p. 52).

Clinical Features.—

(i) Constant backache interrupted by contractions which may be irregular.
(ii) Sometimes rectal or colonic spasm, which may cause desire to bear down.
(iii) Cervix remains thick, only slightly dilated and not well applied to head.
(iv) Very little caput formation.
(v) Retention of urine common.

Treatment.—

(i) Allay fear. Should not be left unattended.
(ii) Keep up strength with light diet and glucose drinks.
(iii) If acetonuria appears, give intravenous glucose drip.
(iv) Chemotherapy if labour in progress for over forty-eight hours.
(v) Sedatives, *viz.* morphia ¼ gr., twilight sleep or pethidine 150 mg.
(vi) Cæsarean section if condition resistant, or if fœtal distress occurs. Especially necessary in elderly primipara.

(2) *Colicky Uterus.*—Upper segment contracts spasmodically and often irregularly.

Clinical features.—

(i) Intense colicky pain, usually in hypogastrium, which precedes and persists after uterine contraction.
(ii) Uterus may become tender.
(iii) Rectal spasm may occur.
(iv) Pains not expulsive so little caput or moulding.
(v) Cervix thick, not drawn up and only slightly dilated.

Treatment.—As for hypertonic lower segment.

(3) *False Labour.*—

Clinical Features.—

(i) Frequent strong and painful contractions.
(ii) Whole uterus contracts. No polarity and no dilatation of cervix.
(iii) Later lower segment stops contracting and labour begins.

Treatment.—Sedatives and rest.

(4) *Contraction Ring.*—Due to spasm of muscle at junction of upper and lower segments, but may rarely occur in upper segment. Forms around neck of child or over a point of slight resistance.

Causes.—

(1) Premature rupture of membranes, especially with malpresentations and malpositions, *e.g.* shoulder presentations and occipito-posterior positions.
(2) Increased irritability of uterine muscle due to delayed labour or excessive manipulations, *e.g.* forceps, version, or turning the head in occipito-posterior positions.
(3) Injection of pituitary or ergot before delivery.
(4) Often preceded by an inefficient uterus.

Clinical Features.—

(i) Severe pain in hypogastrium and sometimes back (may be due to ischæmia of contracted muscle).
(ii) Tender uterus.
(iii) Ring may be seen, or palpated abdominally, during a contraction.
(iv) On vaginal examination—

(*a*) Looseness of presenting part during contraction, with no advance.
(*b*) Cervix is lax during contraction and hangs loosely around and below presenting part.
(*c*) Ring can usually be felt round neck of child.

Prognosis.—Very grave for child (50 per cent. mortality) and grave for mother (15 per cent. mortality).

Treatment.—Deep anæsthesia.

Amyl nitrite or possibly 5 ♏. adrenalin (1–1000) subcutaneously.

Intravenous magnesium sulphate ; either 2 c.c. of a 50 per cent. solution or 10 c.c. of a 20–25 per cent. solution.

Where there is no improvement, morphia may be given to promote rest.

If the ring subsequently relaxes and the cervix is fully dilated, vaginal delivery may be effected by forceps.

Alternatively, Willet's forceps, with a 4–6 lb. weight attached, may be applied to the scalp during sedation, and gradual traction so encouraged.

Cæsarean section may be necessary, the ring having sometimes to be divided before the child can be delivered.

If the child is dead or in extremis, embryotomy may be necessary.

If head is presenting, perforation is followed by the application of Brigg's forceps and gradual traction obtained by attaching a weight (see p. 213).

Deliver placenta immediately after delivery of child, otherwise hour-glass contraction may cause retention of placenta for hours and may be associated with P.P.H.

Tetanic Contractions (Hypertonic Uterus).—(See Rupture of Uterus p. 191.)

(a) Delay in First Stage

Due to Passages

1. **Rigidity of Cervix, or Occlusion of External Os.**—

(*a*) *Spasmodic Rigidity.*—Met with in primigravidæ only, and is more prone to occur in the elderly. Often associated with a high head, early rupture of the membranes and an occipito-posterior position.

Diagnosis.—Edge of cervix thin, but regular in outline.

Treatment.—

(i) Empty bladder and bowels.
(ii) Chloral 15 gr. repeated in three hours.
(iii) Morphia $\frac{1}{4}$ gr. combined with hot douches.
(iv) Spasmalgin or pethidine hydrochloride if os half dilated.
(v) Dilatation if os small, with dilators and/or a finger; if the cervix is half-dilated and not unduly tense, manual dilatation under spinal anæsthesia may be necessary. (Delmas.)
(vi) If the head is low in the pelvis, the cervix may be incised if all other measures fail.
(vii) Cæsarean section will be required if os completely occluded.

(*b*) *Organic Rigidity.*—Generally due to cervicitis, the result of previous lacerations.

May be due to malignant infiltration.

May be intractable.

Diagnosis.—Edge of cervix thick, hard, and irregular.

Treatment.—As in spasmodic. Small incisions may be necessary.

2. **Obliquity of Uterus.**—Anteversion of pendulous belly prevents the powers acting in their proper axis.

Treatment.—Put the patient on her back and retain the uterus in proper axis by applying a tight binder.

3. **Impaction of Anterior Cervical Lip.**—

Treatment.—Push lip up during pains.

Anæsthesia is generally indicated as this manipulation is painful.

4. **Contracted Pelvis** (causing high presenting part). (See p. 174.)

Due to Passenger

1. **Excess of Liquor Amnii.**—May prevent contractions and over-distends the lower uterine segment. Can usually be recognised by feeble, long pains occurring at lengthy intervals.

Treatment.—Rupture membranes and allow presenting part to act as dilator.

(*N.B.*—Early escape of liquor amnii (dry labour) is often stated to give rise to delayed labour. This, however, is *not* the experience of the authors, who have found that labour is usually more rapid in such cases, provided there is no definite cause for the early rupture such as malposition, malpresentation, contracted pelvis, etc., in which cases the delay is due to these factors and not to the early rupture of the membranes.)

2. **Adhesion of Membranes to Lower Uterine Segment.**—

Treatment.—Separate with finger as in artificial dilatation.

3. **Sausage-shaped Presentation of Membranes.**—Due to the presenting part not being closely grasped by the pelvis and thus failing to form a plug whereby the forewaters are cut off from the general amniotic cavity and its contents.

This is chiefly met with, therefore, in contracted pelvis and malpresentations; early rupture is the usual sequence. If rupture does not occur and the dilating power of the membranes is lost, rupture membranes artificially.

4. **Malpresentation and Malposition.**

(*b*) Delay in Second Stage

Delay Due to Secondary Powers.—

1. From paralysis of abdominal muscles.
2. Pain from peritonitis, full bladder, etc.
3. Distension of the abdomen, from—
   (*a*) Ovarian tumours.
   (*b*) Ascites, etc.

4. Chest affections, by preventing fixation of the diaphragm.

5. Stoutness, especially associated with feeble or divaricated recti muscles.

6. Nervous and excitable women ; best treated by administration of twilight sleep.

Treatment.—

(i) Remove the cause if possible ; if not, apply a tight binder and put patient in the dorsal position.

(ii) Forceps.

Due to Passages

1. **Rigidity of Soft Parts.**—Vagina, perineum, vulva.

Causes.—

(1) Tonic rigidity, from want of vital dilatation in muscular primigravidæ and premature labours.

(2) Secondary rigidity, from long labours. Parts are hot, dry and congested.

(3) Malformations of vagina and hymen.

(4) Old cicatrices, ulceration, etc.

Treatment.— *Vaginal.*—

(1) Examine as seldom as possible.

(2) Hot douching.

(3) Ironing vagina.

(4) Forceps.

Perineum.—

(1) Deep anæsthesia.

(2) Distension by De Ribes' bag.

(3) Ironing.

(4) Forceps.

(5) **Episiotomy.**

Types.—

(*a*) Central.

(*b*) Postero-lateral. (Least satisfactory as small artery frequently cut.)

(*c*) J-shaped, beginning centrally and curving outwards.

Uses.—

(1) Replaces an irregular perineal laceration with a clean incision.

(2) Prevents third degree tears.

(3) Allows head to be delivered spontaneously if delayed only by perineal rigidity.

(4) Prevents excessive downbearing during the perineal stage, which would stretch the ligaments of the bladder and uterus unduly and might lead to a future prolapse.

(5) Allows more freedom of manipulation in a primiparous breech delivery to the advantage of both child and mother, as it allows an easier delivery of the child without undue pressure on head and permits complications to be rectified more easily and quickly ; for the mother it prevents gross perineal lacerations.

Varieties of Torn Perineum.—

(1) Partial.
(2) Complete.
(3) Central.

Partial—where the tear does not extend through the sphincter ani.

First Degree—Rupture of fourchette and anterior margin.

Second Degree—Tear of perineal body, but not through sphincter ani.

Complete (Third Degree)—where the tear extends through sphincter ani into rectum.

Central—rare, a button-hole opening forms in the perineum.

If the Perineum is Torn.—Put in stitches immediately after the child is born if patient is under anæsthetic for delivery. If not then wait until after third stage and repair under local anæsthesia. Stitch vagina first from apex downwards with continuous No. 1 (20 day) catgut, then stitch perineum with deep sutures of No. 1 or 2 (20 day) catgut, or silkworm gut, being careful that the deep part of stitch is buried at the base of the wound. The suture nearest the anus should be inserted first and that next the vagina last. (The muscles may be sutured independently with No. 1 catgut buried and the skin separately, but the authors have not found any benefit by so doing and excess of catgut seems to make perineum more prone to infection with subsequent breakdown.)

Do not pull stitches tight ; by this means much unnecessary pain is saved and inconvenience avoided. Parts become œdematous and, if tight, the stitches just cut through later.

Tight stitches are a common cause of urinary retention.

If silkworm sutures are used the ends should be left long and tied together to prevent short ends irritating patient.

In Complete Tears stitch the rectal tear first from above downwards, then stitch the sphincter ani and lastly the vagina and perineum as usual.

After-care.—The perineum should be attended to every time the vulval pad is changed and after micturition or defæcation. The part is first sprayed with hydrogen peroxide solution and is then swabbed gently with methylated spirit. This cleanses and hardens the perineum, and healing is usually rapid and complete. If silkworm gut sutures are used, they should be cut between seventh and tenth days.

Dangers of Perineal Tears.—

(1) Liable to become septic.
(2) Damage to perineal body and levatores ani muscles.
(3) May be starting point of rectocele.
(4) May favour prolapse if healing inefficient.
(5) May cause retention of urine and its sequelæ.

2. **Distension of Rectum.**—A most potent cause of delay, but should never occur if rules of management are attended to.

3. **Distended Bladder.**—Prevents secondary powers from acting. May prolapse before the head and may thus be mistaken for impacted anterior lip cervix.

Treatment.—Draw off the urine ; pass a male rubber or gum elastic catheter far in, as the bladder is pulled up during the second stage and urethra elongated. Can often be aided by putting patient in the genu-pectoral or left lateral position.

4. **Prolapse of Anterior Vaginal Wall.**—Frequently associated with full bladder.

Treatment.—Draw off urine, if any, and if swelling remains, push up between pains. (Anæsthesia greatly assists this manipulation.)

5. **Tumours of Soft Canals.**—Very rare.

6. **Contracted Pelvis** (see p. 174).

Due to Passenger

1. **Toughness of Membranes.**—A common cause ; occasionally the bag of forewaters may protrude from the vulva. Therefore the membranes should always be ruptured when full dilatation of the cervix is completed.

Rupture should be performed during a pain.

In rare cases the head may be born enveloped in the membranes. This is named *born with a caul,* and is popularly supposed to be a sign of luck !

2. Large Size of Fœtal Head.—

(*a*) *Natural.*—

(1) From premature ossification.
(2) From protracted gestation.
(3) In a large fœtus.

The mechanism is analogous to that of a normal-sized head in a justo-minor pelvis, viz., extreme flexion.

(*b*) *Unnatural.*—**Hydrocephalus.**—Due to the increase of cerebro-spinal fluid in the ventricles.

Occurs 1 in 1000 labours.

Diagnosis.—Large head felt above symphysis.

Uterus tends to become hour-glass in shape owing to distension of lower uterine segment.

Vaginally.—Broad sutures and large fontanelles felt with small thin bones in their midst (" islets of bones in a sea of membranes ").

Frequently present by breech owing to large head not fitting into lower uterine segment or pelvis. Can often be diagnosed by birth of small, puny body and yet great difficulty is experienced in delivery of head.

X-ray may help, *but it is not wise to diagnose by X-ray alone,* as sometimes the head seems to be unduly large by X-ray and is found to be quite normal at birth. This is expecially likely to occur when the head is at the fundus.

Dangers.—Rupture of the uterus from inability of the cervix to become retracted over the large head (15 per cent.). Post-partum hæmorrhage not uncommon.

Treatment.—Head presentation—perforate head and leave to nature ; if delay in expulsion extract by forceps or cranioclast.

Breech presentation.—Either perforate head through posterior fontanelle or incise into spinal canal and pass gum elastic catheter up canal through foramen magnum to drain cerebro-spinal fluid.

3. Shortness of Umbilical Cord.— *Actual.*—Rare under 8 in.

Acquired or Relative.—From coiling round the fœtus.

Dangers.—Inversion.

Early separation of placenta.

Rupture of Cord.

Diagnosis of Short Cord.—Signs.—

(1) Funic souffle.
(2) Recession of the presenting part in the intervals between pains.

(3) Variability in the position of head within narrow limits.

(4) Discharge of some blood after each pain.

Treatment.—Cut the cord, if accessible, and deliver rapidly.

4. **Malformation of Fœtus.**—

Hydrothorax.
Ascites.
Distended bladder or cystic kidneys.
Tumours.

Treatment.—If such cause delay after the head is born, make out by external palpation and perforate any part within reach per vaginam (evisceration).

5. **Prolapse of Hand or Arm below the Vertex** (*Compound Presentation*).—Occurs 1 in 400 cases and is due to any condition hindering the engagement of head.

Treatment.—If at the side of the head, the prolapsed member is usually easily replaced, but if across the back of the head, this is difficult and, as it seriously impedes labour, version should be performed.

6. **Malpresentations and Malpositions.**

CHAPTER X

CONTRACTED PELVIS

This condition may result from under-development, disease in childhood or accident. The types most commonly met with are due to rickets or under-development.

Diagnosis.—

1. From history of rickets in childhood.
2. From small stature.
3. From obvious deformity.
4. Abnormal prominence of abdomen in primigravidæ.
5. From difficulty at previous labours.
6. From small or abnormal pelvic measurements found at ante-natal examination or by X-ray.
7. High position of the head at the brim.
8. Inaccessibility of the presenting part per vaginam.

General Effects of Contracted Pelvis

During Pregnancy.—

1. May have no effect. On the other hand—
2. A retroverted uterus may become incarcerated in the pelvis.
3. " Pendulous belly," a characteristic sign of contracted pelvis in a primigravida, may be present.
4. Malpresentations due to the inability of the head to accommodate itself to the ovoid of the lower uterine segment, under normal conditions within the pelvic brim.
5. Lightening does not occur and the head, if presenting, does not fix in the pelvis during last month of pregnancy.

During First Stage of Labour.—

1. Head is slow to engage and may remain movable at the brim.
2. Membranes apt to be sausage-shaped.
3. Early rupture of membranes from inability of the head to descend and form a plug between liquor amnii and fore-waters. Cord may prolapse.
4. Escape of all liquor amnii.
5. Slow dilatation of cervix.
6. Delay throughout.

During Second Stage of Labour.—

1. Cord may prolapse.
2. Child may be subjected to much compression.
3. Caput succedaneum is very large and head moulding is exaggerated.
4. The skull bones may be indented or fractured through pressure.
5. The anterior cervical lip may be nipped between the head and pelvic brim.
6. Soft parts may be lacerated.
7. The lower segment may rupture.
8. There may be delay because of pelvic contraction or malpresentation.

During Third Stage of Labour.—Delay, with risk of post-partum hæmorrhage from inertia following a long tedious labour.

Mechanism of Labour.—Materially changed and varies according to the type of contraction.

Prognosis.—To Mother—Mortality increased. The prognosis differs with the degree of contraction and is influenced by—

1. Exhaustion.
2. Rupture of uterus.
3. Sloughing of soft parts from prolonged pressure in second stage with subsequent fistula formation.
4. More frequent forceps delivery, with increased morbidity rate. Craniotomy may be required in some cases.
5. Post-partum hæmorrhage from uterine inertia.

To Child.—Very grave, from—

1. Faulty presentations.
2. Escape of liquor amnii resulting in greater compression of the child.
3. Greater pressure on fœtal skull with occasional indentation fractures of the cranial bones and intra-cranial hæmorrhage.
4. Prolapse of the cord.
5. Craniotomy in some cases.

TYPES OF CONTRACTED PELVES

1. Symmetrically contracted.—
   Æquabiliter justo minor.

2. Flattened.—
   (*a*) Rachitic.
   (*b*) Non-rachitic or simple flat.
3. Combination of (1) and (2).
4. Irregularly contracted.—
   (*a*) Malacosteon or osteomalacic.
   (*b*) Pseudo-osteomalacic (rachitic).
   (*c*) Thorny pelvis (multiple exostoses).
5. From spinal deformity or abnormality.—
   (*a*) Lordosis.
   (*b*) Scoliosis.
   (*c*) Kyphosis.
   (*d*) Spondylolisthesis.
   (*e*) High assimilation pelvis.
6. Mal-developed pelves.—
   (*a*) Nægele's (obliquely contracted).
   (*b*) Roberts' (transversely contracted).
   (*c*) From unilateral hip-joint disease (obliquely contracted).
7. Android and anthropoid.

Pelvis Æquabiliter Justo Minor

Is simply an undersized pelvis, all the diameters of brim, cavity and outlet being equally contracted.

Diagnosis.—All diameters shortened, but proportionately so.

Head overlaps at brim and is movable.

Mechanism.—Extreme flexion of head which enters in the oblique diameter, the posterior fontanelle being very easily reached.

Treatment.—(See p. 183.)

Flat Pelves

Are characterised by a diminution of the conjugate, with relative increase in the transverse diameters of the brim. They are of two varieties—rachitic and non-rachitic.

Rachitic Flat.—Is due to a rotation of the sacrum on its transverse axis, so that the promontory is approximated to the symphysis pubis.

It is thus specially characterised by diminution of the conjugate at the brim only, all the other diameters being increased.

Due to softening of the bones from rickets, some minor characteristics are present, principally—

1. "Flaring out" of the ilia so that the interspinous approximates to the intercristal diameter in length.
2. Flattening of sacrum transversely.

Non-rachitic Flat.—The result of a sinking forward of the sacrum en masse and characterised by a diminution in the antero-posterior diameters of the brim, cavity and outlet, with relative increase of the transverse.

Extreme contraction is uncommon.

The rachitic and non-rachitic resemble one another in—

1. Diminution of conjugate at brim.
2. Increase of transverse throughout.
3. Wide pubic arch.

They differ chiefly—

Rachitic.—

1. Increase of all diameters except the conjugate at brim. (Non-rachitic—all antero-posterior diameters are diminished.)
2. Relative increase of interspinous to intercristal diameter. (Non-rachitic—normal relationship.)
3. Flattening of sacrum transversely.
4. Crests of ilium less sinuous.
5. Pelvic inlet kidney-shaped.
6. Ischial tuberosities further apart and everted.
7. Acetabula directed more anteriorly.
8. Promontory of the sacrum more easily reached.
9. Posterior superior spines approximated.

Special Effect on Mechanism.—

(*a*) *Anterior-parietal Presentation—Anterior Asynclitism.*—Head enters the brim with the occipito-frontal diameter in the transverse of pelvis.

The head moves laterally to the side of the pelvis occupied by the occiput, allowing the wide biparietal diameter more room, the bitemporal diameter engaging in the true conjugate.

The two fontanelles may lie on the same level (Michaelis' obliquity), *i.e.*, the head is partly extended.

The anterior parietal bone enters the pelvic brim first, the sagittal suture facing the promontory (Nægele's obliquity). This allows the super-subparietal diameter ($3\frac{1}{2}$ in.) to displace the biparietal ($3\frac{3}{4}$ in.). The posterior parietal is then squeezed past the promontory.

After the head passes the brim in the rickety flat pelvis, labour is completed quickly as the other diameters are increased, the occiput rotating to the front as in a normal pelvis. In the non-rachitic type, however, much delay is still occasioned by the diminished antero-posterior diameters of the cavity and outlet.

Because of the increase in the transverse diameters, internal rotation is sometimes absent, the long diameter of the head being born in the transverse of the outlet.

(*b*) *Posterior-parietal Presentation—Posterior Asynclitism* (rare).—The posterior parietal enters the pelvic brim first, the sagittal suture now looking towards the symphysis pubis (Litzmann's obliquity). The head is usually held up at that level. If a mechanism does occur, however, it is similar to that described above, in this case the anterior parietal being pushed past the symphysis pubis.

Treatment.—(See p. 183.)

MALACOSTEON OR OSTEOMALACIC PELVIS. (Fig. 18)

An irregularly contracted pelvis due to softening of the bones, the result of osteomalacia, an endemic disease in the

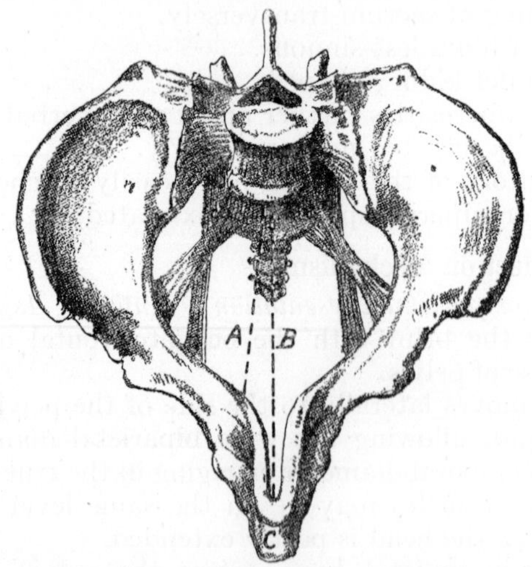

FIG. 18.—MALACOSTEON PELVIS.
A, Available conjugate ; B, Anatomical ; C, Beak-shaped symphysis.

Rhone Valley and North Italy. May be due to deficiency of food (especially calcium and vitamins A and D), bad housing and lack of sunlight. It occurs usually during pregnancy and the puerperium.

Development.—As the weight of the body, when standing, is transmitted from the vertebral column to the heads of the thigh bones through the pelvis, the latter will, if softened, become much compressed and distorted. The contraction will naturally be most marked in the transverse diameter as the heads of the femora drive in the lateral pelvic walls. At the same time, through sitting, the sacrum will be compressed vertically, the promontory being driven downwards and the tip of the coccyx upwards and forwards.

The chief characteristics of the deformity will thus be—

1. Transverse diameters all diminished.
2. Anatomical conjugate (B) at brim lengthened; available conjugate (A) diminished. (Fig. 18.)
3. Forepart of pelvis narrowed (beak shape).
4. Pubic arch narrowed.
5. Outlet diminished in all diameters.
6. Sacral concavities increased.

DIFFERENCES BETWEEN MALACOSTEON AND RACHITIC FLAT PELVIS

	Malacosteon.	Rachitic Flat.
Brim—		
	1. Transverse contracted.	1. Transverse relatively lengthened.
	2. Conjugate lengthened.	2. Conjugate shortened.
	3. Shape-Y. Beak-shaped pubis.	3. Shape-kidney.
Cavity and Outlet—		
	1. All diameters diminished.	1. All diameters increased.
	2. Arch narrowed.	2. Arch widened.
Sacrum—		
	1. More concave.	1. Flattened transversely.

In rachitic flat pelvis the interspinous and intercristal diameters approximate.

Treatment.—Cæsarean section with sterilisation. This should be followed by exhibition of calcium and cod liver oil.

Pseudo-osteomalacic Pelvis

Is a rachitic flat pelvis with osteomalacic characteristics. May be due to rickets prolonged during child life, after the child can stand or walk, or to osteomalacia occurring in a pelvis previously flattened by rickets.

Treatment.—Cæsarean section.

Exostoses. Thorny Pelvis

Danger.—Liable to cause injury to the uterus or child's head during labour.

Treatment.—If marked exostoses, Cæsarean section.

Lordosis

Undue prominence of lumbar convexity preventing the entrance of the presenting part in the axis of the pelvic brim.

Treatment.—A vaginal delivery is usually possible.

Scoliosis

Lateral obliquity of lumbar vertebræ causing asymmetry of the pelvis through encroachment of the promontory on one oblique diameter of the brim. The side of the pelvis corresponding to the spinal convexity is diminished. This deformity is usually due to rickets.

Treatment.—Cæsarean section may be necessary.

Kyphotic Pelvis

This deformity is due to the weight of the body being carried to the promontory of the sacrum in such a manner as to rotate it backwards on its transverse axis. Thus—

1. The true conjugate is increased.
2. The transverse throughout is diminished.
3. All diameters of the outlet are contracted, especially the inter-tuberischial diameter.

It is thus the exact converse of the rachitic flat pelvis and the delay to the passage of the child is most marked at the outlet.

Treatment.—Always examine the pelvic outlet in cases of kyphosis. As the transverse diameter is diminished and the subpubic angle is narrowed, much depends on the length of the posterior sagittal measurement (the distance between the lower end of the sacrum and the mid-point of the transverse diameter). If the outlet measurements, transverse and posterior sagittal, total 5½ in., then vaginal delivery may be accomplished with the patient in the elevated lithotomy position.

In slight degrees of contraction, therefore, spontaneous or instrumental delivery may obtain. In marked deformity, where the inter-tuberischial is $2\frac{1}{2}$ in. or under, Cæsarean section is the treatment of choice. If the child be dead, craniotomy should be performed.

Spondylolisthesis

Where the last lumbar vertebra has slipped down in front of the promontory of the sacrum and so diminishes the conjugate.

Treatment.—If at all aggravated—Cæsarean section.

High Assimilation Pelvis

Here the last lumbar vertebra has taken on the characters of a sacral vertebra and becomes fused to the sacrum. The contraction is in the antero-posterior diameter of the outlet, is usually slight and overcome by instrumental delivery. This abnormality may be present in the anthropoid pelvis.

(*N.B.*—Another form of assimilation pelvis results when the first sacral vertebra assimilates the lumbar variety. This gives rise to a shallow pelvis and generally allows an easy labour.)

NæGELE's Pelvis. (Fig. 19)

An obliquely contracted pelvis due to arrested development of one ala of the sacrum and frequently resulting in

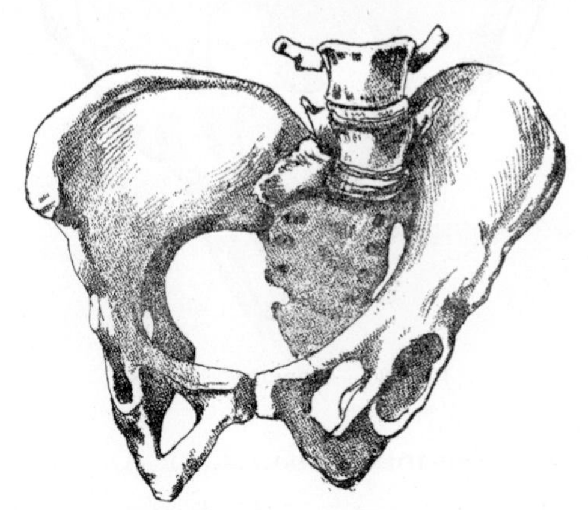

Fig. 19.—Nægele's Pelvis.

ankylosis of a sacro-iliac joint. Results in the diminution of the oblique diameter corresponding to the developed side of the pelvis; thus if the right iliac bone is developed, the right oblique is contracted.

Diagnosis.—Almost impossible from usual measurements, but if suspected the following measurements, normally equal on the two sides, are found to be unequal :—

(*a*) From symphysis to posterior superior spines.

(*b*) From anterior superior spine to posterior superior spine of other side.

(*c*) From last lumbar spine to anterior superior spine of each side.

Treatment.—Cæsarean section or craniotomy, if former is contra-indicated.

Roberts' Pelvis. (Fig. 20)

Is the result of non-expansion of both sacral alæ. It retains, therefore, the infantile shape, viz., transversely contracted.

Treatment.—As for Nægele.

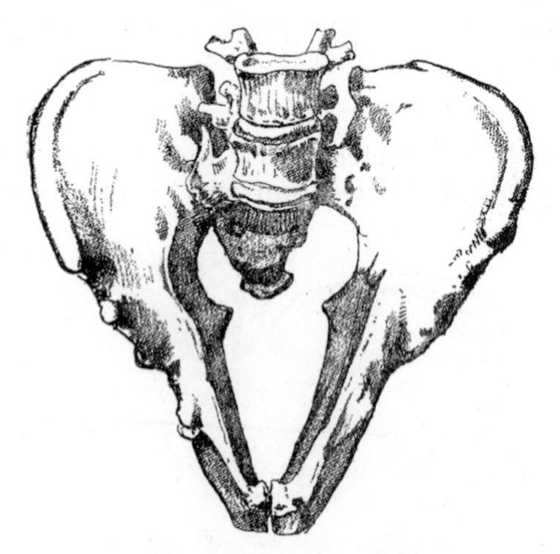

Fig. 20.—Roberts' Pelvis.

Unilateral Hip-joint Disease or Absence of Leg

Here the oblique diameter of the diseased side is shortened. The body weight is taken on the sound limb and therefore that side of the pelvis is pushed inwards. In such cases the pelvis should be measured to discover contraction as in

Nægele's pelvis and the findings acted upon by advising normal labour or Cæsarean section.

Android and Anthropoid Pelves

Caldwell and Moloy have shown that these pelves resemble that of the male and ape respectively. Diagnosis, by ordinary pelvic measurements, may prove difficult.

Android.—

1. The pelvic brim is heart-shaped.
2. The promontory projects forwards.
3. The forepart of the pelvis is narrowed.
4. The pelvic cavity is deepened and the diameters diminish towards the outlet.
5. The sub-pubic angle is narrowed, but increased depth of pelvis may result in the transverse diameter of the outlet approximating the normal.
6. The sacro-sciatic notch is narrow, below two fingers breadth.

Anthropoid.—

1. Forepart of pelvis narrowed, but promontory is not so prominent.
2. Antero-posterior diameter at brim is increased; transverse diameter is diminished.
3. Pelvic cavity is deepened and the diameters lessen towards the outlet.
4. The sub-pubic angle is narrowed, but the sacro-sciatic notch is widened.
5. "High Assimilation" may be present.

In both types of pelvis, occipito-posterior positions are common and no attempt should be made to correct the malposition, as the occiput is occupying the wider posterior part of the pelvis.

Vaginal delivery is usually possible, but, if the outlet is markedly contracted, Cæsarean section or craniotomy may be necessary.

General Treatment of Contracted Pelvis

This can be judged approximately according to the length of the true conjugate.

First Degree.—Conjugate, 4 to 3½ in. With a true conjugate of this length, delivery is usually either spontaneous or can be effected with forceps. The Walcher position can be used with advantage in flat pelves. Very rarely, however, it may be deemed advisable to induce premature labour. Careful examination should be made at weekly intervals during the last month in the doubtful cases and the relative size of head and pelvis estimated. As soon as slight difficulty is experienced in pushing the head into the pelvic brim, labour may be induced.

If contracted pelvis is the indication for induction, this should never be attempted before the thirty-sixth week or with a conjugate of less than 3½ in. Moreover, careful choice of methods is essential. If the membranes are ruptured or bougies introduced into the uterus, there is an increase in the morbidity risk and a subsequent Cæsarean section, if necessary, is prejudiced. There is, therefore, at the present time, an increasing tendency, if medical induction fails, to adopt conservative treatment for this degree of contraction and to allow the patient to have a " test of labour " at term. Should the head show no signs of fixing after 6–12 hours of good labour or when the membranes have been ruptured for one hour, Cæsarean section may be indicated. Again section may be justified where the membranes rupture early, where uterine contractions are weak and ineffective and where there is little dilatation of the cervix after twenty-four hours of labour.

Second Degree.—Conjugate, 3½ to 3 in. Towards the upper limit of this degree, spontaneous or instrumental delivery is possible if the child is small. Usually there is little hope of delivery per vias naturales and Cæsarean section is necessary. As an alternative to this latter procedure, craniotomy is advocated if the child is dead or the mother potentially infected as in failed forceps cases.

Third Degree.—Conjugate, 3 to 2½ in. Here the treatment is Cæsarean section, or if the child is dead or the mother potentially infected, craniotomy.

Below 2½ in. Cæsarean section is absolutely necessary as the mento-nasal diameter of 1½ in., the largest diameter of the ossified skull, cannot be broken by crianoclasm. In actual practice it is unlikely that cranioclasm will result in such a diminution in bulk being approached.

This scheme is satisfactory for both flat and generally contracted pelves. In the latter, however, as the contraction is present at all levels of the pelvis, an extra ¼ in. should be added to each degree, *e.g.*, first degree, 4 to 3¾ in.

Pubiotomy, as a method of treatment in contracted pelvis, is of historical interest only.

ENLARGED PELVIS

Æquabiliter Justo Major

All diameters increased.

Dangers.—Precipitous labour with perineal laceration.

TYPICAL PELVIC MEASUREMENTS FOR COMMON TYPES OF PELVES.

	I.S.	I.C.	I.T.	P.S.	E.C.	D.C.	C.V.
Normal . . .	10″	11″	4″	2½″	7½″	4½″	4″
Justo-Minor . .	8″	9″	3″	2″	7″	4″	3½″
Flat : Rachitic . .	10½″	10¾″	4¼″	3¼″	7″	4″	3½″
Simple . .	10″	11″	4″	2″	7″	4″	3½″
Kyphotic—Anthropoid	9″	10″	3″	2″	8″	5″	4½″
Justo-Major . .	11″	12″	4½″	3½″	8″	5″	4½″

CHAPTER XI

OTHER MAJOR COMPLICATIONS OF LABOUR

POST-PARTUM HÆMORRHAGE

Types.—

1. Primary.—Bleeding during the third stage and in the six hours following delivery.
2. Secondary (puerperal).—Bleeding after that time.

Varieties of Primary.—

(*a*) Atonic.
(*b*) Traumatic.

Normal Hæmostatic Factors in Uterus.—

1. Contraction and retraction of uterus.
2. Contraction of plain muscle of vessels.
3. Clotting at mouth of vessels.

While the uterus is flaccid there is no hæmorrhage showing that retraction alone is sufficient to prevent hæmorrhage. This is, however, assisted by the strong, intermittent uterine contractions, which eventually bring the uterus to such a firm state of tonic retraction that it feels permanently hard. *Dangerous hæmorrhage is thus due to lack of tonic retractility in the organ.*

Primary—(*a*) **Atonic.**—

Causes.—

1. Inertia, from—
   (*a*) Delayed labour with exhaustion.
   (*b*) Too rapid delivery.
   (*c*) Previous excessive distension of the uterus, as in twins, hydramnios, etc.
   (*d*) Artificial delivery during secondary inertia.
   (*e*) Placenta prævia, the placental site being in the relaxed lower uterine segment.

2. Irregular contractions.

3. Partial separation of a morbidly adherent placenta (occurs during the third stage).

4. Disease of the uterine wall, fibroids, etc.

5. Retention of clots or portion of placenta (isolated cotyledons or succenturiate lobe).

6. Large placental site after twins.
7. Mismanagement of the third stage.

Symptoms and Signs.—Hæmorrhage, with the uterus flabby and not contracted.

Frequently in these cases the uterus cannot be felt abdominally.

In some the blood is retained and distends the uterus (concealed variety). Here the uterus will be much enlarged.

Treatment of Inertia.—

1. *Precautionary.*—
   (1) Always express the body of child.
   (2) Deliver the body slowly.
   (3) Control the fundus after delivery.
2. *Active.*—
   (1) Grasp the fundus of the uterus ; rub, knead and compress it.
   (2) *If during the third stage* and bleeding still continues, introduce the hand into the uterus and remove the placenta, if it cannot be expressed by Credè's method. (See p. 190.) If the attendant does not feel competent to remove the placenta manually, ergometrine 0·125–0·5 mgm. may be given intravenously. This should arrest the bleeding and allow time for help to be obtained.
   (3) *If after the expulsion of the placenta,* give a hot intra-uterine douche (120° F.). Get nurse to inject pituitary, 5 units, or ergometrine, 0·5 mgm., intra-muscularly. (Ergometrine, 0·125–0·5 mgm., can be injected intravenously in very severe cases.) Should above treatment fail—
   (4) Insert the right closed fist into the anterior fornix, and with the other hand placed over the abdomen, the uterus can be compressed between the two. (*Bimanual Compression*). This may have to be done for twenty to thirty minutes. If this fails to arrest the bleeding, the right hand should be introduced into the uterus, any clots or retained portions of placenta removed and the uterus compressed between the internal hand and the left hand supra-fundally.
   (5) If the bleeding continues after compression, the uterine cavity must be plugged tightly with gauze.

(6) Compression of the abdominal aorta has been advocated, but this only stops the bleeding whilst the pressure is applied. It is, however, useful in checking the bleeding temporarily until all is ready to perform one of the operations described above.

(*N.B.*—Remember that post-partum hæmorrhage is a very dangerous condition; treatment must be carried out with decision and speed. It is well to have the intra-uterine nozzle sterilised and some boiling water available in case of trouble.)

3. *After-treatment.*—
   (1) Inject ergometrine, 0·5 mgm. intravenously, or pituitary, 5 units, intramuscularly, if not already done.
   (2) Hold the uterus firmly supra-pubically for at least half an hour.
   (3) Keep the patient absolutely quiet.
   (4) Beware of further hæmorrhage.

If Collapse is Severe.—
   (5) Bandage the arms and legs and raise the foot of the bed.
   (6) Rectal, subcutaneous or intravenous salines.
   (7) Transfusion of blood.

(*b*) **Traumatic.**—May arise from—
1. Cervix.
2. Vagina.
3. Vestibule.
4. Perineum.

This may be very profuse but can be differentiated from atonic bleeding by feeling the uterus firmly contracted.

Treatment.—By suture.

By vaginal plug.

To suture the cervix, pull it well down with volsella and push down the fundus supra-pubically. Use catgut sutures.

Secondary Post-partum Hæmorrhage

Causes.—

(*a*) Undue exertion causing detachment of thrombi from the mouths of uterine sinuses; specially to be feared after placenta prævia.

(*b*) Retained products of gestation.

Copious hæmorrhage later than one week after delivery is rare, and is usually caused by—

(*a*) Submucous fibroids or retained products of conception.

(*b*) Placental polypi, formed by deposition of layers of blood round the placental remnant retained.

(*c*) Chorionepithelioma.

(*d*) Retroversion.

Treatment.—In all cases of secondary hæmorrhage the cavity of the uterus should be thoroughly explored and any retained products removed by curettage.

HÆMATOMA

An effusion of blood into the cellular tissue of the pelvis is a type of traumatic P.P.H.

The source of the hæmorrhage may be the vulvar, vaginal or uterine veins.

It may occur during or after labour.

As the blood tends to gravitate, it usually forms a blue-coloured swelling at the vulva, varying in size from an egg to a fœtal head.

The hæmorrhage, if copious, may infiltrate the entire pelvic cellular tissue, bulging the posterior vaginal wall forwards, dividing the layers of the broad ligament and even forming an abdominal tumour (extra-peritoneal hæmatocele).

Symptoms and Signs.—If small—

Pain, swelling and discoloration at the vulva.

If large—

As above, along with the constitutional symptoms of hæmorrhage.

Prognosis.—According to its size.

1. Blood may be absorbed.
2. Hæmatoma may be infected.
3. May rupture and the patient recover.
4. Death may occur from hæmorrhage with or without rupture.

Treatment.—If recognised during labour, deliver as soon as possible.

If the swelling is small, leave it entirely alone.

If the swelling is large, free incision, ligation of bleeding point and drainage.

Incision must always be performed under the most rigid aseptic precautions.

Packing may be required to prevent further hæmorrhage.

Retained and Adherent Placenta

A placenta is said to be *retained* when it is still within the uterus, though separated, one hour after delivery. The cause may be uterine inertia or hour-glass contraction of the uterus.

A placenta is *adherent* when, despite good uterine contractions, it has failed to separate one hour after delivery. This is favoured by placental disease and morbid adherence of the membranes.

Treatment.—Credé's method of expulsion may be attempted if the placenta has been retained for thirty minutes, or before that if the patient is bleeding. The uterus is first rubbed into a contraction and then, with the thumb of the right hand in front and the fingers behind the uterus, the latter is squeezed and at the same time pushed downwards and backwards. This should only be done during a contraction and never attempted more than twice as it is liable to produce shock. It is less shock producing to have the patient lightly anæsthetised while this manœuvre is being carried out. If after one hour the placenta is still retained, it may have to be removed manually. This should be done at once if severe post-partum bleeding is present. The uterus is held with the left hand supra-pubically, the right hand introduced into the uterus and the placenta scraped off, commencing at the upper edge. The entire placenta should be removed and a hot intra-uterine douche at 120° F. given to check the hæmorrhage and cleanse the cavity. Uterine stimulants such as pituitary extract and ergometrine should be administered in addition.

When the bleeding is less profuse the Gabaston-Majin method of injecting warm saline (℥iv to viii) into the umbilical vein often does away with the necessity for manual removal, the placenta being expressed subsequently by Credé's method.

Placenta Accreta.—

Pathology.—Absence of the spongy layer of the decidua, the villi growing into the uterine muscle and obliterating any line of cleavage, the uterine muscle and placenta being one.

Diagnosis.—An adherent placenta which cannot be removed in the usual way.

Dangers.—Hæmorrhage and shock. Nearly all the cases die as they are not recognised and the placenta is removed piecemeal, the uterus frequently being perforated.

Treatment.—Pack the uterus to stop any bleeding and then perform abdominal hysterectomy.

Hour-glass Contraction.—An irregular uterine spasm usually accompanied by pain. May be due to mismanagement of the third stage (overhandling of uterus) or too early administration of oxytoxics.

Best treated by deep anæsthesia, slow introduction of the hand in the form of a cone through the contracted portion and manual removal of placenta or, if there is no bleeding, conservative treatment with morphia may suffice.

RUPTURE OF UTERUS

Occurs in about 1 in 4000 cases.

Site.—The lower uterine segment usually, but the tear may extend upwards to the body of the uterus and downwards through the cervix to the vagina.

The tear may be either vertical as in traumatic, or transverse as in spontaneous, or both combined.

Varieties.—

Complete.—Where the tear involves the entire thickness of the uterine wall.

Incomplete.—Where the muscle is alone involved and the peritoneum is intact.

Rupture may be—

1. Spontaneous.
2. Traumatic.

Causes.—

Spontaneous.—

(*a*) *In Pregnancy.* (*Silent Rupture.*)—

(1) Previous Cæsarean section.
(2) Previous manual removal of placenta.
(3) Perforation with curette at previous operation.
(4) Fatty degeneration of uterine muscle.
(5) Interstitial pregnancy.

(In this group the rupture is usually in the upper uterine segment.)

(*b*) *In Labour.*—

(1) Contracted pelvis.
(2) Hydrocephalus.
(3) Shoulder or brow presentations.
(4) Obliquity of uterus.
(5) Undilatable cervix.
(6) Impaction of anterior cervical lip.

(7) Compression of the uterine wall between the head and pelvis.
(8) Disease of the uterus, viz., cancer, etc.
(9) Previous Cæsarean section.
(10) Degenerative change in uterine muscle.
(11) Administration of pituitary extract and ergot during labour.
(12) Pelvic tumour.

Traumatic.—

(*a*) *In Pregnancy.*—

Fall or blow on abdomen.

(*b*) *In Labour.*—

(1) Intra-uterine manipulations, viz., version.
(2) Prolongation of laceration of cervix into lower uterine segment; may be produced by instrumental delivery or destructive operation.

Symptoms and Signs.—

In *silent rupture* no premonitory symptoms or signs are present; the patient usually experiences sudden pain and shows symptoms of collapse and intra-peritoneal bleeding.

In Labour.—

Premonitory.—

1. Strong painful uterine contractions—tetanic contractions.
2. Due to excessive retraction, the lower uterine segment is very thin and Bandl's retraction ring is felt high above the pubis.
3. Round ligaments are tense.
4. Fœtus is difficult to palpate.
5. Pulse and temperature rise.
6. Lower uterine segment is very sensitive to pressure.

After Rupture.—

1. *If Complete*—

(*a*) *Symptoms.*—

(1) Severe abdominal pain.
(2) Feeling of "something having given way" in abdomen.
(3) Sudden cessation of pains.
(4) Collapse from shock and internal hæmorrhage.
(5) Symptoms of internal hæmorrhage.
(6) Usually some external bleeding.

(*b*) *Signs.*—

(1) Recession of presenting part.
(2) Recognition of rent in the uterine wall (per vaginam).
(3) Fœtus is easily palpated if in peritoneal cavity.
(4) Uterus is felt as a small globular mass beside the fœtus.

2. *If Incomplete.*—

(*a*) Feeling of " something having given way " in abdomen may or may not be present.
(*b*) Gradual but marked decrease in pains.
(*c*) Symptoms of collapse from shock and hæmorrhage.

Treatment.—

1. *Prophylactic.*—

If Rupture Imminent—

(*a*) Procure deep anæsthesia to allay uterine contractions.
(*b*) If the vertex presents—
(1) Correct any uterine obliquity.
(2) Apply forceps and, if immediate traction is unsuccessful, perform craniotomy.
(*c*) If the shoulder presents—decapitate.
(*d*) If there is disproportion—Cæsarean section.

2. *After Complete and Incomplete Rupture.*—The best method of treatment is to open the abdomen.

Thereafter :—

(1) Remove the fœtus.
(2) Stitch the tear if possible.
(3) Remove the uterus by supra-vaginal or panhysterectomy if the tear is too extensive to permit stitching.
(4) Cleanse the peritoneal cavity and drain.

Herbert Spencer has published a series of cases where packing the tear per vaginam has proved effective.

The advantages of laparotomy over more conservative treatment are :—

(1) The exact extent of the damage may be seen.
(2) The damage can be more accurately dealt with.
(3) The bleeding can be controlled.
(4) The peritoneal cavity can be drained.

INVERSION OF UTERUS

1. Acute

Rare occurrence.

Was once common from malpraxis in delivering the placenta by cord traction.

Anatomy.—Invagination of part of the uterine wall into the uterine cavity.

There are three degrees :—

1. Where there is only a dimpling at the fundus.
2. Where the fundus presents at the cervix.
3. Where the fundus is outside vulva (complete inversion).

Causes.—Favoured by fundal insertion of the placenta.

Artificial.—

(*a*) Pulling on the cord in delivery of the placenta.

(*b*) Pushing in a portion of the uterus from above, *e.g.* applying Credé's method of expulsion with a non-contracted uterus.

Spontaneous.—

(*a*) From complete flaccidity of organ. (Atonic.)

(*b*) From partial flaccidity of organ. This is most frequently met with at the placental site.

(*c*) Precipitate labour.

(*d*) Short umbilical cord (relative or absolute) pulling on the placental site during expulsion of the child.

When a portion of the uterine wall becomes invaginated, the rest of the uterus contracts on it and tends to drive it through the cervix, thus increasing the invagination.

Symptoms.—A straining, bearing-down feeling after the birth of the child, associated with hæmorrhage and signs of shock.

If the inversion be partial, much pain is experienced from the contractions of the uterus on the inverted portion.

If complete, there is usually no pain.

Diagnosis.—A soft body projecting through the cervix.

The absence of the fundus uteri supra-pubically or a cup-like depression may be felt in some cases.

Prognosis.—Grave.

Death may occur from shock, hæmorrhage or sepsis.

Treatment.—This consists of cleansing and replacing, the part last inverted being replaced first. A hot intra-uterine douche, fundal massage and uterine stimulants should then be employed. In the second and third degrees the placenta should be removed to lessen the bulk of the body to be returned. If taxis fails, it is just possible that continuous pressure in the vagina by a hydrostatic bag or a pack may succeed. A hot douche with retention of fluid in the posterior fornix has sometimes proved effectve. Shock must be treated either before or after replacement, depending on the degree of shock and the possible difficulty of replacement.

2. Chronic

(*a*) **Ætiology.**—

1. May follow acute, and usually complete (puerperal) inversion, where attempted earlier replacement has failed.
2. May be due to a submucous fibroid arising from the fundus (rarely complete), or
3. A sarcomatous polyp.

(*b*) **Pathology.**—

1. The mucous membrane is first congested, then œdematous and later ulcerated ; if infection occurs, sloughs form.
2. The peritoneal surfaces may adhere and obliterate the depression.
3. The cavity may contain the ovaries and tubes.

(*c*) **Symptoms.**—

1. Irregular bleeding with muco-serous or purulent discharge.
2. Sensation of a tumour in the vagina.
3. A bearing-down sensation in the vagina.

(*d*) **Signs.**—

1. Smooth, reddish tumour in the vagina.
2. Tumour bleeds readily on palpation.
3. The edge of cervix may or may not be felt around the tumour, depending on degree of inversion.
4. On bimanual examination the uterus is not felt in its normal position, but the depression caused by the inversion may be palpated.

(*e*) **Diagnosis.**—

1. From a fibroid polyp :—

Fibroid Polyp.	*Inversion.*
1. Uterus can be felt bimanually.	1. Uterus not felt, or there is a definite depression at the fundus.
2. Sound passes into the uterus which is enlarged.	2. Sound does not pass into the uterus.
3. Little bleeding on palpation.	3. Bleeds readily.
4. Covering is smooth, thin and atrophic.	4. Velvety and thick.
5. Cervix felt around growth.	5. Cervix may or may not be felt.
6. No orifices found.	6. Orifices of the tubes may be found.

2. From carcinoma cervix—uterus is felt bimanually in cancer of the cervix. No friability in inversion.

Method of Reduction.—

1. Anæsthetise the patient deeply and try to reduce the last inverted part first, reducing against the fingers widening the constricting ring through the abdomen. (The obstruction to reduction is caused by the inversion ring rather than the cervix.)

2. If this fails, give vaginal douches, as reposition has occurred spontaneously in this way.

3. Try an Aveling's repositor or by slowly filling a Champetier de Ribes' bag placed in the vagina.

4. *Operations.*—

Conservative : (*a*) *Vaginal*

Spinelli's Operation—

(1) Make a transverse incision in the anterior vaginal wall below the bladder and push the bladder out of the way.

(2) Divide the constriction vertically in the middle line, continuing the incision nearly to the fundus.

(3) Reinvert the uterus, which may be difficult.

(4) Retract the bladder and stitch the uterine wound in layers. Stitch the bladder in position after repairing the cervix.

(5) Stitch the anterior vaginal wall and insert a drain.

(*b*) *Abdominal*

Haultain's Operation—

(1) Make a vertical incision through the constriction on the posterior aspect. Pass two fingers through the incision as an assistant pushes up the fundus per vaginam.

(2) Stitch up the uterine incision in layers and close the abdominal wound.

Radical : Vaginal Hysterectomy

This may be done for inversion caused by tumour formation or when associated with severe sepsis.

OBSTETRIC SHOCK

Obstetric shock is usually associated with a difficult delivery, hæmorrhage, prolonged anæsthesia or great emotional stress, and may prove fatal. The " physiological chill " of labour in the third stage, is a very minor degree of this condition and is probably the result of the sudden lowering of intra-abdominal pressure and chill. Severe shock accompanies concealed accidental hæmorrhage, uterine rupture and inversion.

Where the shock is primary or of early onset, it is thought to be due to a reflex dilatation of the capillaries in the skeletal muscles ; where it is secondary or delayed in onset, it is thought that a toxin, such as histamine, may cause a further capillary dilatation. Such a toxin, according to Miles Phillips, may come from damaged levator ani muscles.

H. L. Sheehan has shown that necrosis of the anterior pituitary lobe, associated with thrombus formation, may be observed in the patient who survives severe post-partum hæmorrhage and shock, and wonders whether the preliminary functional disturbances of the anterior pituitary may be a factor in providing a fatal issue in such cases.

May be followed at a later date by superinvolution, with cessation of menstrual periods and sterility.

Treatment.—

This should be prophylactic in the first place and entails careful supervision during pregnancy and labour. Should shock occur :—

1. Morphia.
2. Remove cold blood-soaked linen and replace by warm blanket.
3. Avoid over-heating, as the patient will already have lost too much fluid.
4. Elevate foot of bed 2 feet. Limbs may be bandaged.
5. Oxygen may be administered.
6. Intra-venous glucose will increase blood volume and is valuable in preventing shock. Lost blood is best replaced, however, by blood, serum or plasma.
7. Adrenalin and cardiac stimulants are not indicated.

PRESENTATION AND PROLAPSE OF THE CORD

Presentation of the umbilical cord—falling down in advance of the presenting part before rupture of the membranes.

Prolapse of the cord—falling down in advance of the presenting part after rupture of the membranes.

Prolapse occurs in about 1 in 150 cases.

May accompany any presentation.

Causes.—

1. Want of complete adaptation of the soft passages round the presenting part. It is met with most frequently in—

   (*a*) Contracted pelvis.
   (*b*) Malpresentations and malpositions. (Breech and shoulder chiefly.)
   (*c*) Sudden rupture of the membranes, especially when woman is in the erect position.
   (*d*) Hydramnios.
   (*e*) Uterine tumours.
   (*f*) Twin pregnancy.

2. Low placental implantation and marginal attachment of the cord.

3. Long cord.

Diagnosis.—Easy. Cord is felt in front of the presenting part.

Prognosis.—

To Mother.—Favourable.

To Child.—Grave.

In cephalic presentations 64 per cent. die.

In other presentations 32 per cent. die.

Death is caused by asphyxia from compression of the cord between the pelvis and fœtus.

Treatment.—Consists essentially in relieving the cord from pressure.

If Vertex Presents

A. **Presentation.**—

1. Preserve the membranes carefully till full dilatation of the os.

2. Vaginal examination should be made with great care to prevent rupture of membranes.

3. Keep patient in bed.

4. Place the patient in the genu-pectoral or Sim's position, as in either position the cord frequently goes up spontaneously.

B. **Prolapse.**—If pulsations have ceased for long, leave alone, as the child is dead.

If Pulsating

(*a*) *Os Slightly Dilated.*—

1. Put the woman in the genu-pectoral position and, between pains, carry the cord up above the presenting part with a finger or repositor—a loop of worsted attached to a catheter.

2. Replace cord by a gauze pack inserted into the lower uterine segment.

3. If replacement is impossible and cord is beating well, Cæsarean section.

(*b*) *Os Partially Dilated.*—

1. Put the woman in the genu-pectoral position and with the fingers carry the cord up, between pains, beyond the retraction ring, and, if possible, hook it round a limb.

2. Bipolar podalic version and bring down a leg.

(*c*) *Os Fully Dilated.*—Deliver by forceps or internal version and extraction.

If Face Presents

Version if possible, and if not, hasten delivery by forceps. Reposition of the cord in these cases is usually impossible.

If Breech or Shoulder Presents

Deliver as soon as the os is fully dilated, in the meanwhile keeping the cord in the sacral concavity to prevent undue pressure on the cord by the presenting part.

ASPHYXIA NEONATORUM

Definition.—Asphyxia of the new-born not incompatible with the continuance of life. (See also p. 383.)

Causes.—

1. Interference with the maternal circulation :—
   - (*a*) Ante-partum hæmorrhage.
   - (*b*) Eclampsia.
   - (*c*) Chest complications.
   - (*d*) Death of mother.

2. Interference with the fœtal circulation :—
   (*a*) Compression of the cord.
   (*b*) Compression of the placenta.
   (*c*) Separation of the placenta.
   (*d*) Cerebral and thoracic compression in—
      Small pelves.
      Face cases.
      Forceps delivery.
      Difficult breech delivery.

3. Interference with sensitivity of respiratory centre :—
   (*a*) Analgesics.
   (*b*) Anæsthetics.
   (*c*) Extreme immaturity.
   (*d*) Inadequate blood supply—hæmorrhage, œdema.

Appearance of Child when Born.—Two types :—

1. Asphyxia livida.
2. Asphyxia pallida.

Asphyxia Livida.—Congested and cyanosed appearance.
Muscular tonicity is present.
Cardiac and funic pulsations are slow, but forcible.

Asphyxia Pallida.—Corpse-like appearance.
Muscular tonicity is absent.
Funic pulsation is absent.
Cardiac beat is frequent and feeble.
Child in condition of shock.

Prognosis.—Asphyxia livida, good, Asphyxia pallida, very grave.

Treatment of Asphyxia Livida.—Remove inhaled fluids and mucus from the mouth and upper air passages. (Mucus extractors are often incorrectly used ; if the sterilised instrument is used for more than one aspiration, then there is the inevitable danger of infection of the baby's throat from that of the operator. This danger can be minimised by using the Aberdeen Mucus Catheter which has an efficient trap and greatly reduces the danger of infection.)

Invert the fœtus, and excite the respiration by cutaneous stimulation by slapping the gluteal region.

Rubbing the chest and wetting the throat or rectum with brandy is often useful.

Sprinkle cold water over the chest.

If treatment is still unavailing, put the child into a warm bath, 100° F.

Perform artificial respiration.—Methods :—

1. *Sylvester's Method.*—Place the child on its back with the shoulders raised.

Fix the feet.

Grasp the arms above the elbow, slowly evert and draw them up to the sides of the head.

Then slowly lower arms and press firmly against the sides of the chest. Can be performed in bath.

2. *Byrd's Method.*—Place the child on hands with its back towards palms.

Slowly bring hands together, thus flexing the child and bringing its feet to its head—this expels air slowly. Unflex the child to full extent—this expands the lungs again.

Can be performed easily in the warm bath.

3. *Laborde's Method.*—Pull tongue in and out rhythmically with tongue forceps.

Mouth to mouth insufflation or administration of carbon dioxide and oxygen.

Treatment of Asphyxia Pallida.—Clear all mucus out of the mouth and upper air passages. Brandy.

Keep as warm as possible by putting in an incubator if available at 90°–100° F. Otherwise wrap in wool or flannel, with protected hot water bottles, in as warm a room as possible.

Rhythmic and gentle compression of chest.

Oxygen.

Injection of alpha lobelin gr. $\frac{1}{20}$ intramuscularly or into umbilical vein. This acts on respiratory centre.

Intra-cardial pituitary or adrenalin (1 to 1000) ♏ii in extreme cases.

Remembering the possibility of intra-cranial hæmorrhage in such cases, it is advisable to give Vitamin K—Kapilon 5 mgm. in aqueous solution, deeply into buttock.

(*N.B.*—The less the child is handled the better, owing to condition of extreme shock.)

CHAPTER XII

OBSTETRICAL MANIPULATIONS AND OPERATIONS

VERSION OR TURNING

THE artificial substitution of one pole of the fœtus for the other.

Varieties.—

Cephalic—substitution to a cephalic presentation.
Podalic—substitution to a breech presentation.

Methods.—

External.
Bipolar.
Internal.

External Version (Cephalic or Podalic).—

Indications.—

1. Breech presentations in primigravidæ; to estimate the size of the head with the pelvis and make labour more advantageous to both mother and child (cephalic).
2. Transverse lie—before or early in labour.
3. Placenta prævia (podalic)—rare.
4. Prolapse of the cord (podalic).

It is only possible when the membranes are intact, the liquor amnii abundant and the presenting part not fixed in the pelvic brim.

In performing external version, place the patient on her back with the knees well drawn up, lay the hands flat on the abdomen and define the breech and head of the fœtus. Press the one down and the other up, turning in such a way as to increase fœtal flexion, but if this fails, rotation in the opposite direction should be attempted.

During uterine contractions desist from active manipulation and confine efforts to holding the fœtus steady in the position already acquired.

Anæsthesia may be necessary.

When version is completed, apply a binder, or if the patient is in labour, rupture the membranes.

Bipolar Version (Podalic). (Braxton Hicks.)—Requires for its efficient performance the membranes intact or just ruptured and the cervix sufficiently open to allow the introduction of two fingers.

Indications.—

1. Shoulder presentation.
2. Placenta prævia—rare.
3. Accidental hæmorrhage—rare.
4. Prolapse of cord.

Preliminaries.—Empty the bladder and rectum.
Anæsthetise the patient thoroughly.
Make certain on which side the back lies.
Place the patient in the lithotomy position.
Cleanse thoroughly the external genital organs and vagina.

Operation.—

1. Introduce the whole hand in the form of a cone slowly into the vagina.
2. Pass two fingers through the os internum.
3. Act only in the intervals between pains.
4. When the presenting part is reached, push it well up to the side of the back and, at the same time, with the other hand on the abdomen, depress the breech; then by a series of short jerking movements between pains, push the two extremities of the fœtus in opposite directions.
5. Feel for a foot and then rupture the membranes, bringing the foot through the vagina to the vulva and securing it by a gauze clove-hitch.
6. Conduct the case according to exigencies, always leaving the expulsion of the child to nature if possible.

Internal Version (Podalic).—By this method the entire hand is introduced into the uterus and thus the os must be half to fully dilated.

It is usually the method of choice after the membranes have ruptured.

Indications.—

1. Shoulder presentation.
2. Brow and mento-posterior cases.
3. Prolapse of cord.
4. Placenta prævia—rare.
5. Accidental hæmorrhage—rare.
6. Persistant occipito-posterior position—rare.

Method of Performance.—

1. Anæsthetise the patient deeply, preferably with chloroform which causes maximum relaxation of the uterus.

2. Place the patient in the dorsal position. Cleanse thoroughly the external genital organs and vagina.
3. Lubricate the gloved hand thoroughly.
4. Introduce the hand in the shape of a cone.
5. Place the other hand over the fundus uteri.
6. If the membranes are intact, rupture them at the lowest part and introduce the hand at once into the uterus to prevent escape of the liquor amnii.
7. Pass the internal hand along the ventral surface of the fœtus and grasp the nearest knee or foot, but during a pain flatten the hand firmly upon the fœtus. As a rule the more accessible foot should be grasped, but in a dorso-posterior transverse lie, the upper foot should be pulled down.
8. Pull on the foot and with the external hand push down the breech.

When the foot and leg are pulled into the vagina, the case should be conducted according to exigencies.

If there is no hurry, leave nature to complete the birth of the breech and conduct the case as an ordinary breech delivery.

If there is danger or delay and the os is fully dilated, complete the labour artificially as in a complicated breech delivery (see p. 152).

Difficulties and Dangers.—If the membranes have been ruptured for a long time and the uterus is firmly contracted on the fœtus, extreme care must be exercised to prevent rupture of the uterus. Never perform internal version if Bandl's ring is very prominent.

General Practical Rules for Version.—

1. If the membranes are unruptured and the presenting part is movable at the brim, try the external method.
2. If the membranes are unruptured and the os uteri is sufficiently open to admit two fingers, try the bipolar method. (If only one finger can be admitted the os can usually be dilated digitally to allow the entrance of the second finger.)
3. If the os is half to fully dilated, perform internal version.

FORCEPS DELIVERY

Since invented by Chamberlen in 1675, the forceps, though maintaining the essential original characteristics, have undergone a never-ending series of modifications. At the present day the perfected instrument is represented by the "Axis Traction Forceps," the principles of which were first suggested by Tarnier.

Axis traction rods are now applied to all the main types of forceps. For practical purposes the Milne-Murray forceps is possibly the best instrument available (Fig. 21).

Advantages of Axis Traction.—

1. Traction can be made in the axis of the pelvis.

With ordinary forceps applied and the head in the cavity, half the traction force is lost against the pubis.

2. The normal mechanism is not hindered. Accommodation and internal rotation can take place during traction.

3. The rules for traction are easier. All one requires to remember is to keep the traction rods parallel with the shanks.

4. These forceps have less tendency to slip.

5. They have greater traction power.

Mode of Action of the Forceps Generally.—

1. As a tractor.
2. As a compressor.
3. Dynamic. Stimulating uterine action.
4. Lever.
5. Rotator—recommended by some for occipito-posterior positions, but must always be used cautiously and only by the experienced. (For this operation the non-axis traction forceps are best.)
6. Dilator of passages.

General Indications.—

1. Where the ordinary powers are unable to complete labour.
2. When speedy delivery is demanded with regard to safety of the mother or the child.

Special Indications.—

1. Abnormality in the powers.
   (*a*) Primary uterine inertia, if persisting in second stage.
   (*b*) Irregular uterine action.
   (*c*) Misdirected force, anteversion, etc.
   (*d*) Absence of secondary powers in paralysis, debility, obesity, etc.

2. Abnormality in the passages.
   (*a*) Rigidity of the vagina and perineum.
   (*b*) Contracted pelvis.

3. Faults in the passenger.
   (*a*) Large well-ossified head.
   (*b*) Malpositions of the head, *e.g.* persistent occipito-posterior.
   (*c*) Malpresentations—
      (1) Face.
      (2) Impacted breech.
      (3) The after-coming head in breech cases (see p. 155).

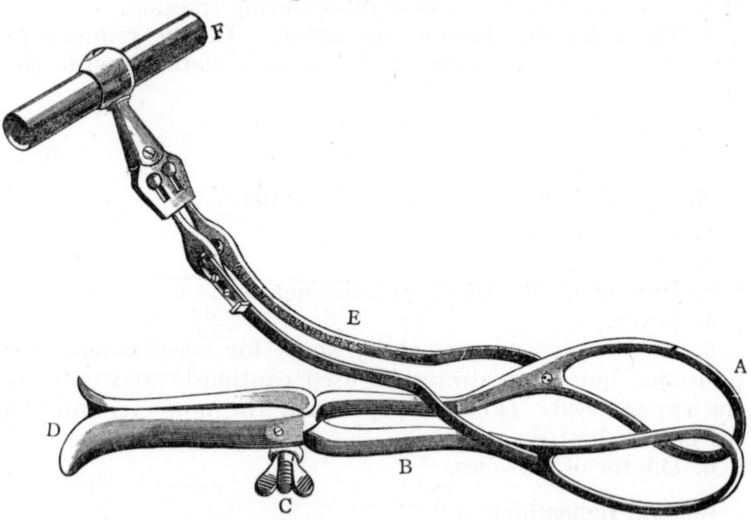

FIG. 21.—MILNE-MURRAY'S AXIS TRACTION FORCEPS.
A, Blades; B, Shanks; C, Fixation Screw; D, Application Handle; E, Traction Rods; F, Traction Handle.

4. Impacted twins.
5. Dangers.
   (*a*) To the mother—
      (1) Pre-eclampsia and eclampsia.
      (2) Heart disease and tuberculosis.
      (3) Rapid pulse and rise of temperature in the second stage, especially if rupture imminent.
   (*b*) To the child—
      (1) Prolapse of the cord.
      (2) Delay in delivery of the after-coming head, with asphyxia imminent.
      (3) Death imminent, shown by irregularity or slowing of fœtal heart below 100.

Method of Operating.—Divided into high, mid and low operations.

High=greatest diameter of fœtal skull above the pelvic brim. **Dangerous and should be done only rarely.**

Mid=greatest diameter between the brim and the ischial spines—in the cavity.

Low=greatest diameter below ischial spines—on perineum.

Rules for Safe Application of Forceps

1. The patient should be anæsthetised.
2. The instruments, after sterilisation by boiling, should be kept in warm lotion.
3. Place the patient in the left lateral position with the hips well over the edge of the bed. Some prefer the lithotomy position. Cleanse thoroughly the external genitals and *catheterise the bladder.*
4. *The cervix must be fully dilated.*
5. *The membranes must be ruptured.*
6. *The head should be in the cavity or at the outlet, in a suitable position and well moulded.*
7. *There should not be undue disproportion between the head and the pelvis.*
8. *The uterus must be contracting.* The use of forceps in secondary uterine inertia is absolutely contra-indicated.

Introduction of the First Blade (patient in left lateral position).—

1. Pass the left hand into the vagina below the fœtal head, with the palmar surface in contact with it.
2. Introduce the left blade first, along the palmar surface of the hand, between pains. Insert in the correct pelvic axis.
3. Once the blade has reached the presenting part, keep the blade closely applied.
4. *The notch should be vertical if correctly applied.*
5. Keep blade in position with the back of the left hand.

Introduction of the Second Blade.—

1. Pass the left hand into the vagina below the fœtal head, with the palmar surface in contact with it.
2. Swing the traction rod forward before the introduction and let it rest on the back of the right hand.
3. Introduce between pains, as with the first blade, along the palmar surface of hand.
4. Glide the blade along the hollow of the sacrum, and

then rotate it over the head by rotating and depressing the handle.

5. When opposite one another the two blades should be locked.

6. If there is any difficulty, do not use force but rather re-apply the blade. If there is still difficulty, examine for malposition.

7. After locking, swing back the traction rod, adjust the fixation screw and apply the traction handle.

8. Feel if the forceps are accurately applied to the head, and make sure that none of the soft parts are included in the grasp.

Traction.—

1. Grasp the traction handle only.
2. Pull during pains or at intervals corresponding to pains.
3. Keep the traction rods parallel with the shanks.
4. Between each pull loosen the fixation screw to minimise compression on fœtal head.
5. Examine occasionally to determine progress.
6. The amount of traction should not exceed the power of the forearms with elbows bent.
7. After the head is crowned, remove the blades and deliver as in normal case.

General Practical Hints.—

1. See that the membranes have ruptured and make certain of the position of the vertex.
2. Apply in multiparæ if the second stage is prolonged over two hours.
3. Apply in primigravidæ if the second stage is prolonged over three hours
4. Always apply the blades *qua* the pelvis (in transverse).
5. *Do not apply until the cervix is fully dilated.*
6. Never touch the application handles during traction.
7. Unless there is danger, do not hurry.
8. After the head is born, always assist delivery of the body by fundal pressure. By this means uterine contractions are favoured and hæmorrhage prevented.
9. If the head rotates through more than a quarter of a circle, as in occipito-posterior cases, the forceps should be taken off and re-applied.
10. If excessive extension of the head occurs before passing the vulva (shown by the application handles becoming thrown up over the abdomen), remove and re-apply the blades.

11. If the forceps slip or if the blades are difficult to lock, take them off and examine for occipito-posterior position before re-application.

12. Never apply if the head is too large for the pelvis or movable above the brim.

Dangers to the Mother.—

1. Laceration of the cervix and perineum. These may be avoided by care and patience.

2. Sloughing of the soft parts from compression, giving rise to fistulæ in some cases. This should not occur if the rules are adhered to, the bladder emptied and too great force avoided.

3. Separation of the symphysis. Very rare.

Dangers to the Child.—

1. Compression of the head.
2. Injuries to the scalp, *e.g.* cephalhæmatoma.
3. Bell's paralysis. Usually disappears soon.
4. Fracture of the cranial bones and intra-cranial hæmorrhage.
5. Little's disease (spastic paralysis). Usually due to the use of forceps when another method of treatment should have been chosen.

CRANIOTOMY

Is the term applied to all operations for the reduction in size of the child's head. The complete operation consists of three stages—

1. Perforation.
2. Comminution.
3. Extraction.

Indications (General).—

1. Where great disproportion exists between the fœtal head and the pelvis, especially if the child be dead or in extremis.

2. Where the prolongation of labour will jeopardise the life of the mother, as in imminent rupture, etc.

Special Indications.—

1. Contracted pelvis—not less than $2\frac{1}{4}$ in. conjugate—when forceps fail or the canal is infected, more especially if the child is not in good condition.

2. Impacted malpositions and malpresentations—child dead or dying.

3. Large head, especially hydrocephalus.

4. Where immediate delivery is required for the sake of the mother and Cæsarean section is contra-indicated.

Now that Cæsarean section, especially the lower segment operation, is being performed with such excellent results, the indications for embryulcia are becoming fewer and fewer.

Method of Operating

(*a*) **Preliminaries.**—

1. Place the patient in the lithotomy position.
2. Anæsthetise deeply.

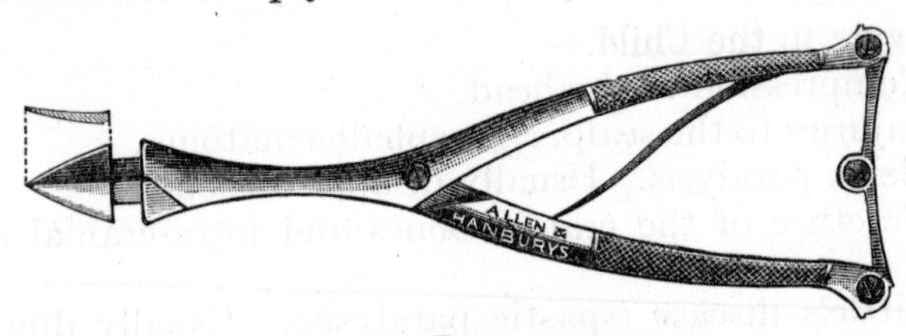

FIG. 22.—PERFORATOR.

(*b*) **Perforation,** by means of perforator. (Fig. 22.)

1. Fix head—by forceps or by supra-pubic pressure.
2. Examine and define edge of the cervix, sacral promontory and position of the head.
3. Introduce the left hand into vagina as a guide.
4. Pass the perforator along left hand to head.
5. Perforate the parietal bone by a boring movement.
6. Push the perforator into the cranial cavity as far as the stop on the instrument, open the blades, then turn the instrument through a right angle and open the blades again.
7. Push the perforator through tentorium cerebelli and destroy thoroughly the base of the brain in case of the child being born alive; the brain matter may be evacuated by douching through a double channel nozzle.

Sites for Perforation.—

1. For vertex presentations—either parietal bone as near the anterior fontanelle as possible.
2. For the after-coming head—through the occiput or roof of the mouth.
3. For a face presentation—through the roof of the mouth or the orbit.

4. For a brow presentation—through the frontal bone.

(*c*) **Extraction.**—

1. By forceps.
2. By comminution—
   (*a*) By cranioclast.
   (*b*) By cephalotribe.
   (*c*) By Winter's combined cranioclast and cephalotribe.
3. By crotchet (after-coming head).
4. By Brigg's forceps and gradual traction, using a weight of 4 lb. or more.

By Forceps.—In minor disproportion between the head and the pelvis, forceps are sufficient for extraction ; if they are unsuccessful, try the cranioclast, etc.

Cranioclast (Fig. 23).—Introduce the solid blade into the cranial cavity and the fenestrated blade over the head, as with forceps. A portion of the cranial vault is thus crushed

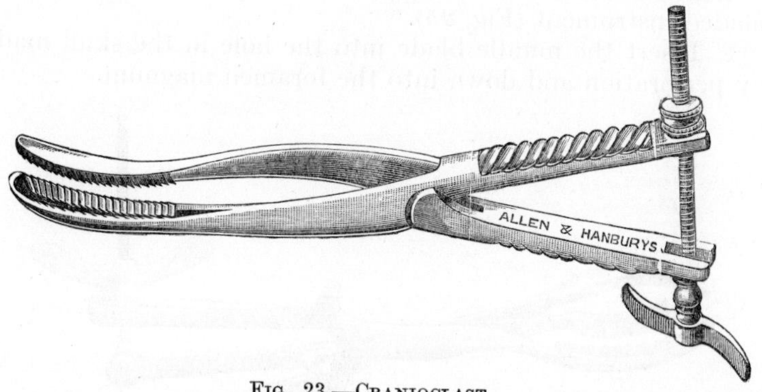

FIG. 23.—CRANIOCLAST.

between the blades and effective traction can be made. It is better, if possible, for the fenestrated blade to pass over the face, as the bones are well ossified here and the grip is firmer.

Cephalotribe (Fig. 24).—Non-fenestrated forceps. Acts both as comminutor and extractor. It is applied in a similar manner to forceps, one blade on either side of the fœtal head. As a simple extractor it is less efficient and more dangerous than the cranioclast, because in being compressed in one diameter the head is elongated in the opposite ; with the cranioclast, moulding of the head to the passages is unhindered.

The head is also very liable to slip from the grasp of the cephalotribe. As a comminutor, however, the cephalotribe is of the utmost service and in some cases, *e.g.* impacteed breech,

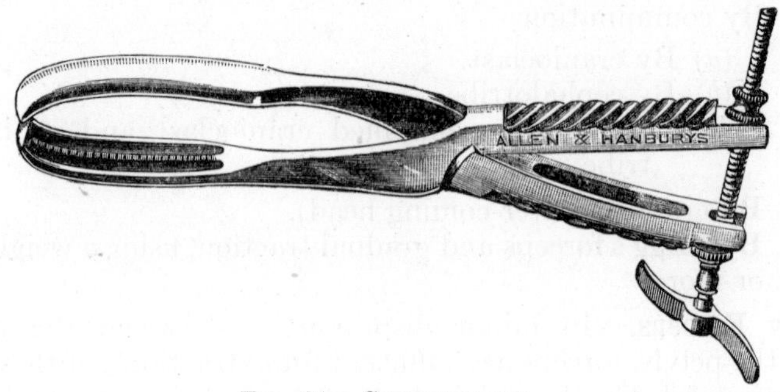

Fig. 24.—Cephalotribe.

was indispensable until superseded by the three-bladed instrument.

Winter's combined Cranioclast and Cephalotribe.—Three-bladed instrument (Fig. 25).

1. Insert the middle blade into the hole in the skull made by perforation and down into the foramen magnum.

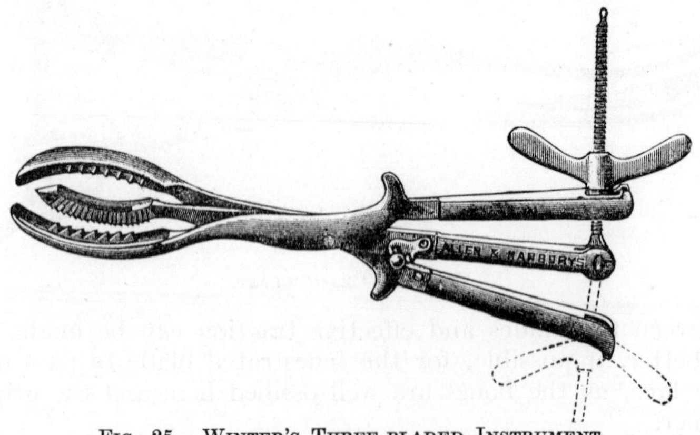

Fig. 25.—Winter's Three-bladed Instrument.

2. Apply one external blade over the face.
3. Fix the external blade to the middle blade by the screw at the handles, thus crushing the anterior part of the head.
4. Depress the catch and thus fix the blade.
5. Apply the other external blade over the occiput.

6. Screw this blade to the middle blade, crushing the occipital end.
7. Depress catch and fix blade.
8. Detach the screw.
9. Extract the head by rotation and traction.

Crotchet.—A sharp, acutely bent hook, much used at one time, but now only used following perforation of the after-coming head or decapitation.

Brigg's Forceps (Fig. 26).—Three or four pairs of these forceps are applied to the edges of the skull bones at the site of perforation. The handles of the forceps are bound together

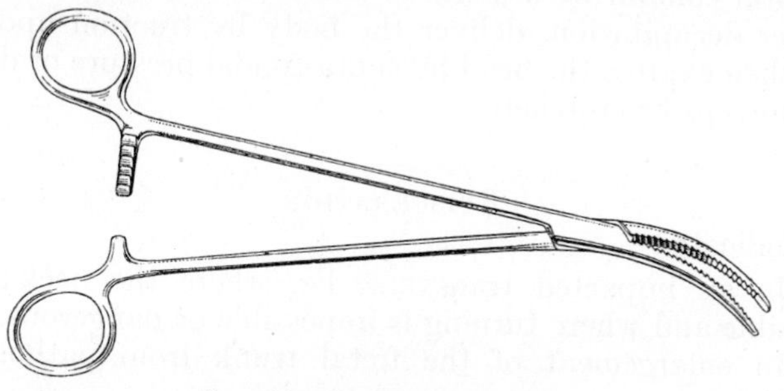

Fig. 26.—Brigg's Forceps.

by gauze to which a 4–6 lb. weight is attached. This weight is allowed to hang over the end of the bed. Gradual traction is provided in this way and the danger of damage to soft parts is very slight compared with other methods of extraction.

Practical Hints for Craniotomy.—

1. If delivery with forceps is impossible, retain hold of the head by the forceps and perforate.
2. After perforation, attempt delivery with forceps again.
3. If unsuccessful, remove the forceps and apply Winter's three-bladed instrument or cranioclast.
4. Do not, for sentimental reasons, delay operating too long, as the safety of the mother must always be the first consideration.

EMBRYOTOMY

Term used for the reduction of the body of the child by mutilation. It includes—

Decapitation.
Evisceration.
Spondylotomy.
Cleidotomy.

Decapitation

Is employed where, in a shoulder presentation with the neck accessible, version is unsafe for the mother. Many special instruments (*e.g.* the sharp hook, decapitating hook, etc.) have been devised for its performance, but if such are not available, it may be most simply and efficiently performed by a long straight pair of blunt-pointed scissors. In operating, pull upon the prolapsed arm to bring the neck well down, guide the sharp hook over the neck by the fingers of the left hand and carefully divide the soft parts and vertebral column by a series of short cutting movements.

After decapitation, deliver the body by traction upon the arm, then express the head by supra-fundal pressure or deliver with forceps or crotchet.

Evisceration

Is indicated—

1. In an impacted transverse lie, where the neck is inaccessible and where turning is impossible or dangerous.
2. In enlargement of the fœtal trunk from pathological conditions.
3. After craniotomy in extreme cases of contracted pelvis.

Operation.—

1. Perforate the chest and divide several ribs.
2. Introduce a hand and eviscerate—first thorax, then abdomen.
3. If the lie is transverse, delivery can now be attempted either by pulling down the breech or by making traction on the arm to expose the neck and allow of decapitation.

Spondylotomy

In some cases of shoulder presentation, where the neck is not accessible, the spinal column may be divided with scissors.

Cleidotomy

Is employed when there is difficulty with the shoulders, the child being dead. It is performed by cutting the clavicles with a pair of long straight scissors, thus decreasing the bisacromial diameter.

INDUCTION OF ABORTION AND LABOUR

Abortion may have to be induced when, if the pregnancy is allowed to continue, the life of the mother is in danger or her future health likely to be impaired. Similarly, premature labour is induced when the continuance of pregnancy causes danger to the mother or child.

The indications for the termination of pregnancy are: (1) General, and (2) Local.

Induction of Abortion.—Indications—

General.—

1. Toxic hyperemesis gravidarum.
2. Acute tuberculosis.
3. Cardiac disease. (Severe.)
4. Chronic nephritis.
5. Rh. incompatability with several fœtal deaths.
6. Chorea.
7. Insanity.
8. Rubella at second month.
9. Essential hypertension (rarely).

Local.—

1. Threatened abortion with severe or persistent hæmorrhage.
2. Missed abortion.
3. Hydatidiform mole.
4. Acute hydramnios in early months.

Although the above list may serve as a guide, it is only in very exceptional circumstances that therapeutic abortion is indicated in those conditions.

A second medical opinion must always be obtained before abortion is induced for any of the general indications.

Induction of Premature Labour.—Indications—

General.—

1. Pre-eclamptic toxæmia.
2. Chronic nephritis.
3. Essential hypertension.
4. Diabetes (some cases).
5. Rh.—patients with antibodies.

Local.—

1. Contracted pelvis—moderate degree. Rarely indicated now as trial labour at term is preferred.
2. Ante-partum hæmorrhage.

3. Acute hydramnios or hydramnios associated with abnormal fœtal development., *e.g.* anencephalic fœtus.
4. Habitual death of the fœtus in the later weeks.
5. Habitual large size of the child.

Induction of labour may be required for post-maturity.

Methods of Inducing Abortion and Labour.

Abortion.—These vary according to the urgency of the indication for induction. In the first three months the cervix may be dilated with Hegar's dilators and the uterine contents removed by sponge forceps and a flushing curette. The operator will soon discover for himself that the much advocated "finger" or ovum forceps cannot be introduced through the cervix without producing trauma—it is often impossible to dilate the cervix sufficiently from zero to allow of an ovum forceps being passed through. Some prefer to do this operation in two stages, especially towards the end of the third month and so avoid risk of excessive hæmorrhage and shock. Two to four laminaria tents are introduced into the cervix and left in situ for twenty-four hours. At the end of that time contractions usually occur or at any rate the cervix should be sufficiently dilated to allow of much easier uterine evacuation.

After the third month uterine contractions may be stimulated by: (1) Tents; (2) a small hydrostatic bag introduced into the lower uterine segment; (3) introduction of male catheter, small stomach tube or small bougies; or (4) rupture of the membranes (not usually advisable as it may fail to produce contractions).

The slow injection into the uterus of an abortifacient fluid such as utus, may be employed up to fifth month of pregnancy and is especially useful when an anæsthetic is not advisable.

Rapid methods of terminating pregnancy at this stage include :—

Abdominal hysterotomy, the steps of which are exactly similar to those of classical Cæsarean section.

Vaginal hysterotomy, where, after the bladder is dissected off the anterior wall of the cervix, the latter is incised up to and including the internal os and the ovum or fœtus and placenta delivered with fingers and ovum forceps.

Of these two operations the abdominal route has definite advantages. There is less shock, less risk of injury to the bladder and better access, while the bleeding can be controlled more readily. The disadvantage of this method is that, in a young mother, the upper uterine segment is being opened into and there is therefore the risk of uterine rupture in a subsequent pregnancy.

Labour may be induced by.—

1. *Rupture of the Membranes.*—The presenting membranes may be ruptured with a finger, volsella or stilette; on the other hand, the point of rupture may be effected high up, by means of a Drew Smythe catheter, so that the bag of waters with its supposed dilating effect is preserved. The escape of the liquor amnii, resulting in a dry labour, is not the disadvantage that was at one time supposed, unless there is a malpresentation or malposition present; the majority of such labours proceed normally. This method should be chosen only if the cervix is patulous and "taking up."

2. *Introduction of Bougies (Krause's Method).*—Two or more gum elastic bougies (No. 18) are introduced between the uterine wall and the membranes. These bougies are 12 in. long and, when in position, only the lower ends should protrude from the cervix. The vagina is packed with gauze. This gauze is removed in twenty-four hours and if no pains start in forty-eight hours, the bougies are removed. It is of advantage to administer a course of pituitary extract while the bougies are in situ if pains do not begin in twenty-four hours. (Not more than three injections of 5 units at intervals of half an hour.) Bougies may be preferred to rupture of the membranes when the cervix is long and closed.

(*N.B.*—If resistance be felt during the insertion, the bougie should be withdrawn and reinserted in another direction; otherwise the placenta may be separated and severe hæmorrhage caused.)

3. *Hydrostatic Bag.*—The lower uterine segment is large enough to accommodate a Barnes bag or rubber balloon. The membranes are preserved and the intra-uterine tension is so increased that labour very quickly ensues. The cervix must admit two fingers before the bag can be introduced. A stomach tube inserted into the lower uterine segment has a similar effect, but both methods may change a favourable position of the presenting part to a malposition and are therefore unpopular.

4. *Medical Induction.*—This method is rarely successful before full-time. It can be done in many ways by the administration of castor oil, quinine and pituitary extract.

The dosage varies with different authorities, but we have found the following to be quite efficient :—

6 A.M.	Castor oil ℥i.
7 A.M.	Quinine bihydrochloride, gr. x.
8 A.M.	Hot bath and enema.
8.30 A.M.	Pituitary extract in 5-unit doses every half-hour until labour starts, or until 3–4 injections have been given.
	It is often advantageous to separate membranes from around internal os before injections of pituitary are given.

Accouchement Forcé

This method of treatment is never indicated in present-day midwifery.

CÆSAREAN SECTION

This means removal of a viable fœtus by abdominal section.

Varieties.—Classical Cæsarean section.
Lower uterine segment Cæsarean section.
Cæsarean hysterectomy.

Indications.—

1. Insurmountable difficulties to delivery per *vias naturales*, viz. :—
   (*a*) Contracted pelvis.
   (*b*) Solid pelvic tumours and cervical fibroids.
   (*c*) Carcinoma cervicis.
2. Severe maternal complications—
   (*a*) Rupture of the uterus.
   (*b*) Central and, in primigravidæ, partial placenta prævia.
   (*c*) Concealed accidental hæmorrhage if more conservative treatment fails.
   (*d*) Cardiac disease (some cases).
   (*e*) Profound pregnancy toxæmia (some cases).
   (*f*) Breech or shoulder presentations in elderly primigravidæ.
   (*g*) History of repeated difficult deliveries with still-births.
   (*h*) Primary inertia (some cases).

3. Where the child is alive and the mother dying or just dead.

4. Previous Cæsarean section (if any abnormality present and likely to cause difficult labour).

The classical operation should not be performed when the genital tract is infected through frequent examinations or attempts to deliver with forceps ; in such cases, if Cæsarean section is indicated, the lower uterine segment route should be chosen. Nowadays the lower segment operation is in practically every case the operation of choice.

1. Classical Cæsarean Section

(*a*) **Period of Operating.**—The most suitable time is the expected day of delivery or soon after the commencement of labour and before the membranes have ruptured.

(*b*) **Preliminaries.**—The preparation is similar to that for any abdominal operation. The bladder must be emptied and the bowel evacuated by aperient or enema.

(*c*) **Operation.**—

1. The abdominal incision should be medial or paramedial and below the umbilicus.

2. The peritoneum is opened in the upper part of the wound as the bladder may be drawn up.

3. When the dextro-rotation of the uterus is undone, the abdominal cavity should be walled off with packs on each side and above the uterine fundus, to prevent contamination of the peritoneal cavity by liquor amnii.

4. The uterine wall is incised in the midline for 4–5 in., stopping short of the lower uterine segment. Bleeding can be arrested by pressure on each side of the incision, or by an assistant grasping the broad ligaments firmly.

5. After rupturing the membranes a hand is introduced and the fœtus extracted by traction on a foot or leg, or by sliding the hand round behind the head and easing it through the uterine incision. If the placenta lies anteriorly, the child must be delivered through the placenta.

6. The cord is clamped with forceps, cut and the child handed to an assistant.

7. Pituitary extract, 5 units, or/and ergometrine, 0·5 mgm., is injected directly into the uterine muscle. Ergometrine 0·25 mgm. may be given intravenously.

8. The placenta and membranes may be delivered through the uterine incision by fundal pressure or extracted manually.

The uterine wall is swabbed with Dettol and any shreds of membrane removed.

9. The uterus may or may not be eventrated and contraction stimulated by the application of hot cloths and by pressure.

10. The uterine wound is closed in three layers—

(*a*) A continuous catgut suture approximates the decidua and deeper portion of the muscle.

(*b*) A continuous catgut suture or interrupted mattress sutures approximate the superficial portion of the muscle, but do not include the peritoneum.

(*c*) A continuous catgut suture (Lembert's) draws the peritoneal edges into apposition.

11. All blood clot and liquor are swabbed out from the peritoneal cavity.

12. The abdominal wall is closed in layers.

The operation may be carried out under general or local anæsthesia as indicated.

2. Lower Uterine Segment Cæsarean Section

Advantages of this route are—

1. Less vascular area to deal with.
2. The edges are thin and are more easily brought into direct apposition.
3. The part is at rest during the puerperium.
4. The wound is stronger and is less liable to rupture in a subsequent pregnancy or labour since lower segment remains passive.
5. The uterine scar is covered by the vesico-uterine fascia, bladder and united peritoneal edges; infection is therefore more securely shut off.
6. Adhesions are less likely to develop.

Operation.—

1. The abdominal incision is paramedial or medial from umbilicus to symphysis pubis.
2. The peritoneal cavity is opened, care being taken not to injure the bladder.
3. The abdominal cavity is shut off by packs.
4. The peritoneum is incised transversely along the line of reflection from the anterior wall of the uterus to the bladder.
5. The bladder is pushed down and the lower uterine segment exposed.

6. The lower uterine segment is incised transversely or longitudinally. If the incision is horizontal, the ends of the incision should be curved upwards with the object of preserving the uterine vessels from damage should tearing occur.

7. In a vertex presentation the head is delivered with the hand, aided in some cases by traction with Willett's forceps or by a blade of the obstetric forceps passed behind it and by fundal pressure. In a breech presentation a foot is grasped or a buttock eased out through the incision.

8. The child is delivered, the cord clamped and cut.

9. Pituitary extract 5 units or/and ergometrine, 0·5 mgm., is injected into uterus. Ergometrine 0·25 mgm. may be given intravenously.

10. The placenta is separated and expelled by fundal pressure or removed manually through the incision.

11. The uterine wound is approximated in two layers and, after the bladder has been replaced, the peritoneal edges are stitched.

12. The abdominal wound is closed in layers.

Sterilisation.—This is usually contemplated when a patient has had two Cæsarean operations or where it is not to her advantage to become pregnant again. It may be accomplished—

(1) By excising a portion of both Fallopian tubes, tying each portion and burying the proximal ends in the broad ligaments.

(2) By excision at the cornua with subsequent peritonisation of both cornua and burying, after ligation, the distal cut ends of the tubes in the broad ligaments.

(3) By crushing loop with a strong clamp twice and passing catgut ligatures around crushed areas. This produces four areas in each tube where the mucosa is so damaged that blockage occurs and sterilisation made fairly certain (Madlener). Tying a loop of tube with catgut and excising loop distal to tie (Pomeroy) has been as effective as other methods. (No method of sterilisation, short of removal of the uterus or ovaries, has been found to be absolutely certain.)

3. Cæsarean Hysterectomy

(*a*) **Supra-vaginal.—Indications—**

1. Multiple fibroids.
2. Inoperable carcinoma cervicis.

3. Uterine rupture, when confined to upper uterine segment.
4. Concealed accidental hæmorrhage. (Rarely.)
5. As a means of sterilisation (in rare cases).
6. If the uterus has been badly infected.

This operation should, if possible, be performed before labour begins, for then the cervical stump will be more easily drawn together. The appendages may be removed or conserved.

Operation.—

1. As in the classical section until the child has been delivered. The broad ligaments may be clamped before incising the uterus to minimise bleeding.
2. The uterus is removed as described in the operation of supra-vaginal hysterectomy. (See p. 360.)

(*b*) **Pan-hysterectomy.**—This means removal of the whole uterus, including the cervix. May be carried out in cases of cervical fibroid, operable carcinoma of the cervix and in uterine rupture where the tear involves the cervix and vagina. (See p. 362.)

Symphysiotomy and Pubiotomy were operations whereby the pelvis was enlarged. They are of historical interest only.

CHAPTER XIII

COMPLICATIONS OF PUERPERIUM

Uterine

Acute Subinvolution of the Uterus.—Delay in the normal decrease in the size of the uterus.

Causes.—

1. Inertia uteri, from—
   (*a*) Delayed labour.
   (*b*) Over-distension (twins, hydramnios, etc.).
   (*c*) Non-lactation.
   (*d*) Multiparity.
2. Retention of portions of placenta or membranes.
3. Local uterine infection.
4. Acute endometritis and salpingitis.
5. Retroversion (tenth to twenty-first day).

Symptoms.—Excess and prolonged duration of red lochial discharge. Fundus higher (early) or uterus larger (later) than normal.

Sometimes fundus is raised by a distended bladder and this may be the case even though the patient is apparently passing water normally. In this case, however, the lochia are not excessive.

Treatment.—

(*a*) Recognised in first ten days after labour—

Liq. ext. ergot ʒ½; ergometrine, 0·5 mgm., or ergotin pills (post-partum pills (see p. 71)) t.i.d.

Hot vaginal douches.

Sit patient up to allow drainage.

(*b*) Recognised after first ten days by persistence of red lochia—

Examine for retroversion, and if present, replace and treat by postural methods to begin with, but should it persist, pessary treatment will be required at a later date (see p. 85).

Hot vaginal douches, 105° to 110° F.

Post-partum pills (see p. 71).

If there is severe bleeding, curettage may be necessary.

After-pains.—Intermittent uterine contractions associated with pains, sometimes of great severity. Seldom last more than twenty-four hours.

If slight, in multiparæ, may be looked upon as practically normal.

In primigravidæ they are at all times abnormal.

If severe, are usually due to incomplete uterine contraction, a loaded rectum or bladder, retained clot and secundines, or commencing inflammation.

May be due sometimes to over-dosage of ergot or pituitary.

Treatment.—Massage uterus.

Empty rectum and bladder.

Liq. Ergot ʒi and hot douches.

Put baby to the breast.

Aspirin gr. x.

Insert a morphia suppository, $\frac{1}{2}$ gr., as a last resort.

Progesterone, 5–10 mgm., will ease pain, but does not cure the cause.

Testosterone, 15–25 mgm., useful if cessation of lactation desired as well.

Abnormalities in Lochia

(*a*) *Sudden Arrest.*—(1) Septicæmia usually, (2) mechanical obstruction—lochiametra.

Lochiametra.—

Rare condition, but may follow Cæsarean section, when undilated cervix gets blocked with clot or piece of membranes. May become infected. Dull pain. Tender uterus, which is subinvoluted. *Treated* by dilatation of cervix with dilators.

(*b*) *Excessive.*—Due to subinvolution. May be associated with early local uterine infection. Later, possibly from a submucous fibroid.

(*c*) *Fœtid.*—Due to retained products undergoing decomposition. Usually associated with local uterine infection, but may, in rare cases, be due to a sloughing submucous fibroid.

Abnormalities of Micturition

Some discomfort may be felt for a few days after labour.

(*a*) **Incontinence of Urine.**—

1. From paralysis of the neck of the bladder due to pressure. Treat with strychnine injections $\frac{1}{60}$ gr. bi-daily, or liq. strych. hydrochlor. ♏iiss, orally, t.i.d.

2. From over-distension of the bladder.

3. From fistulæ—due in the vast majority of cases to sloughing from prolonged pressure and, in such cases, occurring some days after labour (see p. 333).

(*b*) **Retention of Urine.**—Extremely common in primigravidæ.

Causes.—

1. Reflex, caused by a tear in the perineum and tight perineal stitches.
2. Hysteria or nervousness.
3. Swelling of soft parts round urethra from contusion.
4. Paralysis of bladder from previous over-distension.

Treatment.—Try to promote spontaneous evacuation by giving warm sterile "jug douche" over vulva. Allow to get up. As a last resort pass the catheter, but remember that puerperal women are especially liable to urinary infection.

(*c*) **Frequency of Micturition.**—Due to cystitis or irritability of bladder from previous pressure or over-distension.

If simple irritability, treat with potassium citrate, hyoscyamus and buchu internally, and with plenty of demulcent drinks. Wash out bladder with silver nitrate solution, 1–10,000 if more severe.

(*d*) **Pyelitis.**—Usually occurs from seventh day of puerperium onwards, giving rise to practically no symptoms except rise of temperature and pulse rate, and frequency of micturition. Diagnosis is made by presence of pus in urine. Treated as for pyelitis in general (see p. 108).

Venous Thrombosis

May occur during pregnancy, in the puerperium and after operation, especially pelvic operations and Cæsarean section.

Two types (*a*) Thrombo-phlebitis and (*b*) Phlebo-thrombosis.

(*a*) **Thrombo-phlebitis.**—White leg or phlegmasia alba dolens. Primarily inflammatory due to septic infection which may be mild or severe (septic thrombo-phlebitis). May be limited to uterine and femoral veins or, if due to anærobic streptococcal infection, may spread to iliac and ovarian veins.

Pathology.—Inflammation of wall of vein with clot forming on inflamed area. Clot is firmly adherent. Anærobic streptococcal infection may produce pulmonary infarcts later, but hæmolytic streptococcal infections rarely do, as liquefaction of clot occurs. Usually affects left leg though other leg may be affected later.

Clinical Features.—

1. Pain in calf or thigh usually 8 to 10 days after delivery, after which leg begins to swell, reaching its maximum girth in about forty-eight hours' time. Pain is general as leg swells, but abates almost entirely when swelling is at its maximum and leg has then a wooden feeling.

2. Temperature rises to 101° or 102° whilst leg is swelling, and pulse quickens. Temperature usually highest at nights. After swelling is complete, temperature gradually subsides.

3. As leg swells it becomes white and shiny and may not pit on pressure till the acute stage abates.

4. Vein, to begin with, often hard and tender to touch.

5. Red lines may be seen along superficial branches of veins and lymphatics.

6. Constitutional symptoms, such as malaise, headache, constipation, etc., are usually present.

Course.—Acute symptoms abate in the course of ten days, the pain disappearing, tension diminishing and the leg pitting on pressure.

The swelling is seldom entirely reduced for six weeks and may last many months, often returning upon the least exertion.

During convalescence the leg has a stiff wooden feeling; neuralgic twitches occur frequently.

Relapses are frequent after subsequent labours or operations.

Treatment.—As for active treatment of phlebo-thrombosis (see p. 227), but in addition, chemotherapy and/or penicillin will be required.

(*b*) **Phlebo-thrombosis.**—

Causes.—

1. Circulatory stasis due to confinement in bed and immobilisation of limbs.

2. Varicose veins and previous phlebitis.

3. Anæmia and dehydration from excessive blood loss leading to an output of platelets with sticky surface. (Patients who have suffered from post-partum or severe ante-partum hæmorrhage, or from prolonged bleeding from fibroid tumours or severe bleeding during Cæsarean section, are most liable to thrombosis.)

4. Operative trauma liberating thrombo-plastin.

5. Fowler's position or pillow under knees.

6. Cold, by slowing circulation.

Pathology.—Occurs usually in deep veins of calf or sole of foot or in veins of thigh. No phlebitis in early stages so clot loosely attached to vein and there is therefore danger of pulmonary embolism.

Clinical Features.—

1. May be no symptoms till pulmonary embolism occurs.
2. Usually, however, pain in calf or sole 8 to 10 days after confinement or operation.
3. Tenderness in calf on deep pressure may be elicited several days previously; pain in calf may be obtained by sharp dorsi-flexion of the foot (Homan's sign).
4. Pyrexia (mild) may occur later due to mechanical irritation of venous wall by clot; pulse rate also quickens.
5. There is usually slight swelling of affected leg, with pitting on pressure.
6. May spread to thigh, or other leg may become affected.

Dangers.—Pulmonary embolism.

Treatment.—*Preventive.*—Various preventive suggestions have been advocated from time to time without much success, but now the incidence of the condition, and of pulmonary embolism after development, has been greatly decreased by :—

1. Replacing blood loss by blood transfusion.
2. Combating dehydration.
3. Early ambulation.
4. Free movement of knees, ankles and toes hourly.
5. Frequent deep breathing.
6. Avoiding Fowler's position and pillow under knees.
7. Keeping legs warm.
8. Examining daily in expected cases for deep tenderness and Homan's sign.
9. If patient has previously suffered from condition giving heparin prophylactically.

Active.—*Local.*—

1. Wrap the leg in cotton wool, apply a loose bandage and raise on a pillow.
2. Put a cradle over the leg to raise the bedclothes.
3. Do not, under any circumstances, rub the leg as the clot may be detached and pass to the heart or lungs. Handle very carefully.
4. Relieve the pain by saturated solution magnesium sulphate soaks or lead and opium lotion covered with mackintosh. Ichthyol and glycerine or antiphlogistine applications may also be useful.

5. Intramuscular injection of liver extract (pernæmon forte 2 c.c. daily) often prevents any further swelling, if given early.

Anticoagulants.—

Heparin is probably safest, 100 mgms. (10 c.c.). Given by intravenous injection, four-hourly. (The coagulation time should be determined frequently, one hour after an injection, and if over 4½ minutes the dosage should be stopped temporarily and then decreased.)

Lately heparin has been given subcutaneously on alternate days in Pitkin's menstruum into cellular tissue of unaffected thigh, giving 200–300 mgm. heparin sodium in 2–3 c.c. menstruum (ampoules are put up at these strengths).

Paralumbar Sympathetic Block.—

Blockage of regional sympathetic ganglia with procaine hydrochloride, to relax vaso-spasm, may cause quick relief from pain and œdema, and fever subsides rapidly. (5 c.c. procaine (1 per cent.) is injected near the lateral surfaces of each of the first four lumbar vertebræ.)

Absolute rest for a month after acute symptoms have subsided used to be insisted upon, but now, after using heparin, the patient moves her legs freely and may get up or sit on a chair as soon as acute symptoms disappear, usually between 4 to 6 days.

Pulmonary Embolism

Rare, but may occur after a natural delivery. More common after Cæsarean secion or after operation.

Pulmonary embolism is always secondary to a pre-existing thrombosis situated elsewhere, from which a portion of clot has been detached. It may occur any time during the month following delivery or operation.

Symptoms.—Usually sudden in their onset though premonitory pains in chest may have occurred, which are due to smaller emboli and must be treated as such.

1. Pain in the chest over the site of the embolism.
2. Intense dyspnœa.
3. Tumultuous and irregular cardiac action.
4. Quick, feeble pulse.
5. Unimpaired intelligence.
6. Blood-stained sputum (later).

Prognosis.—May be immediately fatal, but if patient survives for half an hour recovery is the rule.

Treatment.—

Complete rest which must be maintained for some time.

Oxygen 100 per cent. by B.L.B. mask.

Atropine, $\frac{1}{75}$ gr., subcutaneously or better, intravenously, and papaverine, $\frac{1}{2}$ gr.

Morphia, $\frac{1}{4}$ gr., intravenously may be a life saver.

Amyl nitrite.

Venesection if much turgidity and cyanosis.

Heparin, after acute symptoms have passed off, to try to prevent recurrence.

LACTATIONAL DISORDERS

Common in the puerperium, especially in the first fortnight; uncommon thereafter. Failure to breast feed successfully is usually due to mismanagement of these early difficulties. Maintain mother's morale, particularly if much pain; optimistic attitude of doctor and nurse essential.

Maternal Difficulties

(*a*) Local

1. **Small Nipples.**—Treat by antenatal traction and by traction before feeds to aid fixing. If baby cannot fix use nipple shield; suckling pulls out nipple and shield can be dispensed with in a few weeks.

2. **Retracted Nipples.**—If nipples will pull out, management same as for flat nipples. If unable to pull nipples out, do not attempt to breast feed and suppress lactation.

3. **Fissured Nipples.**—*Causes.*—(1) Lack of antenatal attention; (2) unnecessarily prolonged feeds in first few days; (3) large, strongly sucking infants; (4) baby being detached from breast without first depressing lower jaw; (5) often no apparent reason.

Usually occur in first two weeks.

Usually occur near base and are exquisitely painful during suckling.

May be starting-point of a mastitis.

Infant may swallow considerable amount of blood causing melæna.

Treatment.—If very painful or more than slight, stop suckling for 1–2 or even 3 days, this allows rapid healing by relief of repeated trauma.

Milk is evacuated by manual expression (not by pump) and given to baby by spoon. Stilbœstrol ointment applied after each feed stimulates epithelial proliferation and accelerates healing.

4. **Excessive Breast Engorgement.**—Breasts show enlargement, discomfort, throbbing, tenderness and diffuse induration. If severe, nipples cannot be grasped and suckling may be impossible until engorgement subsides. Lasts 2–5 days. Subsidence may be followed by poor lactation for a week or two, so do not wean too readily.

Treatment.—Support and bind up breasts.

Apply soaks of magnesium sulphate saturated solution.

Important to remove as much milk as possible as excessive tension in alveoli damages secreting cells; therefore maintain suckling if practicable and evacuate as much milk as possible with pump in all cases.

Small doses of stilbœstrol (1 mgm.) may sometimes be given in severe cases, but its action is uncertain and it may possibly aggravate the condition or cause subsequent hypogalactia.

5. **Mastitis.**—Caused by staphylococcus aureus, occasionally by staphylococcus albus.

Predisposed to by stagnation associated with mismanagement or blocked duct, by fissures and by bacteræmia arising from a focus of infection.

Usually occurs in second or third week of puerperium, but not infrequently up to three months and occasionally later. Is not unknown during pregnancy or in puerperium when mother has never nursed.

Clinical Features.—

General: Malaise, rigor, pyrexia, fast pulse, generalised pains, headache.

Local: Throbbing, pain, tenderness, flushing, œdema, induration, pain on moving isolateral arm. Condition usually subsides in one to three days, but may persist or proceed to abscess formation.

Treatment.—

Prophylactic: Never allow knots to form. Always see breast is empty after each feed. Avoid fissures, but if they do occur look after them carefully.

General: Depends on degree of constitutional disturbance.

More severe cases require rest in bed, fluid diet and analgesics.

Local: Continue to breast feed or take milk off regularly; this may be painful but makes more comfortable, eases tension and promotes resolution.

Support breast and apply soaks of cold saturated solution magnesium sulphate, 10 per cent. ichthyol in glycerine, antiphlogistine or boracic.

Radiant heat or short-wave therapy is often beneficial.

Systematic penicillin can be administered when the first flush appears; it may abort the whole process and should certainly prevent further extension. An initial dose of 200,000 units by intra-muscular injection, followed by 100,000 units 12-hourly for 3 to 5 days.

If abscess develops, stop feeding at affected breast; continue breast feeding if enough for baby at other breast, otherwise suppress lactation.

Incise freely, break down loculi boldly with finger and drain through a counter incision; keep incision well away from nipple and collecting ducts.

Breast feeding in subsequent pregnancies not jeopardised after free incisions, as most of breast secreting tissue is renewed in each pregnancy.

6. **Delayed Lactation.**—Persistence of flaccid breasts and poor lactation beyond the fourth or fifth day does not necessarily mean that breast feeding will fail, yet infants are often weaned in these circumstances.

Chief causes are illness or exhaustion of mother following a prolonged or difficult labour, premature labour, Cæsarean section, but often there is no apparent cause.

Treat by ensuring a good nutritious diet with ample milk and fluid. Porridge, gruel, ovaltine, Horlick's milk, lactagol and stout are good milk stimulants.

Insist on regular and complete evacuation of breasts by giving both breasts to the infant three-hourly and expressing any residual milk.

Bathe breasts with hot and cold water alternately.

Complement with cow's milk, but try to maintain mother's faith in breast feeding.

If little improvement in ten days, stop breast feeding.

7. **Deficient Lactation.**—After the establishment of lactation, whether at the normal time or later, an inadequate amount of milk for the needs of the baby is very common, particularly in the first two or three weeks.

Milk yield often falls temporarily when mothers return home; many babies are needlessly weaned then.

Treatment.—Try giving baby both breasts at each feed starting each successive feed from alternate breasts. Complementary feeding. It is better practice to complement (follow each breast feed by artificial feed), than to supplement (substitute some feeds by artificial feed) because regular evacuation of breasts is such an important stimulus to lactation. Complementary feeding can often be discontinued before the end of a month.

Bathe breasts with hot and cold water alternately.

Good nutritious diet as in delayed lactation (p. 231).

Liver injections or iron by mouth are often beneficial when anæmia is present.

(*b*) General

1. **Lack of Pre-requisites of Successful Lactation.**—*e.g.* malnutrition, overwork, worry.

2. **Physical Illness.**—

(*a*) Associated with pregnancy or labour.

(*b*) Not associated with pregnancy or labour, and either chronic or acute.

3. **Psychological Factors.**—Prejudice, ignorance, subnormal maternal instinct, mental deficiency, insanity.

Infantile Difficulties

(*a*) Local

1. **Congenital Defects of the Mouth.**—Tongue-tie, hare-lip, cleft-palate, short lower jaw, nasal obstruction, facial paralysis, congenital œsophageal atresia.

Tongue-tie (true) is rare, easily treated by snipping frænum.

Others often preclude suckling and feeding has to be by spoon or pipette, or with a large teat.

Use mother's milk in early weeks at least, especially if weakly.

(*b*) General

1. **Prematurity.**—The commonest infantile cause of abnormal breast feeding. Those of about 5 lb. or over are usually strong enough to feed normally. Smaller premature babies are seldom strong enough to nurse at the breast until a weight approaching 5 lb. is attained.

2. **Disinclination of Infant.**—Some infants lack the usual instinct to fix at the breast and to suckle. Education in breast feeding may be difficult and prolonged. Patient supervision of feeds ultimately overcomes difficulty.

3. **Illness.**—Most neo-natal illnesses interfere with feeding.

Worst degrees of anorexia occur in alimentary infections and hepatic dysfunction (jaundice).

4. **Mental Defect.**—Slow in learning to fix at the breast and feed properly, *e.g.* mongols.

Insanity of Pregnancy and Puerperium

Includes insanity of pregnancy, puerperium and lactation. Forms about 10 per cent. of all forms of insanity in females.

Relative Frequency.—During pregnancy, 18 per cent.

During puerperium, 47 per cent.

During lactation, 35 per cent.

Insanity of Pregnancy.—May be either mania or melancholia. The latter is more frequent.

Elderly primigravidæ are most often affected. It seldom manifests itself before the fourth month of gestation and generally continues until after delivery.

The prognosis is favourable, 70 per cent. recovering within six months after delivery. Recovery before delivery seldom occurs.

Puerperal Insanity.—May be mania or melancholia. More frequently the former.

Is considered puerperal if originating within a month after delivery.

Mania usually develops within sixteen days. Melancholia later.

Causes.—

(*a*) Heredity.

(*b*) Exhaustion.

1. From prolonged labour.
2. From excess of hæmorrhage.
3. Too rapid and frequent pregnancies.

(*c*) Shame and fear of exposure if pregnancy illegitimate.

(*d*) Fear.

Occasionally, during delivery, as the head passes the perineum, the excessive pain causes a transient delirium, during which the mother may destroy her child; a point of great importance medico-legally.

Symptoms: Premonitory.—Restlessness.

Sleeplessness very characteristic.

Rapid pulse and elevated temperature.

Causeless dislike of husband, friends, child or attendants.

Actual.—Varies according to the type of insanity. A sudden noisy delirium characterises mania, while a gradual development of deep depression, accompanied by morbid delusions and suicidal tendencies, are the conditions met with in melancholia.

Insanity of Lactation.—Chiefly melancholia.

Causes.—Same as puerperal insanity, to which add exhaustion from excessive lactation.

Prognosis less favourable than other puerperal varieties; 12 per cent. become permanently demented.

With regard to further details and treatment a textbook on psychiatry should be consulted.

CHAPTER XIV

PUERPERAL SEPSIS

B.M.A. Standard of Morbidity.—All fatal cases and all cases when the temperature rises to 100° F. or more on any two occasions from twelve hours after labour till the end of the eighth day, the temperature being taken morning and evening.

Department of Health Standard.—Any febrile condition occurring within twenty-one days after labour or abortion, in which a temperature of 100·4° F. or more has been sustained over a period of twenty-four hours or has recurred during that period.

All such cases should be notified as **Puerperal Pyrexia.**

In Scotland, if the infection is proved to be due to a specific organism, then the condition is notified as **Puerperal Fever.**

Types.—

1. *Local Uterine Infection* (*Sapræmia*).—Infection of uterine cavity by organisms limited thereto. Toxins liberated by such organisms pass into blood-stream.

2. *Septicæmia.*—Organisms enter blood-stream and circulate therein (bacteræmia). May or may not be found on blood culture.

3. *Septic Thrombo-phlebitis* of uterine, pelvic and ovarian veins.

4. *Pyæmia.*—Circulation of septic clot dislodged from septic thrombo-phlebitis, giving rise to metastatic abscesses.

5. *Parametritis* (*Pelvic Cellulitis*).—Lymphangitis and cellulitis arising in pelvic cellular tissue, causing local inflammatory swelling.

6. *Acute Salpingitis.*—Acute infection of tubes, which may spread to ovaries—*salpingo-oöphoritis.*

7. *Pelvic Peritonitis* (*Perimetritis*).—Infection of pelvic peritoneum, either following acute salpingitis or by lymphatics from a septicæmia. Serous effusion at first, which becomes purulent later and causes loose matting of pelvic organs and bowel.

8. *General Peritonitis.*—May result from pelvic peritonitis or be primary, due to lymphatic spread from septicæmia.

9. *Septic Endometritis.*—Present in local uterine infection when endometrium is shaggy.

10. *Acute Vaginitis and Vulvitis.*—Due usually to infection from lacerations, but may follow uterine infection.

Ætiology.

Infection may be caused by organisms permitted to enter vagina from without (heterogenetic infection), which is usual, or by organisms carried to generative organs from foci already present in patient (autogenetic infection).

Heterogenetic infection may be due to numerous causes.—

(*a*) From imperfect antisepsis and asepsis—

(1) Imperfect cleansing of hands.
(2) Imperfect sterilisation of instruments.
(3) Imperfect cleansing of vulva—antiseptics used not being of sufficient strength.

(*b*) From attendant due to—

(1) Imperfect cleansing of hands.
(2) Contact with another septic case, the infection being carried from the septic case to the healthy one.
(3) Attending midwifery case with septic finger or after dressing septic wounds without gloves.
(4) Spray infection from nose or throat of attendant.

(*c*) From direct contact with a septic case in a hospital ward or labour ward.

(*d*) From infected bedclothes or bed pans.

(*e*) From sexual intercourse during last months of pregnancy.

Autogenetic infection may be due to—

(*a*) Organisms already present in vagina, *e.g.* gonococci, B. coli, etc.

(*b*) Imperfect emptying of rectum and bladder before delivery.

(*c*) Organisms borne by blood or lymphatics from a septic focus elsewhere, viz., chronic appendicitis, chronic tonsillitis, pyorrhœa, decayed teeth, etc.

(*d*) Auto-infection by patient's own hand with septic sore or hand which has been in contact with a septic focus from her own body, *e.g.* nasal or pharyngeal secretion.

Infection is favoured by the alkalinity of the lochia in the puerperium, and thus any organism introduced flourishes and gains entrance through raw placental site.

Retained products, *e.g.* membranes or, more especially, pieces of placenta are always potential sources of danger, as organisms flourish on such tissues.

Lacerations of the cervix, vagina or perineum are also

potential sources of danger, as organisms may gain entrance through them.

Cases, in which general resistance has been lowered by toxæmia, hæmorrhage, trauma or difficult delivery, are specially liable to infection.

Chief Organisms Concerned and their Pathological Effects.—

1. *Hæmolytic Streptococcus.*—

Commonest organism in severe cases, causing a septicæmia. Group A is most dangerous.

Causes very little inflammatory reaction and spreads easily through tissues to cause blood stream infection, and in some cases, peritonitis.

Smooth decidua, not thickened, has a "clean" grey appearance though it oozes a serous fluid. Minute foci of pus may be seen in uterine wall, under placental site, in severe cases.

2. *Anœrobic Streptococcus.*—

Often cause of local uterine infection, growing on retained membranes, piece of placenta or blood clot. Often associated with saprophytes.

Decidua is greatly thickened and shaggy and has a dirty appearance, exuding a foul-smelling discharge.

Considerable tissue reaction, so spread of infection is slow and is usually confined to uterus and its proximity.

Thrombo-phlebitis common owing to organism, flourishing in blood clot, gaining access to vessels through retro-placental sinuses and from there to uterine and pelvic veins.

In mild cases firm clotting occurs and organisms disappear. In severe cases infected emboli are frequently cast off and cause abscesses in other parts of the body, especially lungs, the patient developing pyæmia.

3. *Staphlylococcus Aureus.*—

Mild infection round perineal tears or episiotomies.

May cause acute infection after Cæsarean section.

Uterine wall then studded with small abscesses, from which organisms enter blood stream and cause metastatic infections (pyæmia).

4. *B. Coli.*—

Responsible for a number of localised infections in birth canal with little tendency to invasion unless tissues traumatised.

May cause gas formation in uterus.

In rare cases blood stream is invaded.

5. *B. Welchii.*—

Lives on devitalised tissues and is found chiefly after delivery of a fœtus, which has been dead in utero for some time.

May be very fulminating, disseminating gas-forming organisms all over body, the uterine wall, liver and muscles being honeycombed with bubbles of gas. Patient dies in twenty-four to forty-eight hours.

More often is confined to the uterus, along with other bacteria, when it is much less virulent.

6. *Gonococcus.*—

Rarely cultured as causative organism, but is probably quite a frequent cause of sepsis.

Causes endometritis, salpingitis and pelvic peritonitis by ascending infection.

Infection very seldom fatal but often causes chronic pathological pelvic conditions.

7. *Pneumococcus, B. Tetanus, B. Typhosus, and Aerogenes Capsulatus.*—

Very rare but may give rise to very virulent infections.

8. *Saprophytes.*—

Anærobic putrefactive organisms, many of which produce gas. Tend to remain localised to uterus and disappear after dead tissue is removed.

May be cause of local uterine infection and be associated with anærobic streptococci.

Investigation of Causative Organisms.—

High vaginal smear—a sterile test tube containing a sterile swab attached to a long handle is inserted into the vagina, the swab is then pushed from the test tube into the posterior fornix to obtain secretion and then withdrawn into test tube, which in its turn is removed from the vagina.

This smear is cultured and, if a hæmolytic streptococcus is present, grouping is done.

Such a method is just as efficacious as a cervical or intra-uterine smear and is less likely to add to the infection. There may be difficulty at times in culturing the streptococcus if anærobic and a special anærobic technique may be required.

Local Uterine Infection (*Sapræmia*)

Due in most cases to anærobic streptococci and/or saprophytes thriving on some retained products of conception or blood clot. Leucocytes under necrotic layer prevent invasion of germs into blood-stream. Endometrium shaggy, and acute endometritis may develop.

Clinical Features.—

1. Rise of temperature usually to 100° to 102° on third or fourth day of the puerperium and may be ushered in by a rigor. Pulse rate slightly raised.
2. Headache and general malaise.
3. Lochia increased in amount and at first are heavy in odour, but later become fœtid.
4. Uterus subinvoluted, rather boggy in consistence and often tender.

Treatment.

1. In the less severe cases treat as for subinvolution, viz., hot douches, ergot, and sit patient up to allow free drainage.
2. If more severe or no improvement within twenty-four hours, inject glycerine, 30 to 40 c.c., into uterus through a rubber or gum elastic catheter. (If the condition is severe the catheter should be stitched into cervix and glycerine injected every two to three hours; in the less severe cases a daily injection may suffice.)
3. Removal of retained products of conception with finger, followed by thorough irrigation of the uterus. There is always the danger of the germs entering the blood-stream through the raw area left after removal of the retained products and causing a general, instead of a local, infection. This is especially the case if curettage is done and therefore the finger only should be used. If, however, one is sure some placental tissue remains in utero and it can be felt, removal followed by irrigation will produce the quickest cure.
4. Sulphathiazole, 1 grm. four-hourly.
5. Penicillin, 30,000 units three-hourly, or 100,000 units six-hourly.

Prognosis.—Rapid improvement usual after early treatment and no bad results follow; but if neglected, septic thrombo-phlebitis, septicæmia or pyæmia may occur; failing that, chronic subinvolution may cause intractable menorrhagia at a later date.

Septic Thrombo-Phlebitis (see p. 225)

Starts usually from a local uterine infection with similar clinical features. Later, pain develops in iliac fossæ and there is tenderness on palpation and also on vaginal examination at sides of the uterus and more laterally.

Pyæmia

Period of Onset.—Usually after the first week of the puerperium, frequently following a septic thrombo-phlebitis.

Symptoms.—A series of sudden and intense rigors of a prolonged nature, accompanied by high fever and ending with profuse sweating. Fever is intermittent and pulse is fast.

Secondary febrile conditions, the result of metastatic abscesses situated in the liver, lungs, etc.

Emaciation as disease progresses.

Prognosis.—Extremely unfavourable, death usually resulting in the second or third week; the patient may linger however, for months, with occasional periods of apparent convalescence, which are apt to raise false hopes of recovery.

Staphylococcal cases most favourable if patient is able to withstand prolonged nature of disease.

Treatment.—Sulphathiazole or sulphadiazine as in septicæmia. Penicillin 30,000 units three-hourly.

Septicæmia

Commonly known as "**Puerperal Fever**" and is due to germs passing into, and circulating in, the blood-stream.

The most common causative germ is the hæmolytic streptococcus, and the Group A variety is the most virulent.

The leucocytic barrier, if present at all, is thin and allows germs to enter the blood-stream. The endometrium is thin and the whole interior of the uterus greyish in colour. The myometrium and parametrium are often infiltrated with seropurulent fluid, which may ooze into uterine cavity and through vagina.

Period of Onset.—May occur within twenty-four hours after labour, but usually occurs between the second and fourth days, and, if infection occurs at labour, not later than the fifth day of the puerperium. Infection may, however, occur during the early days of the puerperium, when symptoms occur at a later date, usually from seventh to ninth day.

Clinical Features.—May be ushered in by a severe rigor.

Increased pulse rate always present—100 to 120, rising as disease progresses to 140 or more.

High temperature, 102° to 106° F., which may be subject to marked remissions, but rarely descends to normal.

Insomnia, restlessness and headache.

Profuse sweating, with rapidly increasing prostration.

Transient delirium may occur later.

Lochia decreased or may be absent. Milk also suppressed.

Uterus usually involutes fairly well and is not tender.

Tongue becomes dry, red and cracked.

Diarrhœa with or without abdominal distension is a later symptom and usually denotes peritonitis.

Eyes are bright and the patient often states she feels well (bad sign).

Usually there is *no pain.* (Pain usually means that there is a local rather than a generalised infection.)

Prognosis.—The earlier the onset the worse the prognosis. The faster the pulse the worse the prognosis. A great number of rigors affects prognosis adversely. A dry and red tongue is a bad prognostic sign, whereas a moist, clean tongue is a good one.

The earlier the patient begins to get better the quicker is the convalescence, and the less likely is her health to be impaired afterwards.

Some cases die within forty-eight hours of the onset of the infection, but, if fatal, death occurs, as a rule, from seventh to twenty-first day. Some cases become subacute and may die at a later date from sheer exhaustion, whereas if such cases recover, they may never regain really good health again.

Since discovery of the sulphonamide drugs and later of penicillin, prognosis has improved very considerably. (Death rate dropped at Queen Charlotte's Septic Block Hospital from 24·5 per cent. to 3·5 per cent. after use of Prontosil for one year (1936).)

Treatment.—

Prophylactic.—

1. Quinine, gr. ii, twice daily for last fortnight, and vitamins A and D may help general resistance.

2. Routine calcium sulphide, gr. ii, thrice daily for first five days of the puerperium lowered morbidity appreciably at Royal Maternity Hospital, Edinburgh in 1936.

3. Routine sulphanilamide lowered the morbidity rate still further in 1937. Not advisable, however, as a general routine as it may increase patient's resistance to sulphonamide, if required at a later date and cause toxic manifestations when given then. Very useful, however, as a prophylactic, if patient has had a difficult labour and is thought likely to be infected. Penicillin may be used instead in such cases.

4. Efficient antisepsis, as much asepsis as possible, and taking all precautions to prevent the causes of sepsis.

Active.—Good nursing, fresh air and a stimulating diet of eggs, milk, chickentea, etc.

In streptococcal cases, sulphanilamide, sulphadiazine, sulphathiazole or sulphamezathine are effective.

In mild or moderate cases, 1 gm. four-hourly **day and night** is usually sufficient.

In severe cases endangering life, and especially if developing acutely early in the puerperium, 2 gm. can be given as an initial dose intravenously and 1·5 gm. orally followed by 1·5 gm. four hourly for two days, 1 gm. four hourly for two days and then six hourly for two days. In a moderately severe case an initial dose of 2 gm. is followed by 1 gm. four hourly for two days, six hourly for two days and then eight hourly for two days. (Nightly administration must be given, if scheduled, even if patient has to be wakened to receive pills.) Sodium sulphathiazole, sulphadiazine or sulphamezathine are recommended for intravenous administration and should be given, dissolved in 10 c.c. water, very slowly.

In staphylococcal cases sulphathiazole and sulphadiazine are the sulphonamides of preference, as is also the case in infections due to B. Welchii.

All seem to have action accentuated by giving an alkali mixture such as pot. cit. and soda. bicarb. as well.

Action is due to the sulphonamide limiting the organism the use of para-amino-benzoic acid, which it requires in order to exist.

More latterly penicillin has also proved to be very effective ; it may be given in conjunction with sulphonamides, but, as all the organisms causing puerperal sepsis are penicillin-sensitive, penicillin alone should suffice. The drug is non-toxic in its administration. It is important to obtain an adequate blood-level of penicillin, and therefore intramuscular injection of 30,000 units 3-hourly can be given, or 100,000 units 6-hourly. This should be continued for a minimum of 5 to 6 days and until temperature has been normal for 48 hours.

Blood transfusion may be of use in obstinate and prolonged cases, where there is anæmia.

Dangers of Sulphonamide Treatment.—

If sulphathiazole or sulphadiazine are used, care has to be taken that crystals are not deposited in the kidneys, and therefore plenty of fluid must be drunk and the urine output must be satisfactory.

The drug should not be given for more than seven days at a time and the blood should be examined from time to time for agranulocytosis. Should this occur the drug must be stopped at once and pentonucleic acid given.

Prolonged administration may give rise to a skin rash or in some cases to marked rise of temperature, which continues as long as the drug is persisted in.

Cyanosis may occur with sulphanilamide and sickness may develop ; the former is best treated with methylene blue and the latter by nicotinic acid.

Inflammation of Cellular Tissue—Parametritis, Pelvic Cellulitis

Definition.—Lymphangitis and cellulitis arising primarily in the cellular tissue and forming a local inflammatory swelling.

Anatomy.—See cellular tissue of pelvis (p. 10).

Physiology.—All cellular tissue becomes much increased during pregnancy and thus inflammation at this time will cause great thickening.

Ætiology.—

(*a*) Usually due to streptococci or, sometimes, staphylococci. Bacillus coli and gonococci do not produce the condition alone, but may be found associated with one of the former.

(*b*) Entrance is usually effected through a laceration of the cervix or vagina at labour, and the laceration may be large or microscopic, as in a whitlow.

(*c*) Sometimes due to infection at a Wertheim operation, after removal of a submucous sloughing fibroid or amputation of the cervix, all of which open up the cellular tissue.

Pathology.—

(*a*) Hyperæmia, small cell infiltration and effusion.

(*b*) A soft swelling forms, which later becomes hard, due to the fibrinous exudate.

(*c*) Usually confined at first to the base of one broad ligament.

(*d*) Resolution may now occur or the mass may extend in the pelvis, either to the antero-lateral pelvic wall and iliac fossa, or backwards along utero-sacral ligaments to the para-rectal and para-vertebral fascia. Less commonly, it spreads to the base of the bladder and anterior abdominal wall or it may spread by any of the anatomical exits.

(*e*) Resolution may yet occur or suppuration may take place, only one abscess cavity being usual.

(*f*) The abscess is usually seen just above Poupart's ligament, but it may appear at the side of the bladder or in anterior abdominal wall, reaching the surface about midway between the symphysis and the umbilicus, or at any of the anatomical exits. It sometimes appears just above the iliac crest.

(*g*) Rupture into the peritoneal cavity practically never occurs; but if it did, general peritonitis would be rare, as there is always some slight local peritonitis, which, causing adhesions, would shut in the abscess.

(*h*) The abscess rarely opens into the bladder, rectum, or vagina.

(*i*) If pointing occurs, it usually does so from the seventh to the twelfth week after the beginning of illness. Area of pointing is usually above centre of Poupart's ligament, but abscess may spread up anterior abdominal wall and point midway between symphysis and umbilicus, or it may point through any of the exits of the pelvic cellular tissue (see p. 11).

(*j*) The pus may be thick and odourless, foul-smelling or sero-purulent.

(*k*) Sometimes a remote parametritis occurs, absorption having taken place around uterus, but not distally.

(*l*) After thorough evacuation the cellulitic exudate rapidly disappears, and the abscess closes.

If a sinus persists it is due to communication—

(1) With a viscus.
(2) With a suppurating mucous tract, *e.g.* pyosalpinx.
(3) With a cavity having a non-collapsible wall and a pyogenic lining, *e.g.* ovarian abscess.
(4) With dead matter or bone.

Symptoms.—

Usually causes symptoms from seventh to tenth day of puerperium.

Raised temperature and pulse rate with morning remissions. Rigors are rare.

Pain is not marked, but if cellulitis is extensive, it may be present on movement, shooting down the legs and going into the groin.

Painful defæcation and dysuria may occur, and diarrhœa or cystitis may be present if rectal or bladder walls infected.

Sleeplessness, thirst, headache, malaise and constipation are usual.

Symptoms usually disappear in seven to ten days, but, on the patient getting up, slight rise of temperature may occur.

Signs.—

(*a*) To begin with, there is increased resistance at one side and then a hard mass running antero-laterally from the uterus can be felt. This becomes harder and more fixed as times goes on and causes a depression in the vaginal wall.

(*b*) Vagina cannot be moved over mass, which is fixed to the pelvic wall.

(*c*) Uterus is fixed and is pushed over to unaffected side.

(*d*) Mass usually enlarges forwards, but may go backwards.

Diagnosis.—

(*a*) *From matted appendages due to tubo-ovarian inflammation.*—

(1) History—cellulitis being excluded if cellular tissue has not been opened up.

(2) History—cellulitis being excluded if it is present three to four months after labour and resolution or abscess formation has not occurred.

(3) Cellulitis is unilateral, diseased appendages are usually bilateral.

(4) Uterus and mass are more fixed in cellulitis.

(5) Mass is at the base of the broad ligament in cellulitis, at the apex in peritonitis.

(6) Mass usually extends forwards in cellulitis, but backwards into pouch of Douglas in peritonitis.

(7) Fluid can be present in the pouch of Douglas only in peritonitis.

(8) Abdominal pain, tenderness, distension and rigidity show peritoneal infection.

(9) Temperature is higher in cellulitis and the pulse is relatively lower.

Prognosis.—

(*a*) Favourable, there being no serious after-effects.

(*b*) The minority suppurate; pus is suspected by a continued temperature after three to four weeks, dry tongue, sallow complexion, anæmia, leucocytosis, etc., but even then prognosis is favourable, though convalescence is lengthy.

Treatment.—

Prophylaxis—asepsis and stitch any tears immediately.

General treatment—fresh air, etc.

Plenty of fluids to assist elimination.

Hot vaginal douches (112°) b.i.d., and hot fomentations to hypogastrium. Pack vagina with ichthyol and glycerine (8 to 10 per cent.).

Penicillin 100,000 units eight-hourly.

As the disease becomes more subacute, pelvic diathermy helps resolution.

If abscess rises into the abdomen, apply fomentations and radiant heat.

Do not incise till pointing occurs, as it may give rise to fresh infection if done too early. Furthermore, resolution may occur at any time.

When definite pointing does occur, incise, break any adhesions and insert drainage tube.

If a sinus persists, look for some other condition.

Acute Salpingitis, Endometritis, Vaginitis and Vulvitis (see next chapter)

The likeliest cause of an *initial* temperature during the lying-in period is as follows :—

First day.—Reactionary temperature, septicæmia.

Second day.—Septicæmia.

Third day.—Septicæmia, local uterine infection, breast congestion.

Fourth day.—Septicæmia, local uterine infection.

Fifth day.—Salpingitis, local uterine infection.

Sixth day.—Salpingitis, pyelitis.

Seventh day.—Pyelitis, mastitis.

Eighth day.—Pyelitis, mastitis.

Ninth day.—Mastitis.

Tenth day.—Pelvic cellulitis, white leg, mastitis.

CHAPTER XV

INFECTIONS OF GENITAL TRACT

FALLOPIAN TUBES

Acute Salpingitis

Ætiology.—

1. Direct spread upwards from vagina, cervix and uterus, *e.g.* gonococcal infection, post-abortal and post-operative sepsis.

2. *Via* lymphatics of broad ligament from uterus, cervix and vagina, *e.g.* puerperal streptococcal infection.

3. By blood-stream, *e.g.* tuberculosis, scarlet fever in children.

4. By contiguity from adjacent structures, *e.g.* acute appendicitis, diverticulitis.

Common organisms are gonococci, streptococci, staphylococci, anærobes, tubercle bacillus and B. coli ; rarely pneumococcus.

Pathology.—Gonococcal infection does not ascend to tubes till succeeding menstrual period. Most amenable to chemotherapy before period occurs.

Fimbriæ are drawn in and swollen in gonorrhœal cases but do not invert in tuberculosis where the ostium remains patent but is plugged with caseous material.

Streptococcal infection causes little tissue reaction and therefore rupture is liable to occur if a pyosalpinx developes.

Ovary usually resistant to all forms of infection, and usually only surface is involved. If infection invades ovary it enters through a ruptured Graafian follicle.

In gonococcal cases, separation of adhesions usually easy ; in acute septic cases underlying cellulitis occurs and if subacute stage is protracted line of cleavage may be entirely lost. In tuberculous cases adhesions are always bloody on separation and lines of cleavage are lost. Separation of bowel adhesions very dangerous owing to sub-peritoneal infiltration. If bowel is opened, a permanent fistulous tract is not uncommon.

Clinical Features.—

Puerperal.—

1. Rise of temperature usually occurring from fifth to seventh day of puerperium. Fast pulse.
2. Pain and rigidity in both sides of abdomen.
3. Distension of lower part of abdomen.
4. Increase of red lochia.
5. Malaise and sometimes sickness.

Non-puerperal.—

1. Sudden onset of high temperature (101°–103°) and fast pulse.
2. Pain in lower abdomen, especially in iliac fossæ, associated with rigidity and some distension of the lower part of abdomen.
3. Vaginal bleeding may occur. Often purulent vaginal discharge.
4. On vaginal examination, there is tenderness and fullness in both fornices, though no definite swelling is felt.
5. Great pain is elicited on movement of the cervix.

Diagnosis.—In non-puerperal cases acute salpingitis must be differentiated *from acute appendicitis* and, though in some cases this is by no means easy, the following diagnostic points are of value.

1. Careful history.
2. Presence of vaginal discharge or bleeding not due to menstrual period.
3. Diffuse tenderness and rigidity over whole hypogastric and iliac regions.
4. No definite tenderness over M'Burney's point.
5. Movement of cervix causes great pain.
6. On bimanual examination most pain is felt with abdominal hand just above symphysis to one or other side. In appendicitis the maximum tenderness is higher up.

(*N.B.*—If any real doubt, then laparotomy must be done, as it is more dangerous to leave an acute appendicitis than to operate on acute salpingitis. If the latter is found, a drain into the abdomen is the only treatment required and the abdomen should be closed forthwith.)

End Results of Acute Salpingitis.—

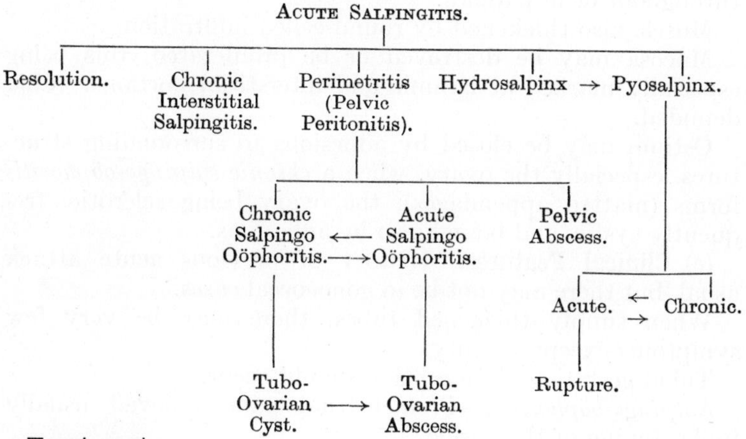

Treatment.—

Puerperal.—

1. Sulphonamides and penicillin as in septicæmia.
2. Hot fomentations to abdomen.
3. Morphia.

Non-puerperal.—

1. Complete rest.
2. Ice-bags or hot fomentations to lower abdomen.
3. Morphia.
4. Fowler's position.
5. Sulphathiazole, especially if gonococcal.
6. Penicillin 100,000 units followed by 50,000 four-hourly for five days.
7. When temperature settles, as it usually does in three to four days, hot vaginal douches.
8. If laparotomy is done for diagnosis *never remove* tubes, but only at most insert drain into pelvis. (Removal of tubes is a mutilating and unnecessary operation, as majority of cases get well quickly and tubes often function normally at a later date. It may also be a dangerous operation, as the septic area must be cut through, if only tubes are removed, and a generalised peritonitis may be substituted for a pelvic peritonitis.)

CHRONIC SALPINGITIS

(*a*) **Cause.**—

1. Previous acute attack.
2. Due to attenuated organisms causing chronic inflammation.

(*b*) **Pathology.**—Tubal wall thickened by fibrosis, either throughout or in patches.

Muscle also thickened by round-celled infiltration.

Mucosa may be destroyed or be proliferated, this being especially marked at isthmic and interstitial portions. Cilia denuded.

Ostium may be closed by adhesions to surrounding structures, especially the ovary, when a *chronic salpingo-oöphoritis* forms (matted appendages), the ovary being sclerotic, frequently cystic, and bound also by adhesions.

(*c*) **Clinical Features.**—History of previous acute attack usual, but there may not be in gonococcal cases.

When simply thickened tubes, there may be very few symptoms except sterility.

Tubal gestation if conception should occur.

Salpingo-oöphoritis.—Premenstrual pain, relieved usually by beginning of the period.

Menorrhagia, due to the accompanying endometritis and metritis.

Leucorrhœa, due to endometritis and endocervicitis.

Dyspareunia and sterility.

Constipation is usual.

Frequency of micturition, which may be associated with cystitis, often occurs.

General health is poor (headache, backache, malaise, loss of appetite, etc.).

(*d*) **Signs.**—Per vaginam—thickened tubes felt, which may be tender.

Salpingo-oöphoritis.—Uterus often retroverted.

Uterus may be fixed.

Swellings at sides or behind uterus, the swellings being usually somewhat tender and feel like bag of hard worms.

(*e*) **Treatment.**—

1. *Palliative.*—
   - (*a*) Rest in bed.
   - (*b*) Hot douches b.i.d., with vaginal pluggings nightly for ten to fourteen days (ichthyol and glycerine 8 to 10 per cent.).
   - (*c*) Short wave therapy.
   - (*d*) Diathermy.
   - (*e*) Elliott's bag. (Distribution of heat to pelvis through bag filled with hot water (temp. 128° F.) in vagina.)

If conservative methods fail and symptoms persist.

2. *Operative.*—
   (*a*) Salpingo-oöphorectomy.
   (*b*) If both tubes and ovaries are involved, as is usual, and require removal, it is best to do a hysterectomy as well.

Hydrosalpinx

(*a*) **Cause.**—Due to closure of the ostia by catarrhal salpingitis, the abdominal ostium being closed by retraction and adhesion of the fimbria, and the uterine ostium by œdema of the mucosa due to catarrh. The secretion is thus retained in the tube.

(*b*) **Appearance, etc.**—
1. Looks like a retort—broad ampulla and narrow isthmus.
2. Fluid is thin, cloudy and serous or mucoid.
3. Wall is very thin indeed.
4. May empty itself through uterus—*hydrops tubæ profluens.*
5. Adhesions to intestine, uterus, etc., may form.

(*c*) **Complications.**—

1. A cystic ovary is a common accompaniment, and a tubo-ovarian cyst may form at a later date, due to interconnection owing to adhesions.

2. If fresh infection occurs, a pyosalpinx may form.

(*d*) **Clinical Features.**—

1. History of salpingitis.

2. Chronic pain due to adhesions if present, but symptoms often very few and not marked.

3. Distended tube, or tubes, felt per vaginam.

(*e*) **Treatment.**—Remove the tube, and ovary, if affected.

Pyosalpinx

Causes.—

1. May be acute following acute salpingitis due to streptococci, gonococci, or B. coli; takes three to seven days to develop.

2. Chronic much more common, following an acute or chronic salpingitis or infection of a hydrosalpinx. In the former cases secretion accumulates in the tube owing to adhesions of fimbriæ blocking abdominal ostium, whereas the uterine ostium is blocked by hyperplastic mucosa.

3. A chronic pyosalpinx may become acute, if general resistance is lowered in any way, *e.g.* by cold, constipation, etc., or by sexual intercourse, fresh infection, instrumentation or intra-uterine radium.

4. Commonest site of genital tuberculosis in the female.

Pathology.—Tube is retort-shaped. Fimbriated extremities thickened and adherent, due to denuding of epithelium. This closes ostium and is aided by protective adhesions to surrounding structures.

If pyosalpinx is quickly formed, as in puerperal, post-abortal and streptococcal cases, the wall is thin ; but as it is usually slowly formed, the wall is thick and consists chiefly of fibrous tissue. Peritoneal coat is rough and covered with adhesions, and mucosa is almost completely replaced by granulation tissue.

In chronic cases, pus usually sterile. In tubercular cases, caseating matter is found, whereas in puerperal and gonococcal cases the pus is thick, creamy and yellow. Secondary infection by B. coli and saprophytes is common, when pus is foul-smelling.

Clinical Features.—

Acute.—High temperature and rapid pulse.

Pain, tenderness and rigidity in lower abdomen.

Vaginal bleeding common, often profuse.

On vaginal examination, tender, retort-shaped, fixed swellings are found in postero-lateral fornices or in pouch of Douglas.

Movement of cervix causes pain.

Blood sedimentation rate very rapid.

White blood count high.

Chronic.—As in salpingo-oöphoritis, but usually more pronounced.

May have acute or subacute exacerbations.

Per vaginam findings as in acute cases, but tenderness not so marked.

Treatment.—

Acute.—As for acute salpingitis until temperature has been normal for a week, then plugging the vagina with ichthyol and glycerine (10 per cent.) daily may be combined with hot douching twice daily.

Pelvic diathermy or short wave therapy often causes rapid absorption of pus.

Rarely, operative treatment may be required if—

(1) General condition deteriorates.
(2) Pyosalpinx grows.
(3) Sedimentation rate is persistently rapid or becomes more rapid despite treatment.

These signs may indicate that rupture, which must be prevented at all costs, is imminent; most liable to occur in post-abortal cases due to streptococcal infection.

Chronic.—Douching and plugging, diathermy or short wave therapy.

If conservative treatment of no avail and symptoms are constant and cause persistent ill-health, or if frequent acute exacerbations occur, then hysterectomy should be done, with removal of both tubes and ovaries. (The uterus is infected also and is best removed with the appendages.)

(*N.B.*—Before operation is undertaken, the acute stage must be over for at least fourteen days so as to allow the pus to become sterile, as rupture of the tube during removal is frequent, owing to the necessity of breaking down many adhesions before removal. If pus is infective, a peritonitis may result. Good practice is not to operate till the sedimentation time is beginning to approach normal, which shows that the acute stage is over.)

Tuberculous Pyosalpinx

May occur at any age either in nulliparæ or multiparæ; may be associated with tuberculous abdomen, but usually peritoneum not involved.

Practically always secondary to infection elsewhere.

Infection burrows, producing thick walled tube, with tubercles throughout musculature.

May progress along tubes forming hard nodules at irregular intervals. (*Salpingitis isthmica nodosa.*) Acute tuberculous tubes may disseminate disease and cause tuberculous peritonitis. Ovary is fairly resistant, but is involved in 15–30 per cent. of cases, usually a cold abscess resulting through invasion of Graafian follicles.

Uterine mucosa is infected in vicinity of cornua by direct invasion and near internal os by stasis and retention of secretion.

Usually does not cause such marked symptoms as occur with other types of pyosalpinx and often the only symptom is some menstrual irregularity, *e.g.* menorrhagia; iliac-ache may be present as well.

General health often affected, the patient being listless, tired and losing weight.

May become acute at any time, when symptoms arise as in acute pyosalpinx due to other infections.

May have lung lesions, or acute attacks may cause spread to lungs.

Treatment.—Conservative treatment, heliotherapy, radiotherapy and pneumo-peritoneum of little avail in majority of cases.

Streptomycin 1–2 gm. daily may be tried, but toxic effects, such as vertigo, may be severe and permanent.

Best treated by supra-vaginal hysterectomy with removal of both tubes and ovaries. (If only one tube is involved, which is rare, then the offending tube only should be removed. When both are involved, the ovaries are better removed as well, as they are infected in quite an appreciable proportion of cases and give rise to symptoms at a later date, necessitating further operative treatment. The uterus is often (60 per cent.) site of tuberculous endometritis and condition may be diagnosed for certain by a diagnostic endometrial biopsy.)

Other Tubercular Infections of Tubes

(1) Tubercles may be found studded over peritoneal surface in association with a general peritoneal infection.

(2) *Salpingitis Isthmica Nodosa.*—Small nodules which on section show tubercular changes are present involving muscle wall of tube.

First described by Chiari in 1890 and was thought at one time to be adenomyoma, but is now considered to be tubercular.

No treatment necessary unless causing symptoms, viz. menorrhagia and pain, when removal is required.

Acute Tubo-ovarian and Ovarian Abscess

Usually unilateral, though opposite appendages also show infection; caused by streptococci or mixed infection with gonococci.

Abscesses may be multiple, or the whole stroma may be destroyed, giving rise to a large pus-sac lined by unhealthy granulation tissue, the cavity frequently joining that of tube.

May become very large.

Gives rise to acute local and general symptoms.

Swelling is fixed, tender and, if large, fluctuant.

Drain through the vagina if possible, as the pus, when acute, is full of streptococci ; when the acute stage is over, remove the tube and ovary abdominally.

If not accessible per vaginam, removal must be carried out by laparotomy, the abscess removed and a drain inserted.

Mumps sometimes give rise to acute oöphoritis, but very rarely to an abscess.

Pelvic Abscess

May follow acute salpingitis, ruptured pyosalpinx (rare), or appendix abscess.

Confined to the pelvis by adhesions separating the abscess from the general peritoneal cavity.

High temperature, especially at nights. Pulse rate raised. Usually pelvic pain, but this is not constant and there may be only a feeling of fullness and discomfort.

Dysuria and possibly retention of urine in some cases.

Lower abdominal tenderness and resistance.

On vaginal examination a fluctuant swelling is felt in the pouch of Douglas, pressing on the vagina and possibly trying to point in that situation.

Diagnose by passing a needle into the swelling through the posterior fornix and withdrawing pus.

Treat by posterior colpotomy—opening into the pouch of Douglas through posterior fornix as soon as pointing is apparent. Drainage per vaginam. Fowler's position.

OVARY

Chronic Oöphoritis

This is usually the result of acute inflammation, the interstitial tissue being most involved. The microscopic appearances are those of chronic inflammation. There is marked hyperplasia of the stroma and thickening of the tunica albuginea. This latter may prevent ovulation and the ovary may be riddled with small cysts.

Clinical Features.—

1. Vague discomfort, backache and iliac-ache, worse before menstruation.

2. Menorrhagia is common.

3. Intermenstrual pain (Mittelschmerz) at definite time each month (twelfth to sixteenth day), probably due to ovulation through a thickened tunica albuginea.

4. Ovaries are normal in size or slightly enlarged, and may or may not be tender to touch. (In some cases the ovary is small and cirrhotic ; these patients seem to have most pain.)

Treatment.—

1. General, *i.e.* tonics, laxatives, etc.

2. Douching and plugging or pelvic diathermy.

3. If no improvement, open the abdomen and examine the ovaries and appendix, removing the ovary if wholly diseased or performing a partial resection.

Tuberculosis of Ovary

Rare but may be associated with a tuberculous pyosalpinx. A primary cold abscess may develop in the ovary when symptoms similar to a subacute pyosalpinx are caused. The ovary is enlarged in either case and in cold abscess is very thickened round small abscess cavity.

UTERUS

Acute Endometritis

May spread and cause cellular and purulent infiltration of the entire thickness of the organ (metritis).

Associated with local uterine infection after abortion or labour.

Symptoms.—Fever, ushered in by chilliness, about the third day after delivery. Pulse is quickened.

Intermittent hypogastric pain.

Signs.—Uterus is subinvoluted and tender on pressure.

Cervix is œdematous and bleeds easily.

Lochia increased, often purulent and fœtid.

Treatment.—General treatment. Hot fomentations applied to hypogastrium. Antibiotics and sulphonamides.

Chronic Endometritis

Endometritis may be an infection caused by streptococci, staphylococci, gonococci or the tubercle bacillus and may follow abortion or full-time delivery.

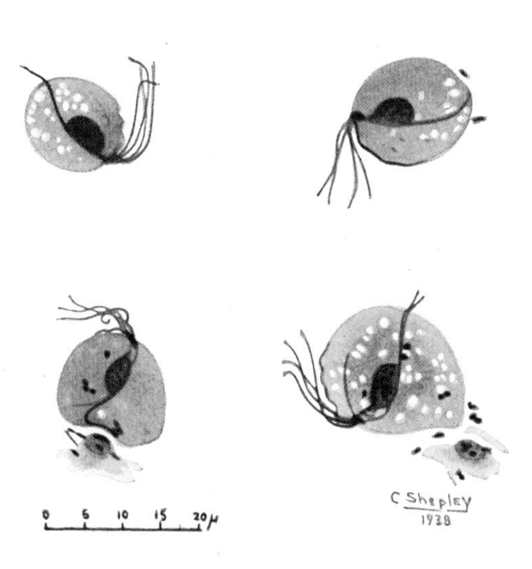

PLATE II.—TRICHOMONAS VAGINALIS.

facing p. 256

Endometritis may accompany sub-mucous and interstitial fibroids or endometrial polypi.

What was formerly called " chronic hyperplastic glandular endometritis " is now no longer recognised as a pathological entity, and only one type of chronic endometritis is described —Chronic Interstitial Endometritis.

Chronic Interstitial Endometritis.—

This condition may occur at any time in the reproductive period and after.

Pathology.—

(1) Round cell infiltration. Polymorphonuclear cells are present in large numbers—(*a*) round the glands, sometimes entering the lumina, and (*b*) under the surface epithelium. The more polymorphonuclear cells, the more sub-acute the condition.

(2) Plasma cells—present in abundance. The more chronic the condition, the more plasma cells are formed.

(*N.B.*—Both (1) and (2) occur in small numbers in normal endometrium, and it is the abundance which denotes a chronic inflammation.)

(3) Fibroblast formation.

(4) New blood vessels.

(5) Granulation tissue areas.

(6) Distortion of the glands ; exudate rarely seen.

Signs and Symptoms.—

(1) Leucorrhœa—from an associated cervical infection.

(2) Menstruation—in mild infection menstruation is unaffected, but in the more severe endometritis, according to Novak, the endometrial responsiveness to the ovarian hormones is impaired and abnormal menstrual rhythm or loss may occur.

(3) Sterility is common, and if pregnancy occurs, abortion is frequent.

Treatment.—

The downhill drainage from the uterus and the monthly desquamation of the endometrium are responsible for spontaneous cure in many cases.

(1) Uterine curettage may effect a cure ; (2) if very persistent, small doses of radium, 800–1,000 mgm. hours may be required ; (3) if patient over forty years, an artificial menopause may be produced by radium, 1,800–2,400 mgm. hours, or by X-rays ; (4) in some cases, hysterectomy may be necessary.

Senile Endometritis.—

This is a form of Chronic Interstitial Endometritis.

(1) Occurs usually many years after the menopause, and is predisposed to by the altered vaginal flora.

(2) Endometrium is thin; infiltrated with round and plasma cells; shows patches of squamous metaplasia; shows surface ulceration.

(3) Uterus is small with thin and atrophic walls.

(4) There is slight bleeding and foul-smelling purulent discharge.

(5) Stenosis of the cervix may follow desquamation of the epithelium, leading to pyometra.

(6) Diagnose from cancer of the body of the uterus by microscopic examination of scrapings.

Treatment.—

The cervix is dilated and, if pyometra is present, the uterine cavity should be swabbed out with some antiseptic and may be drained for several days by the intra-uterine injection of glycerine. The uterus may then be curetted.

Tuberculous Endometritis.—

This condition is another example of chronic interstitial endometritis, but invasion may occur into subjacent muscular tissue.

(1) Infection almost always from the tubes; very rarely a blood-borne infection from the lungs.

(2) Cullen has described small yellowish areas in the mucosa near one or other cornu.

(3) Endometrium thickened; glands proliferate and enlarge; small round cells, giant cell systems and areas of caseation are present.

(4) Uterus usually slightly enlarged.

(5) Enlarged tubes may be felt.

(6) May cause no symptoms except sterility, but usually leucorrhœa and menorrhagia are present. In some cases amenorrhœa or oligomenorrhœa occur.

(7) Diagnosis is made by microscopic examination of uterine scrapings.

Treatment.—

If the only evidence of tuberculous infection is that discovered by curettage, treatment should follow the lines of a sanatorium regime. Should there be evidence of pelvic tuberculosis, *e.g.* enlarged tubes, with no evidence of a pulmonary lesion, operation should be undertaken and the uterus and tubes removed.

Streptomycin 1–2 gm. daily may prove beneficial.

Chronic Metritis

According to Fletcher Shaw, chronic metritis accounts for only 1 per cent. of all cases of enlargement of the uterus associated with uterine bleeding. Usually results from puerperal or gonococcal infection.

Pathology.—

(1) Fibrous tissue excessive. Muscle much diminished. Elastic tissue unchanged.

(2) Round and plasma cell infiltration.

(3) Chronic interstitial endometritis is often present.

(4) Endometrium is thin.

(5) Uterus is enlarged; thickness of wall is twice the normal.

Symptoms.—

(1) Menorrhagia.

(2) An inter-menstrual dragging pain in the lower abdomen and back, probably due to the weight of the enlarged uterus.

(3) Leucorrhœa from an associated endometritis and cervicitis.

Treatment.—

Curettage for diagnostic purposes. Rarely curative.

Intrauterine radium, 1,800–2,400 mgm. hours or X-ray if patient over forty years; in a younger woman hysterectomy with conservation of one or both ovaries, may be required.

Chronic Subinvolution—Fibrosis Uteri

This condition is associated with puerperal infection, retained products and retroversion following childbirth. Goodall and Fletcher Shaw believe that subinvolution is characterised by an excess of elastic and fibrous tissue; Wilfrid Shaw, on the other hand, considers the amount of elastic tissue to be dependent on parity and attributes the large uterus of subinvolution to a delayed involution of the muscle cells.

Pathology.—

(1) Elastic tissue excessive, especially round blood vessels and between muscle bundles. Fibrous tissue excessive. Muscle much diminished.

(2) New vessels formed in lumina of old.

(3) Endometrium in early stage is thickened, but later becomes atrophic.

(4) Uterus is enlarged and hard.

Symptoms and Treatment.—

Similar to chronic metritis.

CERVICITIS

Lacerations of the cervix at childbirth predispose to cervical infection, but they may not necessarily be present. The infection may be acute, occurring after childbirth or gonorrhœal exposure, but is more usually chronic.

1. Inflammation of the cervical mucous membrane results in—

(*a*) Round and plasma cell infiltration beneath the columnar epithelium and around the glands.

(*b*) The columnar epithelium proliferates.

2. There is desquamation of the epithelium on the vaginal surface, usually adjacent to the external os, with the formation of an ulcer. This area is later covered by a downgrowth of the columnar epithelium to give the appearances of a true **erosion.** This must be differentiated from eversion of the edges of a cervical laceration exposing the reddened mucous membrane of the cervical canal.

The same pathological changes take place when infection occurs in a deep laceration of the cervix, the edges becoming everted and exposed to the acid vaginal secretion.

Characters of an Erosion.—

(*a*) A single layer of columnar epithelium under which are aggregations of inflammatory cells.

(*b*) A tendency to heal, the squamous cells replacing the columnar. Nabothian follicles are produced by this process of cure, the squamous epithelium and contracting fibrous tissue closing the mouths of the glands.

Clinical Features.—

1. Leucorrhœa—white to yellow, very tenacious and often irritating to the skin; most profuse before and after a period.

2. Pain in the lower abdomen and back, worse before and during menstruation.

3. There may be frequency and dysuria from a spread of infection to the bladder.

4. There may be menorrhagia from an associated endometritis.

5. Chronic ill-health, *e.g.* rheumatoid arthritis, etc.

On Examination.—

1. Redness and swelling of the cervical mucous membrane.
2. Velvet-like to the touch.
3. Occasionally slight bleeding on touch but no friability.
4. External os often patulous.
5. Mucous polypi may be attached to the margin of the external os.
6. Cervix thickened with, in long-standing cases, the presence of Nabothian follicles.
7. Production of pain by moving the cervix and so stretching the infected pelvic cellular tissue.

Diagnosis.—

1. From tuberculosis of the cervix which gives a dull red coloration, is softer, more velvety and bleeds more readily.
2. From syphilis—other manifestations of syphilis are present.
3. From cancer which is friable and bleeds freely, while the cervix is dull red in colour, hard and irregular. If any doubt exists, a cervical biopsy must be carried out.

Treatment.—It is only in early cases that success obtains by a course of vaginal douching (1/5000 perchloride of mercury) and ichthyol and glycerine tamponage.

Dilatation of the cervix, cauterisation of the endocervix and erosion with the thermo-cautery yield excellent results; diathermy is satisfactory in gonorrhœal infection.

A torn cervix may be repaired.

Where the cervix is hypertrophied, amputation of the cervix or a conical excision of the eroded area and lower half of the endocervix may be done.

Occasionally pan-hysterectomy may prove necessary.

Tuberculosis of Cervix (Rare)

1. May occur in multiparæ or nulliparæ.
2. Usually associated with tuberculosis of uterus and tubes.
3. May occur in vaginal portion of cervix, in canal or together.

4. Types.—
   (*a*) Ulcerative—single or multiple ulcers round os.
   (*b*) Proliferative—papillary outgrowths round external os giving a dark red appearance and velvety feel.

5. Cause vaginal discharge often tinged with blood, or slight bleeding.
6. Diagnose from cancer and syphilis by microscopical examination.
7. Treated by pan-hysterectomy, especially if tubes and uterus involved; if cervix alone is involved, a high amputation may suffice.

VAGINA

Acute Vaginitis

(*a*) Puerperal.—

Usually follows acute endometritis or may be due to septic tears.

Mucosa swollen and small ulcers are often present.

Discharge is excessive and is usually purulent and later fœtid.

Dysuria and dyschezia as condition progresses.

Treatment.—Syringe vagina frequently with alum solution (ʒi to pint). Cauterise any ulcers present with silver nitrate or pure carbolic acid.

(*b*) Non-puerperal.—

Inflammation is very rarely primary on account of (1) the lactic acid bacillus, (2) the absence of glands and (3) the many-layered squamous epithelium. It is usually secondary, therefore, and is due to the vaginal discharge being made less acid by discharge from above, or to the epithelium becoming sodden for some cause, or being subjected to pressure by an ill-fitting pessary, when the barrier against infection is broken down. Some organisms such as trichomonas or monilia, however, seem to infect the vagina in spite of physiological protection.

Causes.—

1. Gonococci, streptococci, trichomonas vaginalis or yeast (monilia).
2. Misfitting pessaries and foreign bodies.
3. Too frequent, too strong or too hot douching.

4. Threadworms in children.
5. Fistulæ, necrotic and malignant tumour growths.

Clinical Features.—

1. Throbbing pain and burning heat.
2. Dysuria.
3. Mucous membrane is red and roughened.
4. Surface tender and papillæ may bleed.
5. Vulvitis is usually present as well.

Treatment.—Douching in acute stage with alum (ʒi to pint), then lactic acid pessaries.

Pathological Vaginal Discharges (Leucorrhœa)

Causes.—

1. May come from the vagina, cervix, uterus, tube, bladder, rectum, urethra, peritoneal cavity, or cellular tissue.
2. May be due to gono-, strepto-, staphylo-, or pneumococcus, Bacillus coli or diphtheriæ, the vaginal bacillus being absent and the discharge less acid.
3. May be due to trichomonas vaginalis or yeast (monilia) infection (see p. 89).
4. May be non-infective, due to general causes.
5. May be due to constipation—usually offensive.

Types.—

(*a*) *Leucorrhœal.*—
1. Normal excess, especially pre- and post-menstrually.
2. Due to congestion caused by pregnancy.
3. Anæmia or bad general health.
4. Vaginitis (chronic).

(*b*) *Ropy and mucoid*—endocervitis and erosions.

(*c*) *Purulent.*—
1. Vaginitis (acute or subacute).
2. Pelvic abscess.
3. Endometritis (senile).
4. Pyometra.
5. Senile vaginitis.
6. Gonorrhœa.

(*d*) *Offensive.*—
1. Ulcerated malignant tumour, *e.g.* cancer of cervix.
2. Neglected pessary.

3. Local uterine infection following labour or incomplete abortion.
4. Sloughing submucous fibroid.

(*e*) *Watery.*—
1. Ruptured cyst (vaginal).
2. Intermittent hydrosalpinx.
3. Tubal cancer.

(*f*) *Brown.*—
1. Carcinoma cervix.
2. Dead ovum (missed abortion).
3. Ectopic gestation (some cases with tubal mole).

(*g*) *Urinary*—from bladder or ureter.

(*h*) *Fœcal*—from rectum.

Physiology of Vagina

Vagina is kept clear of infection by the lactic acid bacillus (Döderlein's) which keeps the *p*H about 4·4 or less.

If Döderlein's bacillus is absent, then vagina becomes less acid, *p*H 4·8 to 6·8 and organisms can then flourish.

Döderlein's bacilli are activated by glycogen produced by the action of œstrone on the vaginal mucosa and thus in some cases (senile vaginitis) organisms get into vagina owing to atrophy of vaginal cells.

When treating cases of vaginal discharge the normal physiology should be kept in mind.

Occurrence of Discharge.

1. Before puberty.
2. During child-bearing period.
   (*a*) In married women.
   (*b*) In virgins.
3. After menopause.

1. Before puberty.—Rare.

May be due to—
(*a*) Gonorrhœa.
(*b*) Dirt.
(*c*) Threadworms.
(*d*) Irritation of vaginal mucosa.

Vaginal cells inactive and no Döderlein bacilli present to resist infection.

Treat with œstrogenic pessaries and small doses œstrogen or sulphathiazole orally.

2. During child-bearing period.—
   (*a*) In married women.

(1) Due to infection by streptococci, diphtheroids, etc., causing an excess of white secretion, which may occur only before or after period, or become constant and profuse.

Treatment.—

(i) In milder cases—

(*a*) Lactic acid pessaries (one morning and evening).

(*b*) Lactic acid douching (1-500).

(*c*) Sour milk douching, diluted with equal part water.

(ii) In more severe cases—make vagina sterile by insufflating daily with an inert powder, such as dermatol (bismuth subgallate and zinc oxide), subsequent to painting vagina with 2½ per cent. picric acid and thereafter swabbing dry. This prevents any organism thriving.

After about ten days' treatment, lactic acid pessaries or sugar pessaries, consisting of lactose, glucose and boric acid āā gr. v, can be inserted to encourage growth of lactic acid bacillus, thus preventing further infection.

(2) Due to Infection by **Trichomonas Vaginalis.**

The Trichomonas is an oval flagellate organism which moves by amœboid movements and by means of its flagellæ (Plate II). It can readily be seen microscopically in an ordinary vaginal smear, in a hanging drop slide or in a smear stained with Leishman's stain.

It is not known where the infection comes from in first instance, but re-infection may occur from organisms under prepuce of penis or from prostate, the husband being infected by wife and harbouring organisms.

Trichomonas are smallest, most active and numerous, at end of menstrual period and probably multiply at that time.

Clinical Features.—

(*a*) Either mottled or general redness of vaginal mucosa and vaginal portion of cervix.

(*b*) Thin yellow frothy discharge with characteristic odour.

(*c*) May cause irritation of vulva and inside of thighs.

(*d*) May cause great discomfort, soreness and irritation.

Treatment.—

(*a*) Dry vagina thoroughly and insufflate with picragol powder (silver picrate) or stovarsol vaginal compound powder.

(*b*) Insert one picragol pessary or two (or more) stovarsol pessaries nightly for a week.

(*c*) Repeat insufflation.

(*d*) This routine may have to be continued for 3 to 4 weeks to effect a cure and is best followed by course of sugar pessaries to stimulate growth of Döderlein's bacilli.

(*e*) Milder cases, may be treated with stovarsol or devegan pessaries alone, two to be inserted twice daily to begin with and then gradually decrease dose.

(3) Due to monilia (yeast) infection. (See p. 89.)

(*b*) In virgins.

(1) May be due to general condition, *e.g.* anæmia, etc. Take *p*H of secretion and if 4·4 or under then not due to infection, so treat general condition.

(2) May be due to constipation. Discharge slightly offensive. Treat constipation.

(3) May be due to *Congenital Erosion of Cervix.*

This is a circular erosion around external os due to overgrowth of columnar epithelium and causes a mucous secretion from cervix, which is prevented exit by intact hymen.

Causes irritation of vaginal mucosa, and vaginal discharge, which sooner or later seeps over hymen to give rise to continuous whitish-yellow discharge.

Probably commonest cause of discharge in girls from 16 to 18 years.

Treated by cauterisation of erosion and, if hymen is very tight, by excision of hymen and perineotomy, so as to allow free drainage.

(4) The discharge may be due rarely to trichomonas or monilia.

3. After Menopause.

(1) **Senile Vaginitis.**—Due to atrophy of vaginal cells and absence of Döderlein's bacilli, so that any infective organism can gain entrance into vagina.

Clinical Features.—

(*a*) Purulent discharge, sometimes blood-stained and offensive.

(*b*) Reddening of vaginal mucosa and vaginal cervix, usually mottling.

(*c*) May be associated with kraurosis and give symptoms of discomfort, irritation and sometimes dysuria.

Treatment.—

Intensive œstrogenic therapy. Stilbœstrol, or its equivalent, (see p. 354), 5 mgm. twice daily for 10 to 14 days, and œstrone pessaries one daily from fourth to fourteenth days.

Œstradial benzoate, 50,000 I.B.U., can be given twice weekly for five injections, and 1,000 I.U. œstrone thrice daily orally instead of stilbœstrol.

(*N.B.*—**If discharge is tinged with blood, or if it does not clear up quickly with œstrogenic therapy, or should it recur after the treatment is over, then uterus must be curetted as discharge may be due to, or be present along with, a carcinoma of the body of the uterus.)**

(2) Infections by trichomonas and monilia are treated as already described, but some œstrogenic therapy should be given, after cure is effected, to prevent recurrence.

Tuberculosis of Vagina (Very Rare)

1. Usually accompanies tuberculosis of cervix.
2. May follow tears at labour.
3. Miliary or ulcerative.
4. Fistulæ may form in ulcerative type.
5. Causes discharge, possibly stained with blood.
6. Pruritus and often dysuria.
7. Treatment difficult. Excision if possible. Radiotherapy.

VULVA

Acute Vulvitis

(*a*) *Puerperal.*—

Usually follows acute endometritis or may be due to septic tears.

Mucosa swollen and small ulcers are often present.

Discharge excessive and is usually purulent and later fœtid.

Dysuria and dyschezia as condition progresses.

Treatment.—Syringe vagina frequently with alum solution (ʒi to pint). Cauterise any ulcers present with silver nitrate or pure carbolic acid.

(*b*) *Non-puerperal.*—

May be gonorrhœal, rarely tuberculous, gangrenous or diphtheritic in origin. Filth or irritating fluids may be underlying cause. Often associated with vaginitis due to trichomonal or monilial discharge. In all cases of vulvitis the urine should be examined for sugar.

Treatment.—This should aim at removal of the cause. General antiseptic measures.

Tuberculosis of Vulva (Very Rare)

1. Usually occurs as small ulcers.
2. Causes pruritus, discharge and, sometimes, dysuria.
3. Prognosis bad.
4. Treated by excision of vulva.

CHAPTER XVI

DISPLACEMENTS OF THE UTERUS

(A.) FORWARD (ANTEFLEXION)

THE normal position of the uterus is anteversion, but in some cases anteflexion exists, which may cause symptoms.

Ætiology.—

1. *Congenital.*—The uterus is usually not well developed and this is often associated with a conical cervix and pinhole os. (See " Dysmenorrhœa," p. 286.)

2. *Pathological.*—Due to chronic inflammation of the utero-sacral ligaments—*chronic utero-sacral cellulitis*—which, being shortened, pull the isthmus uteri back, thus causing marked anteversion.

Congenital.—

Symptoms.—

1. Spasmodic dysmenorrhœa (first day of the period) due often to weak musculature of the uterus.
2. Scanty menstruation.
3. Sterility.

Treatment.—Dilate the cervix. (Pregnancy cures the condition.)

Chronic Utero-sacral Cellulitis.—

Probably two types.—

1. Due to a spasm of the unstriate muscle fibres in the cellular tissue of the ligaments. This spasm results from irritation caused by an endocervicitis and, though it is most common in parous women, it is frequently present in nulliparæ. When the patient is examined under anæsthesia the tenseness of the ligaments disappears; when patient is examined vaginally without anæsthesia, the ligaments are tense and there is marked tenderness (Young).

(*N.B.*—These cases may therefore not be discovered, if examination is carried out only under an anæsthetic.)

2. True utero-sacral cellulitis; caused by tears or punctures of cervix, being similar to other pelvic cellulitis. Ligaments tense when examined with or without anæsthesia.

Clinical Features.—

Constant backache and often iliac-ache, with premenstrual exacerbations.

Viscid leucorrhœal discharge, worst pre- and post-menstrually.

Abdominally.—Tender spot or spots about one inch below and lateral to umbilicus, there being no tenderness elsewhere (Young).

Per Vaginam.—The uterus is anteverted, often acutely.

Great tenderness on movement of cervix.

Very tender and tense ligaments running back from cervix. (Often only one ligament is affected.)

Treatment.—

Type 1. Dilatation and cauterisation of cervix to cure endocervicitis and thus remove the causal factor. The cure in such cases is immediate.

Type 2. Dilatation and cauterisation of cervix. This removes focus of infection and cures some cases; others require a local anæsthetic such as proctocaine (4 c.c.), injected postero-laterally into cervix to reach ganglia; should pain still persist a course of douching and plugging or diathermy, or both, may be required. These may have to be given at intervals for several months to obtain softening of ligaments and absorption of cellulitis.

(*N.B.*—Some cases resist all such conservative treatment and become chronic invalids with constant backache and associated pelvic pain. In such cases, if over thirty-five years and multiparous, pan-hysterectomy may be required to produce an effective cure: if under thirty-five years or anxious to have children, presacral sympathectomy will give patient freedom from pain, and conception and labour are not interfered with.)

(B.) BACKWARD

(Includes Retroversion and Retroflexion)

In Retroversion there is no angle between body and cervix.

In Retroflexion there is distinct angle between body and cervix.

(*a*) **Ætiology.**—

A. *Congenital.*—Occurs in about 20 per cent. of healthy women and produces no symptoms. This is due to a congenital error in development, the genital cord being placed in front of, instead of in the axis of the pelvis, and thus the uterus and vagina lie closer to the symphysis. When growth occurs at puberty, there is no room for the body of the uterus in front and so it has to incline backwards.

Usually causes no symptoms, but if retroflexion is present, dysmenorrhœa may occur as in acute anteflexion, and is treated similarly, but, in some cases, reposition and insertion of a pessary are required as well. Sterility may occur owing to cervix lying too far forwards and upwards, the spermatozoa being unable to gain entrance. If pregnancy does occur in such a displaced uterus, early reposition is essential to prevent possible abortion or incarceration.

B. *Acquired.*—

1. Mechanical—relaxation of the uterine supports, often associated with prolapse.

A retroverted uterus is more liable to prolapse because—

(1) It derives no support from the bladder and surrounding fascia.

(2) The long axis of the uterus is in the long axis of the vagina.

(3) As the lower segment of the uterus lies forward in the pelvis, the essential ligaments are stretched and are thus not so strong; thus when a greater strain occurs, they are not fit for it, and prolapse occurs. Thus a retroverted uterus is more liable to displacement by prolapse, and it is from the descent that symptoms occur.

A prolapsed uterus nearly always becomes retroverted, even if anteverted before, because the utero-sacral ligaments are stretched, and this allows the cervix to pass forwards as well as downwards. As it passes forwards, the fundus must go backwards, the ligaments yielding, owing to increased strain.

2. Puerperal—

(*a*) Subinvolution.

(*b*) Lying in bed for a long period after labour, the heavy uterus gravitating backwards if any tendency to this condition be present.

3. Inflammatory—pelvic peritonitis—the uterus being pulled back by adhesions.

4. Tumours—a fibroid in the posterior wall may cause the uterus to fall backwards, or large tumour may lie in front and displace uterus backwards.

(*b*) **Symptoms.**—

1. *May cause none whatever per se,* but if any prolapse is present—

2. Pain, usually backache, due to irritation of the fourth sacral nerve, or a dragging pain in the iliac regions.

(*N.B.*—If severe, usually denotes adhesions.)

3. Dysmenorrhœa (menstrual) often present, when there is congestion, or (premenstrual) when the ovaries are prolapsed and œdematous.

4. Menorrhagia and leucorrhœa due to an accompanying chronic interstitial endometritis and endocervicitis. This is caused by an impeded return of venous blood, due to pressure on the veins by the utero-sacral ligaments owing to the descent.

5. May cause sterility, dyspareunia and constipation, the sterility being due to the position of the external os or to the endometritis, and the dyspareunia resulting from the prolapsed ovaries, especially if they are congested. If pregnancy occurs, abortion is frequent.

(*c*) **Signs.**—

1. The cervix points forwards and the external os looks forwards and downwards.

2. With the fingers in the posterior fornix the uterus is felt bimanually, nothing being felt by the fingers in the anterior fornix.

3. If difficult to feel, the uterus can be made out by one finger in the rectum, one in the vagina, and the other hand on the abdomen, the body being felt either between the fingers in the vagina and rectum or between the finger in rectum and the hand on the abdomen.

(*N.B.*—Per rectum, be careful not to mistake the supravaginal part of the cervix for the uterine body.)

4. If the ovaries are prolapsed, oval tender bodies are felt in the postero-lateral fornices to the side of or below the uterus.

Treatment.—

None unless causing symptoms.

Always study general conditions and not pelvis alone. Treat bowels.

Pessary

1. During early pregnancy to prevent possible abortion or incarceration.
2. Sterility.
3. Puerperium. Curative often, if inserted four to six weeks after delivery.
4. Pessary test. To see if replacement cures the symptoms.
5. Operation contra-indicated for some reason or other.

Pessary Contra-indicated—
1. Adherent retroversions.
2. With inflammation of the ovary or tube, or parametritis.
3. Future medical care not available.
4. Tender prolapsed ovaries.

Operative

1. When pessary test cures symptoms, which recur after removal of pessary.
2. When other abdominal operation is required, *e.g.* appendicectomy, salpingo-oöphorectomy, etc.
3. When uterus is so large and heavy that pessary is useless.
4. When associated with severe menorrhagia near menopause. (Hysterectomy required in such a case.)
5. When manual replacement impossible.

If menorrhagia due to endometritis be present, the uterus must be curetted before either pessary or operative treatment.

Pessary Treatment.—

(*a*) *Replacement of Uterus.*

1. Put patient in left lateral position and pass two fingers into posterior fornix; push uterus beyond promontory of sacrum.

2. Turn patient on to back and (1) keep on pressing upwards with second finger in posterior fornix, (2) push cervix backwards with first finger in front of cervix and (3) bring body of uterus forward by grasping fundus with other hand through abdominal wall.

(*b*) *Insertion of Pessary.*

1. Pull back perineum with finger of one hand.

2. Insert pessary in long axis of vulval inlet.

3. When two-thirds inserted turn pessary clockwise to a right angle and push in further. (The upper end now lies in front of cervix.)

4. Hook forefinger over upper bar and withdraw bar until it can be pushed up behind cervix into posterior fornix. (The anterior bar should lie against anterior vaginal wall just behind the symphysis pubis.)

Pessary acts by distending posterior fornix and keeping utero-sacral ligaments taut, which in turn keep uterus in anteverted position.

Essentials for Pessary Treatment.—

1. Must keep the uterus in position.
2. Must not cause discomfort or any urinary dysfunction.
3. Should be worn for three months and then be removed. If symptoms recur after being absent when wearing pessary, then operative treatment should be advised. (*Pessary test.*)
4. Patient should douche, when pessary is in situ, if any discharge occurs.

Operative Treatment.—Ventro-suspension of the uterus by means of tightening the round ligaments. A very large number of such operations have been devised, but the most generally performed in this country are: *Gilliam's Operation* or modifications; the *Sling Operation* (Baldy-Webster), the last named being of especial use if the ovaries are prolapsed (see p. 367).

If prolapse requires treatment the uterus can be retained in a position of anteversion by means of Fothergill's operation,

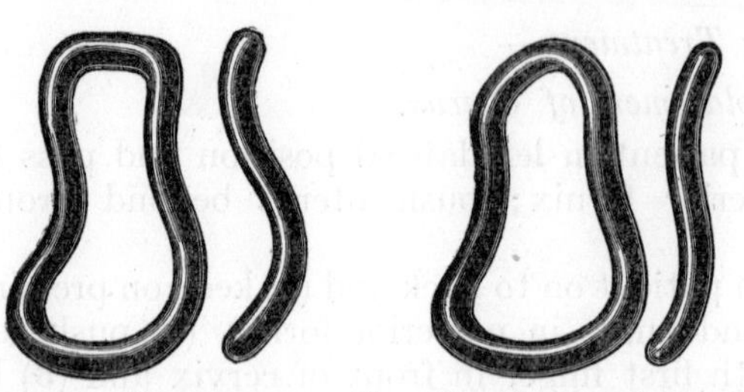

Fig. 27.—Hodge Pessary. Fig. 28.—Albert-Smith Pessary.

the uterus being replaced before the uppermost cervico-vaginal stitch is tied; this brings the transverse cervical ligaments across in front of the cervix and keeps uterus in position (see p. 370).

(C.) PROLAPSE AND RECTOCELE

Definition.—Displacement in part or in whole of the displaceable portion of the pelvic floor (*i.e.* the uterus, bladder, urethra and vagina with the connective tissue), past the fixed portion (*i.e.* the pelvic diaphragm, muscles of the sphincter layer, fascia, fat and skin).

Cause.—

1. *Of Cystocele and Prolapse.*

(*a*) Usually due to excessive involution of the musculo-connective tissue accompanying the vessels, nerves, etc., to the sides of the cervix, bladder and vagina, causing atrophy and degeneration, especially of the unstriate muscle (Fothergill), *i.e.* degeneration of cardinal ligaments of cervix, pubo-vesical ligaments, etc.

This may follow labour, but more commonly takes place at the menopause, when the atrophic ligaments have to contend with increased intra-abdominal pressure due to fat formation, or possibly bronchitis, lifting heavy weights, etc.

(*b*) May be due to excessive bruising, tearing, or prolonged distension of the vagina, cervix and lower uterine segment during labour, the ligaments becoming stretched and degeneration occurring.

(*N.B.*—Often due to mismanagement of labour, *e.g.* application of the forcep before cervix is fully dilated, allowing patient to bear down before cervix is fully dilated or allowing head to be held up for a long time on the perineum with patient having strong pains.)

Prolapse then occurs in post-natal period, and a definite herniation may develop.

The following factors aid prolapse, but do not cause it :—

(*a*) Perineal tears, as they make the descent easier.

(*b*) Retroversion of the uterus.

Pelvic cellulitis and perimetritis prevent prolapse by causing adhesions, fibrous thickening and contraction of the pelvic cellular tissue.

2. *Of Rectocele.*—

(*a*) Torn perineum with infection.

(*b*) Inflammation causes adhesions between the anterior rectal wall and the posterior vaginal wall.

(*c*) With constant straining at defæcation on account of (*b*) the rectal wall is unable to slide upward over the fæcal mass, and is thrust into the vagina (Fothergill).

Types.—

1. *Cystocele.*—

(*a*) The anterior vaginal wall, with the urethra and part of the bladder, bulges into the vagina.

(*b*) The uterus is usually anteverted.

(*c*) On bearing down, the uterus remains anteverted, but the anterior vaginal wall everts from below upwards.

2. *Prolapsus Uteri.*—

Stage 1.—

(*a*) Cystocele accompanied by a downward movement of the uterus on down-bearing.

(*b*) The uterus is nearly always retroverted.

(*c*) As the cervix descends, the posterior wall is inverted from above downwards.

Stage 2.—

(*a*) The cervix is seen at the vulva.

(*b*) The anterior fornix is obliterated due to complete eversion of the anterior vaginal wall.

(*c*) The posterior fornix is shortened, and the junction with the cervix is on the perineum.

Stage 3.—

(*a*) *Complete procidentia*, the vagina being turned inside out and lying outside the vulva with external os at apex of prolapsed mass.

(*b*) The inverted vagina contains the uterus with appendages, urethra, part of the bladder, and maybe small intestine.

(*c*) The rectum does not prolapse, unless rectocele is present.

(*d*) The posterior vaginal wall inverts from above downwards, and the posterior fornix, as well as the anterior, is obliterated.

(*e*) Cervix is elongated, especially the supra-vaginal portion, owing to excessive traction. Cavity may measure 5 to 6 in. from external os to fundus.

(*f*) Vaginal walls or cervix may ulcerate or, if procidentia is of long duration, keratinisation may occur.

3. *Hypertrophy of the Supra-vaginal Portion of the Cervix associated with Inversion of Vaginal Vault.*—

(*a*) The cervix comes down to the vulva with or without straining.

(*b*) The anterior and posterior fornices are shortened by inversion, but are still present.

(*c*) There is no cystocele.

(*d*) The uterus is enlarged, due to elongation of the supravaginal cervix, and is retroverted.

(*e*) Both vaginal walls may be totally inverted, and thus resemble procidentia. Diagnose by replacing the prolapse and telling the patient to bear down, when the cervix will appear at the vulva first, and not the everted anterior vaginal wall, as in the more common prolapse.

4. *Rectocele.*—
   (*a*) May or may not be associated with prolapse.
   (*b*) There is bulging of the posterior vaginal wall on straining, it being everted from below upwards and, should the condition occur with any form of prolapse, it is accompanied by inversion of the upper end of the vagina from above down.
   (*c*) The pouch contains the rectum, the anterior rectal wall adhering to the posterior vaginal wall.
   (*d*) The perineum is deficient.

When the perineum is completely torn, the patient does not strain at stool, and thus a rectocele never results.

(1), (2), and (4) practically always occur in parous women. (3) usually occurs in parous women, but is not rare in nulliparæ.

Clinical Features.—

1. *Cystocele.*—
   (*a*) Feeling of " something coming down."
   (*b*) Frequency of micturition.
   (*c*) Cystitis from residual urine causing increased frequency and dysuria (late).
   (*d*) Incontinence of urine on coughing, etc., due to loss of tone of the involuntary bladder sphincter and loss of support of the pubo-coccygeus muscle which has been damaged at a previous labour (*exertion or stress incontinence*). This condition may occur with urethrocele only and without cystocele formation.

2. *Prolapse.*—

   Stage 1.—
   (*a*) The symptoms of cystocele.
   (*b*) Dragging pain (often), worse on walking and relieved by rest.

   Stage 2.—
   (*a*) As for Stage 1.
   (*b*) Leucorrhœa.

Stage 3.—
(*a*) The inverted vagina hangs between thighs.
(*b*) The vagina becomes hard, excoriated and sometimes ulcerated, as also does the cervix.
(*c*) Congestion and œdema may occur.
(*d*) Difficulty in walking.
(*e*) The urinary symptoms often improve, but retention may occur.
(*f*) Leucorrhœa and, if ulcerated, blood-stained discharge.

3. *Hypertrophy of the Supra-vaginal Cervix.*—
(*a*) A feeling of discomfort in the vagina and of "something coming down."
(*b*) The cervix may be excoriated, ulcerated and œdematous.
(*c*) Leucorrhœa.
(*d*) No urinary symptoms.

4. *Rectocele.*—
(*a*) Backache.
(*b*) A feeling of loss of support in the perineum.
(*c*) Constipation is common, great straining being required for defæcation.

Diagnosis.—

1. Is usually easy, but it may be difficult in the lying position, as the erect posture exaggerates the displacement; on lying down, even on down-bearing, it may be hardly perceptible in some cases.

2. Tell the patient to bear down, and examine vaginally for—
(*a*) Cystocele, bulging of the anterior vaginal wall from below upwards.
(*b*) Descent of the cervix (1) with cystocele; (2) with inversion of the anterior and posterior walls from above downwards.
(*c*) The length of the cervix, vaginal and supra-vaginal portions.
(*d*) Rectocele, bulging of the posterior vaginal wall from below upwards.

3. A cyst on the anterior vaginal wall might be mistaken for a cystocele, but it is readily diagnosed by noting that a bladder sound does not pass into it.

4. Inversion of the uterus is excluded by feeling (1) the external os and (2) the fundus of the uterus.

5. Enterocele—put a finger in the rectum and another into the vagina. Bring the fingers together, when the intestine will escape into the abdomen with a gurgling noise.

Treatment.—

1. A ring pessary, preferably vulcanite, may be used during pregnancy (Fig. 29), if the patient refuses or is unsuited for operation, or in the post-natal period when the tone of the unstriate muscle is being restored by cold douching. A Hodge pessary, with a special double horizontal bar in front, is useful in cases of cystocele, when operation is contra-indicated.

The pessary must be changed every four months if vulcanite, every two months if rubber and douching must be practised frequently, when a rubber ring is in situ. Ulceration must always be looked for when changing the pessary and, if present, the pessary should be removed.

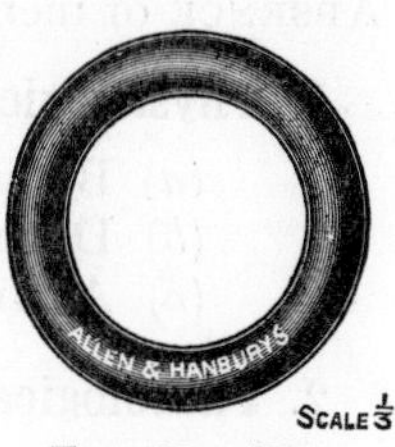

FIG. 29.—RING PESSARY.

2. **Operative** (see p. 369).

Cystocele.—Anterior colporrhaphy, with perineorrhaphy if necessary.

Prolapse.—Anterior colporrhaphy, amputation of part of the hypertrophied cervix, correcting retroversion if required and posterior colporrhaphy and perineorrhaphy.

Elongation of the Cervix with Inversion of the Vagina from Above Downwards.—Amputation of the cervix and obliteration of anterior fornix. Perineorrhaphy if necessary.

Rectocele.—Posterior colporrhaphy and perineorrhaphy.

(*N.B.—Abdominal operations for prolapse, either as an adjunct to the vaginal operation or by themselves, are practically never required, the vaginal operation alone effecting a cure in every case.*)

When a prolapse is associated with menorrhagia, especially near the menopause, a combined vaginal hysterectomy with a pelvic floor repair (Mayo's operation) may be the operation of choice.

Stress Incontinence.—Tightening of bladder sphincter. Various sling operations, *viz.* Millin-Read and Aldridge operations.

CHAPTER XVII

DISORDERS OF MENSTRUATION

1. AMENORRHŒA

ABSENCE of menstruation.

1. **Physiological.**—

   (*a*) Before puberty.
   (*b*) During pregnancy and lactation.
   (*c*) At and after the menopause.

2. **Pathological.**—

   (*a*) *Apparent* (**Cryptomenorrhœa**).

Causes.—

(1) Imperforate hymen—the commonest cause.

(2) Congenital atresia, especially imperforation of the lower end of the vagina.

(3) Acquired atresia, due to tears at labour, sepsis, operations on the cervix, new growths, etc.

Clinical Features.—

(1) Usually none to start with, the case being looked upon as one of delayed puberty. Sometimes menstrual molimina occur, the symptoms becoming aggravated as more secretion accumulates.

(2) The first symptom is usually dysuria or retention of urine.

(3) A tumour can be felt abdominally and the hymen may bulge outwards (hæmatocolpos).

Prognosis.—If the obstruction is low down, the bulging membrane is incised and the retained fluid is allowed to escape. The prognosis in such cases is good.

If the atresia is at a higher level, in the upper vagina or cervix, hæmatometra and hæmatosalpinx are usually present. There is often irretrievable damage to the uterus and tubes which may necessitate their removal.

(*b*) *Actual.*—

(*a*) *Primary.*

Causes.—

(1) Absence or disease of the ovaries before puberty.
(2) Absence or under development of the uterus.
(3) Disease or removal of genital organs before puberty.
(4) Systemic disease, *e.g.* the anæmias.
(5) Unsuitable environment.
(6) Endocrine dysfunction.

(*b*) *Secondary.*

Causes.—

(1) Superinvolution of the uterus. This condition may follow obstetric shock, severe hæmorrhage or prolonged lactation and may be due to damage of the anterior pituitary (see p. 197).

(*N.B.*—The uterus is probably atrophied before the ovaries, as cessation of menstruation occurs before the menopausal symptoms.)

Clinical Signs.—(*a*) Uterine body only ¼ to ½ in. in length. (*b*) Mild menopausal symptoms.

Prognosis.—There is little or nothing that can be done to improve this condition.

(2) Removal of the uterus.
(3) X-rays or radium therapy.
(4) Disease or removal of the ovaries.
(5) Anæmia.
(6) Nervous-emotional strain or severe shock.
(7) Debilitating diseases, *e.g.* typhoid.
(8) Exposure to cold.
(9) Change of environment.
(10) Drugs, *e.g.* morphine or cocaine taken over a long time.
(11) Endocrine dysfunction.

A more perverted function is seen in—

(*a*) Myxœdema.
(*b*) Dystrophia adiposo-genitalis (anterior pituitary deficiency).
(*c*) Acromegaly (anterior pituitary excess).
(*d*) Tumours or hyperplasia of the adrenal cortex.

Treatment.—In some cases the cause may be a definite systemic lesion, and the treatment is then obvious. Benefit may follow attention to general hygiene, diet, non-specific thyroid therapy or X-ray stimulation of the pituitary or ovaries. There is more difficulty, however, when the fault is associated with endocrine deficiency. There are four main possibilities (Sturgis)—

1. *Uterine Amenorrhœa.*—Here the uterine endometrium is atrophic and is incapable of responding to ovarian stimulation. Normally, when œstrogen is given, there is growth of the endometrium and "withdrawal bleeding" some days after the course is stopped. If there is no such bleeding following twenty-one days of œstrogen therapy, the diagnosis of uterine amenorrhœa is established. A non-functioning endometrium follows radiation, and may result from uterine sepsis or disease as in tuberculosis. Menstrual bleeding cannot be induced in those circumstances by any form of treatment.

2. *Ovarian Amenorrhœa.*—The uterine endometrium is relatively inactive because the ovaries fail to respond to gonadotrophic stimulation with resulting deficient œstrogen production. Cessation of œstrogen production by the ovaries is associated with an immediate increase of FSH in the urine. Ovarian amenorrhœa is diagnosed therefore by (*a*) a consistently low level or complete absence of œstrogen, and (*b*) evidence of excessive gonadotrophic stimulation. It is important to differentiate between relative and absolute ovarian failure to produce œstrogen. If 5 mgm. progesterone be given intramuscularly daily for five days, bleeding should occur within seventy-two hours of the last dose if there has been any previous "priming" of the endometrium by œstrogen. There will be no bleeding in absolute ovarian failure. The menopause and ovarian aplasia are examples of such amenorrhœa. If the menopause is precocious and the patient disturbed from the pyschological aspect, monthly withdrawal bleeding can be induced by œstrogen therapy, 2 mgm. stilbœstrol being given daily for four weeks followed by one week without treatment. Where there is a congenital absence of the ovaries, œstrogen may be administered in a similar dosage.

3. *Pituitary Amenorrhœa.*—The amenorrhœa is due to a deficiency of gonadotrophic hormones. The diagnosis is made by determining that the endometrium can be activated by exhibition of œstrogen, by demonstrating a lack of œstrogen production as shown by absence of progesterone "withdrawal bleeding" and by showing a sub-normal level of FSH. Substitution therapy by gonadotrophic preparations is

unsatisfactory but for psychological reasons, "withdrawal bleeding" may be produced by œstrogen.

4. *Hypothalamic Amenorrhœa.*—Greep has shown that active œstrogen is produced only when FSH is supplemented by small amounts of LH, and it is believed that the release of LH from the pituitary is controlled by the hypothalamus. It is suggested, therefore, that in this group of cases there is a disturbance in the hypothalamic-pituitary pathway which prevents release of LH. The diagnosis is made by tests which show that (1) the endometrium is capable of responding to œstrogen; (2) the ovaries are not producing œstrogen (no progesterone withdrawal bleeding), and (3) the FSH is within normal limits. Hypothalamic amenorrhœa may be associated with organic lesions or psychogenic states. In the latter benefit may result from psychiatric investigation and reassurance; hormone therapy is of no value. In the opinion of one of us (C. K.) hormone therapy has proved unavailing in the treatment of amenorrhœa.

2. MENORRHAGIA

Excessive or prolonged flow or too frequent periods. May be due to—

General Causes.—

(*a*) Blood diseases, *e.g.* purpura, pernicious anæmia, etc.
(*b*) Conditions associated with hypertension.
(*c*) Mental derangement—mania.
(*d*) Hot climate.
(*e*) Myxœdema.
(*f*) Endocrine imbalance—ovulation occurs but the secretory phase of the cycle is shortened and there is incomplete progestational development of the endometrium. It is believed that in such cases there is a deficiency of progesterone, incomplete shedding of the endometrium and undue prolongation of a heavy menstrual loss.

Local Causes.—

Conditions which increase pelvic congestion tend to menorrhagia.
(*a*) Infection of the uterus and appendages.
(*b*) Chronic endometritis, metritis and sub-involution.
(*c*) Uterine fibroids—interstitial and sub-mucous types.

(*d*) Uterine adenomyosis.

(*e*) Uterine displacement—in certain cases of retroversion with prolapse, endometritis may also be present.

(*f*) Metropathia hæmorrhagica associated with follicular cysts of the ovary—here the usual history is one of metrorrhagia, but in some patients there may be menorrhagia.

Menorrhagia of Puberty.—

Usually coincides with the onset of menstruation. The bleeding may be continuous or the periods frequent and prolonged.

Causes.—We have seen that menorrhagia is associated with incomplete development of the corpus luteum, a deficiency of progesterone and a slow shedding of the endometrium. Hypothyroidism or blood dyscrasia may, however, be the cause.

Treatment.—Where no organic lesion can be demonstrated, hormone therapy may be tried as follows (Bishop) :—

1. The œstrogen level can be raised above the "bleeding threshold" by—

(*a*) 0·15 mgm. ethinyl œstradiol every two hours.

(*b*) Injections of œstradiol benzoate 100,000 I.U. every four to six hours.

Such a concentrated course is reserved for cases where there is very severe loss, and the bleeding should be controlled within twenty-four hours.

2. Where the endometrium has been primed beforehand by œstrogen, bleeding of a metropathic type can be prevented by giving at four-weekly intervals progesterone—25 mgm. by injection on alternate days for four doses or 30 mgm. ethisterone orally daily for one week. There is the chance with such treatment that menstruation may assume normality.

3. When the bleeding is less severe androgens, by antagonising both ovarian hormones, may prove successful. Methyl testosterone 10 mgm. daily, is advised for two months. A month's interval should elapse before the next course, if necessary, is begun. (The authors consider that this dose may produce virilising changes and recommend 5 mgm. daily instead.)

4. In very severe cases resort may have to be made to curettage, but in the adolescent girl it is obvious that more radical measures must, if possible, be avoided.

Menorrhagia of the Menopause.—

Causes.—

1. Cancer, fibroids, adenomatous polypi.
2. Chronic metritis and subinvolution.
3. Adenomyosis of uterus.
4. Endocrine imbalance.

Treatment.—Where obvious pathology is present the treatment is straightforward. Where no such lesion is demonstrable, the cause very probably lies in dysfunction of the pituitary-ovarian relationship. At this time of life there is not the same argument for a conservative outlook and treatment may resolve into—

1. Curettage.
2. Hysterectomy—including, as a rule, bilateral removal of the appendages.
3. Radium 2,400 mgm. hours or X-ray therapy.

(*N.B.*—**If no definite cause is found for irregular bleeding at the menopause, a curettage is essential to exclude cancer.**)

3. METRORRHAGIA

Bleeding not connected with a period. Due to—

1. Threatened, inevitable, incomplete abortion or hyatidiform mole.
2. Ectopic gestation.
3. Tumours, etc., of the uterus.
   - (*a*) Submucous fibroid polypus.
   - (*b*) Mucous polypi.
   - (*c*) Carcinoma of the cervix or body.
   - (*d*) Chorionepithelioma.
   - (*e*) Sarcoma of the uterus.
   - (*f*) Chronic metritis (some cases).
4. Hyperpiesis (some cases).
5. Acute pyosalpinx (some cases).
6. Torsion of pedicle of ovarian cyst (some cases).
7. Granulosa-cell tumour of the ovary.

Treatment.—This consists in dealing with the primary cause.

Post-menopausal Hæmorrhage

In a series of 937 cases collected in Edinburgh, it was found that the frequency of the different causes of post-menopausal bleeding was as under :—

	Total.	Percentage.
1. Carcinoma of cervix	241	25·7
2. Undiagnosed ; ? ovarian dysfunction, including endometrial hyperplasia	144	15·4
3. Fibro-adenomatous polypi of body and cervix	114	12·2
4. Genital prolapse, including pessary and friction ulceration	97	10·4
5. Carcinoma of body of uterus	93	9·9
6. Fibromyoma of uterus	63	6·7
7. Malignant ovarian neoplasms	32	3·4
8. Cervicitis	32	3·4
9. Urethral caruncle	27	2·9
10. Benign ovarian neoplasms	20	2·1
11. Senile endometritis	20	2·1
12. Carcinoma of vulva	12	1·4
13. Carcinoma of vagina	12	1·4
14. Vaginitis	7	0·7
15. Malignant degeneration in uterine fibroid	5	0·5
16. Benign urethral conditions other than caruncle	4	0·4
17. Sarcoma of uterus	3	0·3
18. Extra-genital malignant conditions	3	0·3
19. Carcinoma of urethra	2	0·2
20. Tuberculous endometritis	2	0·2
21. Fibroma vaginæ	2	0·2
22. Adenomyoma of uterus	1	0·1
	937	99·9

It was interesting to note the percentage of benign and malignant cases, which was as follows :—

		Total.	Percentage.
937 cases	Benign	533	56·9
	Malignant	404	43·1

(*Edin. Obst. Soc Trans*, vol. liii.)

(Since these cases were collected, one of the authors has had two cases of post-menopausal bleeding due to scurvy.)

If no definite cause for post-menopausal bleeding, *e.g.* polypus, cervical carcinoma, etc., **is found, it is absolutely essential that the case be examined under an anæsthetic and the uterus curetted so as to exclude malignant disease of the uterus.** The curettage, besides being diagnostic, may also be curative, as a polypus of the body of the uterus may be removed. **This treatment should be adopted no matter how slight is the post-menopausal bleeding.**

4. DYSMENORRHŒA

Painful menstruation.

Two types are described : (1) primary, essential, intrinsic, idiopathic, functional or spasmodic ; (2) secondary, acquired, extrinsic or congestive.

1. **Primary Dysmenorrhœa.**—

Clinical Picture.—The pain begins at puberty or in the years that follow. It is situated in the lower abdomen and radiates to the back and thighs. It is sharp, colicky and begins a few hours before, or with the onset of, menstruation. The pain reaches its maximum intensity within twenty-four hours and may be accompanied by nausea and vomiting. On occasion there may be a degree of mild shock.

Incidence.—Statistics vary with the standard of the observer, but recent figures show a variation of 8–23 per cent.

Type of Patient Affected.—Primary dysmenorrhœa is more severe in the virgin because the stimulus of normal intercourse has a beneficial effect on the endocrine apparatus and neuro-circulatory system of the generative organs. In married women, pain is less common in the parous patient because tearing of the circular fibres at the internal os during labour causes atrophy of the sensory nerve fibres which are situated there and which are concerned in the transmission and perception of pain. Primary dysmenorrhœa occurs most frequently in asthenic women whose threshold for pain is low and whose generative organs may be functionally faulty. It is more common in the thin, nulliparous, slightly sensitive, mentally alert, apprehensive and self-centred woman.

Causes.—The precise cause is not known, and the search for a common ætiological factor applicable to most cases has, so far, been unsuccessful. There would appear to be four main factors in the causation of primary dysmenorrhœa—

(*a*) **Psychosomatic.**—It is now recognised that hypoplasia of the uterus, which in the past was considered a common cause of dysmenorrhœa, is rarely found in women with ovulatory menstrual cycles. Further, it is of significance that if ovulation is inhibited the succeeding period is painless. This finding suggests that the pain is not psychosomatic in origin but is due primarily to some other cause. The psychosomatic factor, if present, supervenes usually as a result of recurring menstrual pain but may well be induced in the young girl by an over-anxious mother with a wrong outlook on what is, after all, a physiological process. At the time of the menarche, the guiding rule in a girl's life should be to follow as normal and as active a routine as possible.

(*b*) **Acute Anteflexion.**—While there is no actual obstruction of the cervical canal, such flexion may add to the difficulty of passing macroscopic fragments of tissue or small clots which may form when the anti-coagulating substance of the endometrium is relatively inactive.

(*c*) **Œstrogen—Progesterone Imbalance.**—It is known that œstrogen-induced bleeding is painless and that primary dysmenorrhœa is always preceded by ovulation. If the suppression of ovulation promotes painless menstruation, it must be the intervention of the luteal hormone—progesterone —which determines whether menstruation will, or will not, be

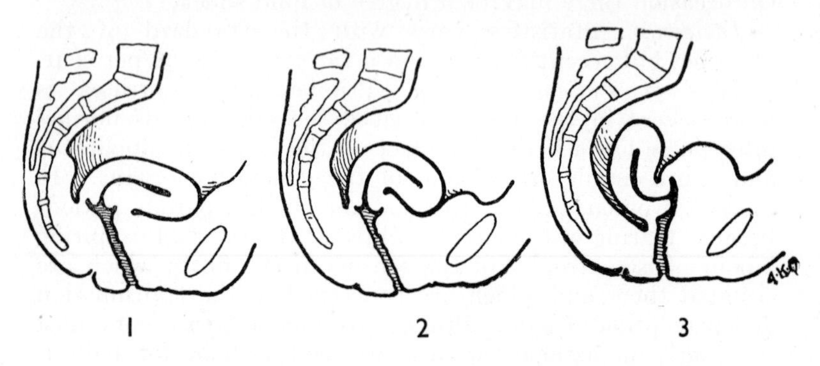

Fig. 30.—Varieties of Anteversion and Anteflexion
1. Anteversion. 2. Anteflexion.
3. Retroposition with anteflexion (cochleate uterus).

painful. As the majority of menstruating women ovulate but do not have dysmenorrhœa it must be inferred that menstruation is painless in those cases because œstrogen and progesterone are in equilibrium and synergistic one with the other. Dysmenorrhœa arises when this synergism is disturbed and as an over-riding action of œstrogen promotes painless bleeding, the imbalance is most probably associated with an over-production of progesterone.

Studies in myometrial activity indicate that menstrual pain is due to an over-activity or inco-ordinate hyper-contractility of uterine muscle, and it is thought that the activating factor in this must be progesterone, a product of progesterone metabolism or some chemical substance elaborated in the secretory endometrium.

According to present physiological concepts, the activity of an organ under autonomic nervous control results from a balance between the parasympathetic and sympathetic nervous systems or between acetylcholine released by the parasympathetic and chemical substances—adrenalin-like in effect—released by the sympathetic nervous system. Reynolds has shown that in the rabbit the administration of œstrogen causes liberation of acetylcholine through inactivation of cholinesterase. The result is hyperæmia and bleeding. It is possible therefore that œstrogens are parasympathetic stimulants, and in so far as œstrogen-induced bleeding is painless, the parasympathetic control of the uterus may be inhibitory, at least to the cervix. If this assumption is correct, progesterone may have the opposite effect and act, under certain circumstances, as a sympathetic stimulant. Over-action of the sympathetic control of the uterus would cause marked vaso-constriction of the vessels and hyperactivity of the musculature, especially in the region of the internal os.

(*d*) **Uterine ischæmia** associated with neuritis of the presacral nerve. Moir showed that the normal rhythmic contractions become stronger before and during menstruation, and that they are exaggerated in primary dysmenorrhœa. He observed, too, that the peak of each contraction coincides with the most intense pain and the disappearance of uterine artery pulsation. Moir postulated therefore the theory of an ischæmia on the same lines as in angina pectoris.

According to Keiffer the highly-specialised sensory nerve corpuscles in the region of the internal os have the property of initiating uterine contractions through a reflex spinal arc, and this viewpoint must make possible, as an ætiological factor, disorders of the autonomic nervous system. According to workers such as Davis, Cotte and Mazer, a sub-acute or chronic neuritis of the presacral nerve is present in a large majority of primary dysmenorrhœa cases, and the pain may be due to exaggeration of motor or sensory impulses passing through a nerve rendered hyper-sensitive by inflammatory change.

Treatment of Primary Dysmenorrhoea.—

(*a*) *Non-surgical Treatment.—*

1. General principles.—A careful investigation of the physical and mental status is essential, removal of chronic foci of infection, a well-balanced diet with special attention to vitamin and calcium content, sufficient mental and physical rest, outdoor exercise, attention to anæmia and sometimes a change of environment, are all important. The B.M.R. should be determined and appropriate treatment

carried out to correct malfunction The sexual habits of the patient must be investigated since sexual excitement without relief, as in coitus interruptus or in masturbation, leads to neuroses, pelvic congestion and dysmenorrhœa.

2. Antispasmodic and analgesic drugs. Atropine, benzyl benzoate, calcium, benzedrine sulphate, pethidine, etc., may all be used. The number of such drugs is legion, attesting to their relative inefficiency in curing this condition. They are of some value, however, in relieving an attack.

3. Endocrine therapy—

(*a*) *Progesterone.*—Most observers are now agreed that progesterone is the principle endocrine factor responsible for painful uterine contractions; its therapeutic use therefore is contra-indicated.

(*b*) *Gonadotrophins.*—Both serum and chorionic gonadotrophins have been employed either to inhibit myometrial activity directly or to stimulate luteal function. The early enthusiastic reports are now received with some scepticism.

(*c*) *Androgens.*—A high dosage of between 300–900 mgm. of testosterone proprionate in a cycle will inhibit ovulation and give complete relief in over 70 per cent. of patients. Smaller doses up to 125 mgm. per cycle which are not sufficient to cause virilisation have been found equally effective in allaying pain. Such a small dose does not inhibit ovulation.

(*d*) *Œstrogens.*—They are used to inhibit ovulation and to bring about painless bleeding. If the pain is thought to be of psychogenic origin an "œstrogen test" may be carried out by giving the patient 2 mgm. of stilbœstrol daily for 14–20 days. Such a course of therapy normally results in withdrawal bleeding with absence of pain, If, however, the patient states that such a bleeding is still accompanied by pain, she may be better dealt with by the psychiatrist than by the gynæcologist. Ethinyl œstradiol 0·05–0·1 mgm. daily or diethyl stilbœstrol 1 mgm. daily may be used as an alternative to stilbœstrol.

4. Low dosage irradiation of the ovaries and pituitary gland. This may be done only in women who have irregular menstruation. At best it is a rather risky form of treatment and not to be recommended.

5. Psychotherapy.—There is a small place for such treatment, *e.g.* the woman who still complains of pain when anovular bleeding has been produced by œstrogens.

Surgical Treatment.—The nerve supply of the uterus comes from the sympathetic and parasympathetic systems. The sympathetic, derived from the 10th, 11th and 12th thoracic nerves reaches the pelvis through the presacral nerve and inferior hypogastric plexus. The parasympathetic supply is through the 2nd, 3rd and 4th sacral nerves—the nervi erigentes. The two systems meet in the cervical or Frankenhauser plexus which lies postero-lateral to the cervix on either side. Some highly-specialised sensory nerve filaments join this plexus from the region of the internal os. Surgical treatment aims at interrupting this nerve pathway at one point or another.

Three surgical procedures deserve mention :—

1. Cervical dilatation.
2. Injection of alcohol into the cervical plexus.
3. Resection of the presacral nerve.

1. Dilatation of the cervix cures a few, but when it is coupled with the introduction of a wide-stemmed pessary or hard rubber tubing for two days, the results are good, due probably to the production of a pressure atrophy of the nerve fibres in the region of the internal os.
2. Injection of 5 c.c. of an 80 per cent. solution of alcohol, by the vaginal route, into the cervical plexus, causes the degeneration of nerve tissue and some report a permanent cure in 60 per cent. This method may well be combined with No. 1.
3. This was devised by Cotte and is now used for intractable pain in advanced genital malignancy. The cure rate in dysmenorrhœa approximates 85 per cent. and the 15 per cent. failure may be explained by incomplete division of the nerve or to the pain being a manifestation of a psycho-neurosis rather than a true dysmenorrhœa.

2. **Secondary Dysmenorrhœa.**—

The pain here is caused by gross pathological lesions within the pelvis—the pain is therefore an incident in a pathological process already present.

Clinical Picture.—The pain is situated in the sides, is constant and gnawing in character, may be present for a varying time before menstruation starts and is relieved by menstruation.

Some Causes of Secondary Dysmenorrhœa.—

1. Chronic inflammatory disease.—May be suspected by a lessened uterine mobility, thickening of the parametrium and adnexal tenderness.
2. Intramural fibroid.
3. Endometriosis.
4. Adherent, and sometimes non-adherent, retroversion.
5. Cystic disease of the ovaries.

When premenstrual pain is unilateral, the possibility of ureteral stricture must be investigated. The premenstrual œdema often renders a symptomless stricture painful because of the greater constriction and consequent back pressure.

Treatment of Secondary Dysmenorrhœa.—The primary cause must be dealt with, and where there is obvious pelvic pathology the surgical approach is best. Where there is ovarian dysmenorrhœa without any palpable pelvic lesion, diathermy and, if need be, ligation and division of the infundibulo-pelvic ligaments with the nerves and blood-vessels contained therein (Browne) yield good results.

Premenstrual Tension Syndrome

This syndrome is characterised by the premenstrual occurrence of insomnia, depression, irritability, emotional disturbance, physical exhaustion, headache, vertigo, nausea and a feeling of tension in the lower abdomen. The exact cause of this syndrome is obscure. Androgens have been found to be the most effective therapeutic agent, 10 mgm. being given daily. This may well be combined with restriction of salt, and ammonium chloride 15–30 gr. daily.

Intermenstrual Pain

The name Mittelschmerz is given to pain occurring about the middle of the menstrual cycle. The cause of this pain is uncertain. It may be associated with the hyperæmia and œdema accompanying ovulation; with the liberation of follicular fluid into the peritoneal cavity at the time of ovulation; with an old chronic inflammation of the ovary resulting in a thickening of the tunica albuginea, prevention of ovulation, formation of cystic follicles and increase in intra-ovarian tension.

Treatment.—

1. Improvement of pelvic circulation.
2. Diathermy and short-wave therapy.
3. Administration of androgens—they reduce hyperæmia and œdema associated with ovulation. Salmon suggests the following course—100 mgm. testosterone proprionate in four divided doses administered during the pre-ovulatory phase of the cycle for two successive months; thereafter 30 mgm. methyl testosterone daily for the first ten days of the cycle for one month and 10 mgm. daily for the first ten days of the cycle for the following two months.
4. Inhibition of ovulation by œstrogens.
5. Division and ligation of the infundibulo-pelvic ligaments, together with the nerves and blood-vessels they contain.

CHAPTER XVIII

DISEASES OF THE UTERUS

METROPATHIA HÆMORRHAGICA

Ætiology.—

This condition is the result of a prolonged action of œstrogen, which presumably follows a dysfunction in the anterior pituitary-ovarian relationship. There is a complete absence of progesterone.

Pathology.—

The ovaries show follicular cystic change and an entire absence of corpora lutea.

The uterus is enlarged and the wall is thickened.

Characteristic appearances are met with in the endometrium, which is hyperplastic and often polypoidal. The glands are irregular and much dilated (Swiss-cheese pattern); the stroma shows areas of œdema, round-cell infiltration and necrosis.

Symptoms.—

Appear most commonly between the ages of thirty-five and forty-five. The most frequent symptom is irregular bleeding, coming on, as a rule, after a period of amenorrhœa.

Diagnosis.—

This is made by microscopical examination of uterine scrapings which are usually profuse.

Treatment.—

1. Curettage for diagnostic purposes ; may be curative.
2. Hormone therapy—
    (*a*) Œstrogen hæmostasis—ethinyl œstradiol 0·15 mgm. two-hourly or injections of œstradiol benzoate 100,000 I.U. every four to six hours. This should arrest the bleeding within twenty-four hours.
    (*b*) Progesterone 25 mgm. daily until bleeding stops. Thereafter the flooding of metropathia can be prevented by giving at regular four-weekly intervals a course of progesterone—25 mgm. of progesterone every second day for four doses or 30 mgm. ethisterone daily for one week.

(*c*) Hamblen advised cyclic œstrogen and progesterone therapy. Œstrogen is given for twenty days and oral progesterone in the last ten days of this treatment. Should bleeding occur before the twenty days of treatment are ended, treatment is discontinued and resumed on the fourth or fifth day of bleeding. The second and subsequent courses of therapy should be identical to the first.

(*d*) Androgen therapy—10 mgm. testosterone propionate three times a week, and in severe cases 25 mgm. twice weekly. Methyl testosterone linguets may be used instead of injections.

3. Where the above treatment has failed there remain hysterectomy or radiotherapy. This latter may be accomplished by intra-uterine radium (2,400 mgm. hours) or X-ray therapy. In the younger patient, hysterectomy with conservation of one or both ovaries is the method to be preferred.

TUMOURS. A.—BENIGN

FIBROMYOMA

Innocent encapsuled solid growths, consisting of unstriate muscle and fibrous tissue arising in the myometrium.

A. **Ætiology.**—Occur more frequently in nulliparous women.

More common in the body of the uterus (92 per cent.), and are usually multiple.

Less common in the cervix (8 per cent.), and are usually single.

B. **Types.**—The tumour may remain in the muscle where it starts—*interstitial.*

The tumour may grow out under the peritoneum—*subperitoneal* or *subserous.*

The tumour may grow in under the mucosa—*submucous.*

C. **Pathology.**—

(*a*) *Naked Eye.*—The tumour is pale and silk-like.

There is a whorled arrangement of interlacing fibres.

The tumour protrudes convexly when the capsule is cut.

(*b*) *Microscopically.*—It consists of plain muscle and white fibrous tissue in varying proportions.

The vessels are variable, depending on the hardness or softness of the tumour.

The capsule contains many vessels.

(*c*) *Other Changes.*—The endometrium is thickened and hyperæmic due to (*a*) the tumour; (*b*) increased ovarian secretion; and (*c*) chronic congestion; most marked with interestitial and submucous types.

(*N.B.*—This gives rise to the menorrhagia so commonly present.)

The uterine cavity is enlarged and the position of the uterus is often distorted.

D. **Degenerations.**—

1. *Atrophy.*—May occur at the menopause, due probably to stoppage of the ovarian secretion. This is, however, exceptional. X-rays and oöphorectomy may also produce atrophy. May occur also after labour.

2. *Hyaline.*—This is the first change to take place; due to malnutrition and common to all types.

It occurs chiefly in the fibrous part which is replaced by a homogeneous substance. The centre, being least vascular, is affected usually first. The pressure on the muscle fibres by the hyaline substance causes them to break up and disappear. (*N.B.*—In some cases the muscle cells become sarcomatous.) Blood-vessels resist the change to the very last.

3. *Cystic.*—A later stage of (2), the hyaline substance liquefying to form cystic spaces. The cysts' walls are lined by hyaline tissue which liquefies later, with consequent enlargement of the cysts. It is most common in the pedunculated subserous tumours.

4. *Fatty.*—Occurs in the muscle, the tumour being more yellow and the whorled appearance becoming indefinite. It is the forerunner of calcareous degeneration which is due to deposition of calcium salts.

5. *Calcareous.*—May occur all through the tumour or only in patches. It is common after the menopause. It occurs in all types, but chiefly in the subperitoneal.

6. *Necrosis.*—Occurs in the centre of the tumour owing to deficient blood supply. It is preceded by either (2) or (4). It is most common in the submucous polypus type where it may pass to gangrene.

7. *Necrobiosis.*—Partial death of the tissues. The tumour is red in colour and has a peculiar fishy odour. The capsule

contains dilated vessels which are often present in the tumour as well. It is preceded by (4). It occurs most commonly either in pregnancy or the puerperium and the tumour may later become cystic or wholly necrotic. The colour is due to staining by soluble blood pigments following hæmolysis which may be caused by lipoid substances circulating in the blood (see p. 114).

8. *Œdema.*—Rare.

E. Complications.—

1. *Axial Rotation.*—Uncommon but may occur in subperitoneal tumours with a long pedicle. The rotation is gradual and hardly ever complete, the symptoms being few. The tumour becomes congested and adhesions form; there is pain and rise of temperature. The pedicle may atrophy beyond the twist; the tumour, then being isolated, adheres to the omentum, peritoneum, etc., and is nourished from these structures—*parasitic fibroid.* The tumour is dark in colour and tender to touch.

2. *Infection.*—Is most common in the submucous variety, the infection coming through the endometrium from the vagina or via the tubes from the abdomen; sometimes the subperitoneal variety is affected through the bowel and adhesions may occur. Suppuration is rare but has been found in the subserous, interstitial and intra-ligamentary types. Sloughing often occurs in the submucous polypus variety due to necrosis.

3. *Adhesions.*—They are not common (3 to 5 per cent.); may occur after degeneration, axial rotation and infection; may be due to inflammation of a neighbouring structure, *e.g.* appendicitis or salpingo-oöphoritis.

F. Malignant Changes.—Endothelioma, carcinoma and sarcoma.

All are rare, sarcomatous change being the least rare.

Sarcomatous.—May occur after hyaline degeneration. If far advanced, it appears as a yellow, homogeneous soft area in the tumour. This area may become cystic, with blood-stained fluid in the spaces. It begins usually in the centre of the tumour and can be diagnosed with certainty only by microscope, the intermuscular fibrous tissue being very cellular in a definite area and the muscle bundles disappearing or being absent. In other cases there is sarcomatous metaplasia of the muscle cells. Thin-walled vessels are also found to be numerous and may be dilated to form blood cysts. Malignancy should be suspected—

1. If tumour grows much after the menopause.
2. If bleeding returns after the menopause.
3. If the tumour becomes soft and is growing rapidly.
4. If there is local pain over tumour, especially after the menopause.
5. If ascites or marked wasting are present.
6. If polypi recur.

G. **Symptoms.**—Often few or none.

(*a*) *Bleeding.*—Menorrhagia is the commonest symptom but is only present in the interstitial and submucous types. The periods become excessive and the intervals become shorter; if this persists, anæmia and debility occur. (*N.B.*—Increased bleeding is due to (1) the increased size of the uterine cavity; (2) the increased congestion of the endometrium; (3) the difficulty of uterine contraction, due to the mechanical obstacle of the tumour.)

The menopause is delayed.

Metrorrhagia or irregular intermenstrual bleeding occurs with submucous tumours. Severe flooding may occur when the capsule is broken through.

(*b*) *Pain.*—Unusual in uncomplicated fibroids, except in the submucous variety when pain is present owing to uterine contractions. Dysmenorrhœa occurs with small interstitial growths, the pain coming with the flow. Pain practically always denotes a complication, *e.g.* infection, adhesions, axial rotation, necrobiosis, etc., and should be viewed with suspicion.

(*c*) *Leucorrhœa.*—Due to endocervicitis. In sloughing submucous fibroids the discharge will be offensive and purulent.

(*d*) *Pressure Symptoms.*—

1. Pain, if the tumour is impacted in the pelvis.

2. Retention of urine, if the tumour is impacted in the pelvis. Frequency of micturition often occurs before the growth reaches the pelvic brim.

3. Œdema of the legs or varix, due to pressure on the veins. Piles may occur also. Varicocele of the broad ligament is common.

4. Intestinal obstruction due to pressure is very rare.

5. Difficulty in breathing, if the tumour is very large.

(*e*) *Sterility* is common, due probably to the accompanying endometritis. If pregnancy occurs, abortion or necrobiosis often results.

H. **Signs.**—The uterus is enlarged, hard and usually nodular, though a single fibroid may cause uniform enlargement. If large, the tumour can be felt abdominally as well as vaginally.

I. **Diagnosis.**—

(*a*) From an ovarian cyst.—

Fibroid.	*Ovarian Cyst.*
1. Tumour usually solid and hard.	1. Tumour cystic.
2. Cervix usually continuous with it. (*N.B.*—Pedunculated subserous type is exception.)	2. Cervix not continuous and does not move with the tumour.
3. Sound in uterus moves tumour mass.	3. No movement of tumour.
4. Uterine cavity elongated.	4. No elongation.
5. Souffle may be heard.	5. Never heard.
6. Menorrhagia usual.	6. No menorrhagia.

(*b*) From pregnancy (see p. 43).

(*c*) From missed abortion—careful history.

(*d*) From hydatid mole with indefinite amenorrhœa—careful history and negative A.Z.R.

(*e*) From subinvolution or chronic metritis, in which cases—

(i) The uterus is regular.

(ii) The uterus never enlarges more than the size of a three to four months' pregnancy.

(*f*) From cancer of the body—by diagnostic curettage. They may occur together.

J. **Differential of Types.**—

	Interstitial.	Subperitoneal.	Submucous.
(*a*) Capsule . .	Present.	Present.	May be absent if polypoid.
(*b*) Thickened endometrium .	Present.	Absent.	Present.
(*c*) Bleeding .	Excessive.	None.	Excessive.
(*d*) Degeneration .	Not common.	Common.	Sloughing common.
(*e*) Size of the uterus .	Enlarged.	Slightly enlarged.	Slightly or moderately enlarged.
(*f*) Elongation of the cavity .	Elongated.	Not elongated.	Much elongated.
(*g*) Pain . .	Slight (dysmenorrhœa).	Nil.	May be severe.
(*h*) Sterility .	Common.	No.	Common.
(*i*) Infection .	Not common.	Not common.	Very common.

Cervical Fibroids

Interstitial.—

1. Found usually on the posterior wall, the anterior aspect being covered by cervical mucosa and the rest by a capsule of cervical wall.
2. Usually single and uniform in outline.
3. The body is elevated on the growth, but not enlarged.
4. The cervical canal is greatly elongated and laterally expanded.
5. The external os is drawn up and may be displaced upwards or laterally.
6. The external os is expanded to form a slit.
7. The uterine vessels and ureters are displaced; they may be stretched over capsule.
8. In large growths the lymphatics and vessels of the broad ligament are enormously dilated and may give rise to much bleeding at operation.

Clinical Features.—Pressure symptoms, the first usually being retention of urine.

(*N.B.*—Bleeding is never a sign of an uncomplicated purely cervical fibroid.)

Treatment of all Fibroids.—

Radiotherapy.—Only indicated in a few cases.

1. Small interstitial fibroids which cause bleeding only and are not complicated by salpingitis or any degeneration.
2. When operation is contra-indicated by some intercurrent disease, *e.g.* diabetes, chronic Bright's disease, Graves' disease, etc.
3. When tumour is not very large.

(*N.B.*—Radium must never be used for submucous fibroids as it causes marked necrosis.)

Operative.

1. Supra-vaginal hysterectomy (see p. 360).
2. Pan-hysterectomy (see p. 362).
   (*a*) This is the most popular method of treatment and it is performed to obviate the rare risk of cancer of the cervix developing later; should always be done if cervix is badly lacerated or unhealthy.
   (*b*) Usually required in cervical fibroids and may be combined with enucleation of tumour from its capsule.

3. Myomectomy (see p. 363).

(*N.B.*—The following facts, taken from Giles, demonstrate the average present-day opinion of myomectomy:

Indications.—

(*a*) If the patient is of the child-bearing age, especially if married.

(*b*) Solitary pedunculated tumours.

(*c*) Solitary interstitial tumours unassociated with severe bleeding.

(*d*) During pregnancy, if the tumour shows signs of degeneration or is going to cause obstruction during labour.

Contra-indications.—

(*a*) Multiple fibroids, after the age of forty to forty-five.

(*b*) If double tubal or ovarian disease is present.

(*c*) If myomectomy is going to leave a battered and useless organ.

(*d*) If there has been excessive bleeding.)

4. Submucous fibroids, in some cases, may be removed by curettage; if polypoidal, treated usually by grasping the pedicle with forceps and twisting until polyp is removed. The uterus must always be curetted after the removal of a polyp so as to cure the coexisting endometritis. If the base of the polypus is very broad, hysterectomy may be required.

Polypi

1. **Fibroid.**—Submucous fibroids which become pedunculated.

They are apt to undergo necrosis or malignant change.

A special type, the *intermittent polyp*, appears at the os only during menstruation, owing to slight cervical dilatation at that time and to the uterine contractions forcing it down; disappears between the periods.

2. **Placental.**—Small portions of retained placenta surrounded by adherent blood clot.

They give rise to severe and frequent bleedings in the puerperium or after an abortion.

They may become infected and give rise to local uterine infection.

Remove with a finger or blunt curette and examine under the microscope so as to exclude chorionepithelioma.

3. **Mucous** (Adenomatous).—

Pathology.—They consist of loose connective tissue in which are numerous glands and retention cysts. The stroma is very vascular. They are covered by an incomplete layer of cylindrical epithelium.

They occur chiefly in the cervical canal.

Two Types.—

(1) Flat, long, tongue-shaped growths, usually single or, at most, two in number. Red in colour. Not usually associated with any cervical catarrh or erosion. Usually occur in nulliparous women at or after the menopause. Arise from endocervix but may be present in body of uterus as well. (*Endometrial polypi.*) They are new growths.

(2) Small, round, pea-like structures attached by short stalks to the external os which shows marked ectropion and erosion. May be multiple and usually occur in multiparæ before the menopause. Caused by inflammation and irritation.

They are pink or red in colour but may become purple if the circulation is interfered with. They are velvety to the touch.

The endometrium is usually thickened.

Symptoms.—

(1) Bleeding—irregular. It may be continuous, but is usually not excessive.

(2) Leucorrhœa.

Diagnosis.—Growths seen or felt on vaginal examination.

Treatment.—

Type 1.—Seize polyp as high up as possible with forceps, crush and twist it off. Curette uterus to treat endometritis and to exclude carcinoma of the body. Cauterise the cervix.

Type 2.—

(1) Remove polypi as in *Type* 1. Curette the uterus and cauterise the cervix.

(2) If very numerous and the cervix very eroded, partial amputation of the cervix along with the polyp-bearing area may be required.

(*N.B.*—All polypi must be examined microscopically to rule out malignancy.)

4. **Sarcomatous.**—Only to be distinguished by microscopical examination. Treated by pan-hysterectomy followed by deep X-ray therapy.

ADENOMYOMA AND ENDOMETRIOMA

Consist of glands surrounded by very cellular connective tissue and muscle.

They occur most commonly in the uterus, but may occur in the tubes, ovaries, recto-genital space, round ligament, ovarian ligament, lymphatic glands and abdominal scars.

Adenomyoma of Uterus

Occurs usually high up on the posterior wall of the body, often starting at a cornu; in some cases involves the greater part of the body but never extends to the cervix. The tumour is formed by the endometrium eating into the muscle, causing great hyperplasia of the muscle and connective tissue from irritation.

Pathology.—Macroscopic. It is like a fibroid but not so white, nor so definitely distinct from the surrounding tissue having no capsule. Cut surface concave in contradistinction to fibroid. It often contains cystic spaces.

Symptoms and Signs.—Difficult to diagnose from myoma.

1. Menorrhagia and dysmenorrhœa are common (pelvic pain and sacralgia), metrorrhagia later.
2. Sterility is very common.
3. The uterus is enlarged and often fixed by adhesions.
4. Fibroids often coexist.
5. The menopause usually is delayed.

Treatment.—Hysterectomy. Curettage is worse than useless.

Endometrioma

Ætiology.—Theories.

1. May develop from Wolffian rests where the Wolffian ducts cross the Müllerian ducts at the cornua; the tumour is apt to develop at the cornua where confluence of tissue might have taken place (Von Recklinghausen).

2. The invasion of existing fibroids by endometrium—Müllerian theory (Cullen).

3. Due to peritoneal proliferation. Serosal theory—Ivanoff.

4. From retrograde menstruation through fimbriated extremity of tube, the endometrial tissue penetrating the ovarian substance and giving rise to a tarry cyst; may form other deposits on surface of uterus, recto-genital connective

tissue, etc.—Endometrial theory (Sampson). Most generally accepted.

1. **Uterine.**—Only found in the body of the uterus.

Usually small sessile subperitoneal growths on posterior wall, often near cornu. Probably due to theory (4).

2. **Round Ligament.**—May be due to theories (1) to (3). Occurs most commonly as a cystic swelling outside the external abdominal ring in the canal of Nuck or near the mons veneris, but may occur in the abdominal cavity. They are usually bilateral and can be diagnosed by their slow increase in size and painfulness during menstruation. Diagnose from hydrocele, enterocele, epiplocele, ovarian cyst and hernia of the ovary.

Treatment.—Excise if pain is caused.

3. **Recto-genital Connective Tissue.**—Due to retrograde menstruation causing endometrial implants. It starts usually as a small growth about the size of a cherry, found above the posterior fornix. It is usually discovered by investigating the cause of dyspareunia. The growth may enlarge and become fixed, involving the rectum, vagina and the adjoining cellular tissue, especially on the left side. Simulates a posterior parametritis. Should the growth involve the rectum and vagina the rectal mucous membrane moves over the tumour, whereas the vaginal mucous membrane is fixed to it, often becoming papillary and bleeding easily. Ulceration may occur and rectal carcinoma must be excluded.

Symptoms and Signs.—

(1) Marked constipation and pain on defæcation result from stenosis.

(2) Dyspareunia.

(3) Blood - stained vaginal discharge, but never rectal bleeding.

(4) Small or large tumours fixed between the vagina and rectum.

Diagnose from diverticulitis.

Treatment.—

There is a present-day tendency to advocate local resection of the ovaries. The condition is rarely discovered in such an early stage as to make this possible and, as a rule, more radical treatment is required. This takes the form of total hysterectomy with, possibly, double salpingo-oöphorectomy.

Where this is difficult, a radium menopause may be induced, with eventual cure of the condition.

4. **Fallopian Tube.**—

Small nodular swellings.

No treatment is necessary unless there are symptoms, viz. pain, menorrhagia, etc., when salpingo-oöphorectomy is required.

5. **Ovary.**—*Endometriomatous Cysts.*—

(1) Often found associated with endometrioma of recto-genital space.

(2) Endometrial stroma consisting of glands, stroma and unstriped muscle is found in the walls of the small cysts. In the larger ones this tissue becomes flattened out and ultimately disappears leaving only a flattened endothelium-like lining ; this is due to the cyst enlarging with each period. The cyst contains tarry material.

(3) This is the only type of endometrioma where unstriped muscle is a new formation. It is not found normally in the ovary.

(4) Lining wall is thick and leathery, but adhesions are so dense that in being removed the cyst usually ruptures.

(5) Probably due to tubal or uterine epithelium passing through the fimbriated extremity of the tube allowing development in the ovary, pelvis, or both (Sampson).

(6) Probably endometrial in origin because they (*a*) react to menstruation, having menstrual phases corresponding with the uterine mucosa ; (*b*) are active only during menstrual life ; (*c*) undergo decidual reaction (Sampson).

(7) Usually bilateral and very adherent, due to perforations, with resulting adhesion formation.

(*N.B.*—These adhesions consist of endometriomatous tissue.)

(8) Dysmenorrhœa is acute for the first day or two of period. This occurs late in sexual life (after thirty years).

(The history of dysmenorrhœa occurring at this age for first time, especially if increasing in severity with each period, is very suggestive of endometrioma.)

(9) Menorrhagia of slight degree is usually present.

If ovaries are found to contain a tarry material at any operation, always look for endometriomata of other organs and especially of the recto-genital space.

Treated by removal of cyst and, if bilateral, of uterus as well.

6. **Abdominal Scar.**—Endometrial implants following operations opening into uterus, *e.g.* hysterotomy, Cæsarean section and myomectomy. Treated by excision.

B. MALIGNANT

CARCINOMA

1. Of the Cervix

Ætiology.—

1. It occurs usually between forty-five and fifty-five years of age, but has been seen by authors in patients as young as nineteen and as old as eighty years.
2. It occurs usually in multiparæ with a large family.
3. It is probably predisposed to by chronic inflammatory eversion and erosion, which become more unhealthy and persistent with each successive labour.

Pathology.—

(*a*) *Naked-eye Appearances.*—

1. It may form a cauliflower excrescence on the vaginal portion of one or other lip. Necrosis is very apt to occur. (*N.B.*—This type is not so malignant, spreading at first by contact alone, *e.g.* affecting the vagina.)
2. It may form in the cervix as a node, giving rise to some increase in size of the cervix. It usually spreads by ulceration, which may eat away most of the wall. It ulcerates usually towards the cervical canal. (*N.B.*—This type is very malignant.) Endocervical type.

(*b*) *Microscopically.*—

1. *Squamous Celled.*—
   (*a*) Much the more common.
   (*b*) May be found in any of the naked-eye types mentioned.
   (*c*) Starts in the deeper layers of the epithelium, and processes are sent into the fibro-muscular layer. In some cases epithelial pearls are present. In cauliflower growths the processes grow outwards and the endocervix is not invaded so soon.
   (*d*) Ulceration is very common, especially in endocervical cases when they are at all advanced.

2. *Columnar Celled.*—
   (*a*) Probably only occurs in cancers arising from the endocervical mucosa.
   (*b*) Many tubules project into the fibro-muscular layer, where they give off buds and branch.

(*c*) The lumen is surrounded by one layer of cells only, but is diagnosed by the tubules projecting into the fibro-muscular tissue. The stroma between the cancer processes is gradually invaded by cancer.

(*d*) Not so malignant as the squamous-celled endocervical type, but more so than the cancers arising on the vaginal surface of the cervix.

(*c*) *Concomitant Changes.*—

1. *Vagina.*—

(*a*) May be invaded by direct extension, or by the lymphatics in its muscular wall.

(*b*) Invasion is most likely when the growth is on the portio vaginalis.

(*c*) The growth may be due to implantation.

2. *Pelvic Connective Tissue.*—

(*a*) Involved early by permeation and later by infiltration.

(*b*) In permeation, the nodules of growth are at first discrete, but later expand and coalesce.

3. *Pelvic Peritoneum.*—It is affected fairly early, sometimes even when the uterus is mobile.

4. *Bladder.*—It is usually involved fairly early, especially if the anterior lip of the cervix is diseased; the mucous membrane, usually at the trigone, is involved later.

5. *Ureter.*—

(*a*) Frequently affected, either by the pressure of the growth or invasion of its walls from without, through permeation of the lymphatics.

(*b*) Obstruction of the ureters may cause hydronephrosis, with subsequent pyelonephritis.

(*c*) Uræmia may be caused, due to renal insufficiency.

(*d*) Complete suppression though rare may occur.

6. *Rectum.*—It is not invaded till late, when the growth spreads along the utero-sacral ligaments.

(*d*) *Dissemination.*—

1. The glands are only involved late and, sometimes not at all; the glands affected being the middle chain of the external iliac, internal iliac, and sacral glands (see Lymphatics, p. 9).

2. Metastases are but rarely found, but when present are usually in the liver, spleen and lungs; may be caused by emboli in the blood-stream.

Signs and Symptoms.—Usually none at the very beginning, then—

1. Bleeding—slight and irregular; may occur only after coitus. (When the disease is advanced and ulceration occurs, the bleeding may be severe.)

(*N.B.*—**Bleeding caused by vaginal examination is always suspicious of cancer of the cervix.**)

2. Discharge—
   (*a*) Slight, constant, yellow or brown.
   (*b*) Usually occurs later than the bleeding.
   (*c*) Becomes offensive and increases as the disease advances.

3. Pain—
   (*a*) A relatively late symptom due to infiltration or infection of the connective tissue.
   (*b*) Usually low backache with acute exacerbations. Not relieved by lying down and rest.

4. Cachexia and loss of weight, anæmia, etc. Late symptoms.

On Examination.—

1. Per vaginam—
   (*a*) A raised indurated patch, cauliflower excrescence, or ulceration may be felt.
   (*b*) The area is friable and bleeds easily.
   (*c*) There is an irregularly thickened cervix.

2. By speculum—
   (*a*) A definite area of growth is seen.
   (*b*) The area is dull and dark in colour.

3. Curettage—
   Curette the cervix or cut out a wedge and examine it microscopically. (The only certain method if any doubt regarding the presence of a carcinoma exists.)

Diagnosis.—

(Early diagnosis is of the utmost importance and any case of irregular bleeding, especially at or after the menopause, must be thoroughly investigated and not treated empirically with drugs.)

1. From erosion, by—
   (*a*) The hardness and roughness of the growth.
   (*b*) The darkness and dullness of the area.
   (*c*) The friability and ease by which bleeding is obtained.

(*d*) Schiller's test.—If cervix is painted with Lugol's iodine, carcinomatous area remains white.
(*e*) Examination for cancer cells of scrapings removed from cervix by a wooden spatula. (Ayre.)
(*f*) Examination for cancer cells of vaginal secretion aspirated by a bulb and pipette. (Papanicolaou.)
(*g*) Ring biopsy of junction of squamous and columnar cells area.
(*h*) Wedge biopsy of any suspicious area.

2. From chancre—
(*a*) No early secondary symptoms found.
(*b*) The Wassermann is negative.
(*c*) No spirochætes are found in the scraping.

Staging (as used at Holt Institute, Manchester; Royal Infirmary, Edinburgh, etc.).—

Stage O.—Pre-invasive carcinoma or carcinoma in situ.

Stage I.—The tumour is entirely confined to the cervix. (Approximately six to eight weeks after first symptoms.)

Stage II.—The mucous membrane of the vagina is not involved beyond the fornices.

And/or the parametrial induration is confined to the medial half on one or both sides.

Endocervical carcinomata, otherwise limited as above, are placed in this Stage. (Approximately two to six months after first symptom.)

Stage III.—The mucous membrane of the vagina is not involved beyond the upper half.

And/or the parametrial induration has extended beyond the medial half and may extend to the wall of the pelvis on one side, but must not extend to the walls of the pelvis on both sides. (Approximately three to twelve months after first symptom.)

Stage IV.—The mucous membrane of the vagina is involved beyond the upper half.

And/or there is parametrial induration extending to the walls of the pelvis on both sides.

And/or there is involvement of the bladder as determined cystoscopically.

And/or there is involvement of the rectum.

And/or there are distant metastases.

Prognosis.—

Best for squamous celled cauliflower type growing from

vaginal portion of cervix, and worst for squamous celled endocervical type.

Early diagnosis very important to prevent development of more advanced stage.

Thus, if Stage I is treated efficiently, the five years' survival rate is about 80 per cent.; in Stage II it is about 60 per cent., and in Stage III about 30 per cent., whereas if seen first in Stage IV the prognosis is almost hopeless. (Hurdon.)

Complications.—

1. Pyometra.
2. Vulvitis and intertrigo due to discharge.
3. Cystitis and pyelonephritis.
4. Fistulæ into bladder and rectum.

Pyometra.—May be associated with carcinoma cervicis or corporis, or may occur without any malignant condition being present.

May be associated with senile endometritis.

Retention may be due to obstruction, *e.g.* carcinoma, or to lack of tone of muscle wall.

Puriform fluid consisting of epithelial debris, but not pus. Fluid varies in amount up to a pint and is usually offensive.

Uterine wall usually thin and endometrium atrophied.

May cause no symptoms for a long time, but later causes discharge, often offensive and frequently tinged with blood. A sense of discomfort in hypogastrium often present.

Treated, if not associated with a carcinoma, by dilating the cervix, gently curetting uterus to exclude carcinoma corporis; then either apply pure carbolic acid to the interior of the uterus or inject glycerine into the uterus. Both treatments may require to be repeated.

Treatment.—

1. *Radium.*—Many cliniques have evolved special detailed radium treatments, viz. Paris, Brussels, Stockholm, etc. *Heyman* (*Stockholm*) *Method* (see **Fig. 31**).

The cervix is dilated and an intra-cervical applicator containing 50 mgm. radium is inserted into the cervix, which is surrounded in the vagina by three flat applicators (often hinged together) containing 20 mgm. each; thus cross radiation of the growth itself is effected and the parametrium is also radiated by the applicators in the lateral fornices. This dosage is retained for twenty-four hours and is repeated in a week's time and again three weeks later. Some advise deep X-ray therapy as well as radium, but though theoretically it should improve the prognosis, there is some dubiety as to its efficacy. If given, it should be administered before radium treatment so as to kill outlying metastases in glands and parametrium and thus limit spread before destroying main growth with radium.

Radium treatment practically always improves symptoms and prolongs life, even if a permanent cure is not effected.

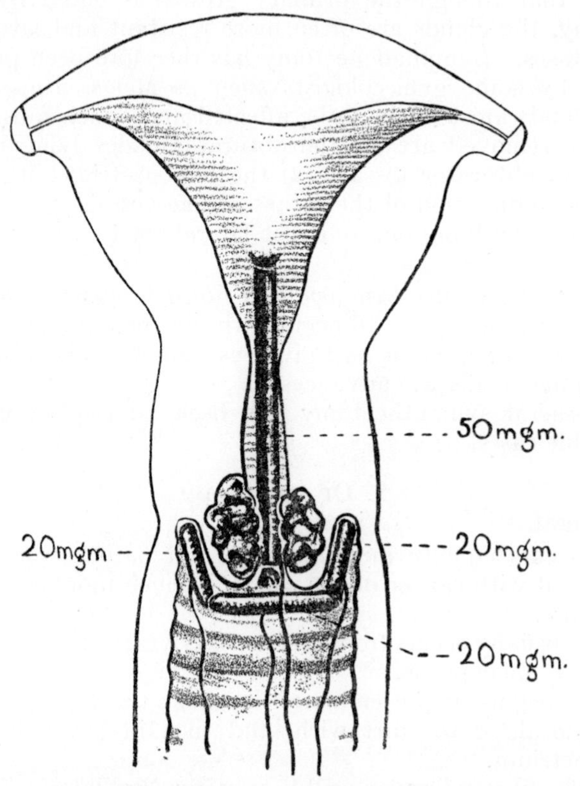

FIG. 31.—DIAGRAMMATIC DRAWING ILLUSTRATING RADIUM TREATMENT OF CARCINOMA CERVICIS (STOCKHOLM TECHNIQUE).

Bleeding is stopped and discharge ceases, but pain may persist or even be aggravated, if previously present. The general health improves markedly also.

2. *Operative* (Wertheim's Hysterectomy).—Removal of whole uterus with adnexæ and upper third of vagina along with as much parametrial tissue as possible and pelvic glands.

This is only possible in Stage I and Stage II. This operation which used to give a high primary mortality rate is now, in the hands of experts and with present-day operative aids such as blood transfusion, chemotherapy, antibiotics and better anæsthesia, much safer, and is being practised much more frequently than it was five years ago. Whether the survival rate is higher than with radiotherapy has still to be proved.

3. *Lymphadenectomy following Radiotherapy.*—It has been found that though the primary growth is cured by radiotherapy, the glands are often more resistant and later cause metastases. Lymphadenectomy has therefore been practised lately by some gynæcologists such as Meigs, Taussig, etc. The glands most likely to be affected and which must therefore be removed are (1) the obturator nodes lying in fatty tissue in obturator fossa ; (2) the hypogastric, lying in the angle of bifurcation of the common iliac vessels ; and (3) the external iliac lying on, and just lateral to, the external iliac vessels.

4. *For pain after treatment has failed to effect a cure*—try aspirin, veramon, etc., to begin with, but before long morphia will be required, and is best given as a suppository, in increasing dosage as disease advances.

Pre-sacral sympathectomy has been advised in very intractable cases.

2. Of the Body

General.—

1. Occurs equally in nulliparous and parous women, but compared with cancer of the cervix is much more common in nulliparæ.

2. It usually occurs from fifty to sixty years of age, following a definite menopause.

3. It begins in the endometrium near the fundus, usually being localised to start with, and then involves the whole endometrium.

4. The fibro-muscular wall is only involved later.

Pathology.—

Types.—

1. *Naked Eye.*—

(*a*) Nodules growing in and from the cornua and then later filling the uterine cavity—*nodular*.

(*b*) Small polypoid projections attached to the wall by a small base—*polypoid*.

(*c*) Long thread-like processes projecting into the cavity—*villous*.

2. *Microscopically.*—

(*a*) *Tubular*—

(1) Irregular and branching tubules practically take the place of the stroma.

(2) The tubules are lined by many layers of columnar epithelium.

(3) It extends slowly into the muscular coat.

(*b*) *Alveolar*—

(1) Gland lumina are filled with many layers of irregular and different-sized columnar cells.

(2) It is more malignant than (*a*).

Concomitant Changes.—

1. *Endometrium.*—

(*a*) Mucous polypi are often present.

(*b*) The endometrium is sharply defined from the tumour, and may even be overlapped by it, the tumour spreading by proliferation of the tumour cells, and not by malignant conversion of the endometrium.

2. *Muscle.*—Usually thinned.

3. *Peritoneum.*—

(*a*) Remains smooth and shining till late.

(*b*) When invasion occurs, white or yellow patches appear, it loses lustre and adhesions form.

4. *Cervix.*—Invasion is late and occurs through the lymphatics and not to direct invasion. Mucous polypi may be present.

5. *Ovaries.*—The commonest seat of metastases; conveyed either by the peritoneum, lymphatics, or blood-vessels.

6. *Fallopian Tubes.*—They may be invaded by direct growth along the mucous membrane or muscular wall, or by lymphatics.

7. *Fibroids.*—They are often present (22 per cent.—Norris), and may be invaded by the growth.

Dissemination.—

1. There is slow infiltration of the uterine walls and lymphatics.

2. The lumbar and inguinal glands are the first to be affected, but this only occurs in advanced cases.

3. The peritoneum and adjacent cellular tissue become infiltrated late.

4. Metastases only occur when the disease is very advanced, if then; commonest in the ovaries, omentum and liver.

Signs and Symptoms.—

1. There are few or none to begin with, the symptoms appearing at an even later stage than in cervical cancer.
2. The patient may complain of slight bleeding when straining at stool.
3. Discharge—slight, pale, watery, blood-stained, sometimes offensive.
4. Bleeding—slight and irregular to begin with, but becoming more constant and profuse. Usually follows a period of amenorrhœa.
5. Pain may be present, but is usually represented by a sense of heaviness in the pelvis, unless later, after adhesions have formed, when it is severe.
6. The uterus is slightly, and uniformly, enlarged and softened. It is movable until late, when it becomes fixed by adhesions or extension to the cervix and pelvic tissue.
7. Patients are often very stout.

Diagnosis.—All cases of post-menopausal bleeding or persistent purulent vaginal discharge, whether tinged with blood or not, must be curetted and the scrapings examined microscopically.

Complications.—

1. Pyometra.
2. Mucous polypi.
3. Vulvitis and intertrigo.
4. Suppurating inguinal glands.
5. Cystitis and pyelitis.

Treatment.—

1. Pan-hysterectomy and removal of appendages.
2. If for any reason inoperable, intra-uterine radium (total dose, 6000–7000 mgm. hours) may effect a cure.
3. Pre-operative X-ray or radium therapy has been found by some authorities (Norman Miller, etc.) to help the prognosis, but it is doubtful whether post-operative X-ray is of any advantage.

SARCOMA OF THE UTERUS

A rare occurrence. It is usually found in the body of the uterus; five times more common in parous women and three times more frequent after menopause; it may occur in infants, adolescents or at any age.

Pathology.—

Types.—

1. Usually *intramural* and circumscribed, being seen as a solitary circumscribed homogeneous yellow growth consisting of mixed cells, spreading later to invade the uterine wall. Is apt to become cystic or to necrose. At first it is interstitial, but may become subserous or submucous; if the latter occurs, inversion may follow.

2. May be *endometrial* and (*a*) Diffuse.—Arising from the fundus and spreading all over body of uterus. Soft and friable, pieces often being found in the vaginal discharge. The endometrium is thickened and shaggy. The uterus is enlarged uniformly and is soft.

Or (*b*) Circumscribed.—Solitary nodule growing into the cavity to form a polyp and liable to cause inversion.

3. *In Fibroids* (see p. 297).—

(1) Is most common in the interstitial type.

(2) Is the least malignant of uterine sarcomata.

4. *Cervical.*—Very rare. Occurs in the form of small cysts, like a bunch of grapes, arising from the cervical canal or the vaginal portion, and filling the vagina. Each cyst is surrounded by columnar epithelium and inside are round or spindle cells separated by clear spaces due to œdema. Growth is very rapid.

Dissemination.—

1. By the blood-stream to the lungs and liver.
2. To adjacent organs, *e.g.* bladder, ovaries, etc.
3. Along the endometrium.
4. Growth is slow to start with but becomes rapid, when deposits occur.

Signs and Symptoms.—*Of Body.*

1. Bleeding; irregular and then continuous; becomes more rapidly continuous in the endometrial type. No floodings.
2. Discharge; watery, blood-stained and offensive.
3. Pain; occurs early in intramural, late in endometrial type, being specially marked with polypi.
4. The uterus is usually symmetrically enlarged, unless a subserous sarcoma or fibroid is present.
5. The uterus is soft, and pregnancy has to be excluded.
6. Infection is very liable to occur, with septicæmia.
7. A uterine souffle is often heard, especially in telangiectatic growths.

Of Cervix.—

1. Sarcoma of the cervix usually gives rise to no symptoms, and is often found accidentally.

2. Bleeding and a watery discharge may occur, but pain is late and indicates parametric involvement.

3. The mass may be mushroom-shaped, polypoid or grape-like.

Diagnosis.—Diagnose from tuberculous and senile endometritis, and chorionepithelioma by microscopic examination of the scrapings.

Diagnose cervical cases from cancer of the cervix, or, if grape-like, from hydatidiform mole, by microscope.

Prognosis.—

1. Is grave even after removal, as usually metastases have formed.

2. Is best in sarcomatous change in a myoma, then in endometrial type.

3. Is worst in a round-celled sarcoma.

Treatment.—Pan-hysterectomy, with removal of adnexæ, or radium as for carcinoma.

CHAPTER XIX

DISEASES OF OVARY AND FALLOPIAN TUBES

OVARY

Distention Cysts.—

1. *Follicular Cysts.*—Due to non-rupture of a Graafian follicle; degeneration occurs in the ovum and membrana granulosa, increasing the liquor folliculi with subsequent cystic distension. The cause may lie in a disturbed endocrinal control or in the presence of a chronic infection of the appendages with thickened tunica albuginea or adhesions preventing ovulation. May be single or multiple, the latter in many cases being converted into the former by absorption of septa. They contain a pale serous fluid often rich in œstrogen. There may be no symptoms; occasionally there is iliac fossa pain and menorrhagia or irregular bleeding may occur.

Treatment.—None may be required. Rupture may occur and a spontaneous cure result. Treatment is necessary where the cystic ovaries are associated with metropathia hæmorrhagica (see p. 294) or are causing menorrhagia, when resection of the cysts will often effect a cure.

2. *Lutein Cysts.*—Two types are described:—

(*a*) Corpus luteum cyst—accumulation of fluid in what is apparently a normal corpus luteum.

(*b*) Theca-lutein cyst—where fluid gathers in the cavity of an atretic follicle in which the granulosa cells have undergone lutein change. This type is associated with hydatidiform mole and chorionepithelioma.

Lutein cysts are usually single and about the size of a walnut; where they accompany hydatidiform mole, they are larger and bilateral. They contain a thin fluid, occasionally blood, when they are known as blood cysts or hæmatomata of the corpus luteum. The fluid comes partly from the lutein cells which give a yellow colour to the cyst wall, and may be the result of exudation from vessels in the zona vasculosa.

There may be excessive and irregular bleeding, with, in addition, lower abdominal pain. Should the cyst rupture, serious intra-peritoneal bleeding is possible and may necessitate laparotomy.

TUMOURS OF THE OVARY—CLASSIFICATION

Innocent

1. **Epithelial Origin.**—
   (*a*) Single and multilocular serous cysts.
   (*b*) Pseudo-mucinous cystadenoma.
   (*c*) Papillomatous cystadenoma.

2. **Connective Tissue Origin.**—
   Fibroma.

3. **Mixed Tissue Origin.**—
   Cystic teratoma (Dermoid).

4. **Endometrial Origin.**—
   Endometrioma.

Malignant

1. **Epithelial Origin.**—*Primary*—
   (*a*) Malignant papillomatous cystadenoma.
   (*b*) Malignant pseudo-mucinous cystadenoma.
   (*c*) Solid carcinoma.

Secondary.—Metastatic carcinoma (Krukenberg).

2. **Connective Tissue Origin.**—
   (*a*) Sarcoma.
   (*b*) Endothelioma.
   (*c*) Perithelioma.

3. **Mixed Tissue Origin.**—
   Solid teratoma.

INNOCENT TUMOURS

Epithelial

(*a*) **Serous Cysts.**—

1. Usually unilateral.
2. Contain serous fluid.
3. Lined by flattened cubical or columnar ciliated epithelium.
4. Occur usually after twenty years of age.
5. Often one loculus, but may be multiple.

(*b*) **Pseudo-mucinous Cystadenoma.**—

1. Most common ovarian tumour.

2. Largest benign ovarian tumour.

3. Usually is pedunculated, the pedicle consisting of the broad ligament, the infundibulo-pelvic and ovarian ligaments, the tube and blood-vessels.

4. Multilocular.

5. Loculi contain thick glairy fluid, whitish yellow or green in colour. The fluid consists of desquamated epithelial cells and larger cells filled with yellow pigment, and is derived from the epithelium and vessels in the walls.

6. Loculi often communicate by fluid bursting through the fibrous septa.

7. Cyst wall is smooth, white and glistening, but there may be elevations due to distension of individual loculi.

8. Three definite layers are present in the wall—(*a*) Outer—tunica albuginea; (*b*) Middle—glandular depressions and connective tissue; (*c*) Inner—columnar epithelium with many goblet cells which may project as papillary ingrowths, but the ingrowths have no pedicles as they have in papillomatous cysts.

9. Epithelium secretes pseudo-mucinous fluid and, if rupture occurs, the epithelium may be detached and become attached to peritoneum, etc.; there it still continues to secrete fluid which causes the peritoneum to thicken from chronic inflammation, the condition being known as pseudo-myxoma peritonei. (Rare.)

Pseudo-myxoma Peritonei.—

(1) Usually arises from pseudo-myxomatous cysts, but may arise from mucous cysts of the appendix.

(2) Peritoneum is thick and opaque, shaggy adhesions occurring where it is in contact with pseudo-mucin, and nodules like miliary tubercle may be found.

(3) Mucinous secretion may be due to (*a*) chronic inflammation or (*b*) myxomatous degeneration.

(4) Repeated laparotomies may be necessary, due to implantation metastases occurring and the epithelial cells forming new gelatinous masses.

10. May occur at any age and grows fairly rapidly to a large size.

(*c*) **Papillomatous Cystadenoma.**—Excrescences from cyst wall project into the cavity of the cyst, but are attached by definite pedicles. Excrescences may be large or small.

Papillomatous and pseudo-mucinous cysts compared :—

Papillomatous Cysts.	Pseudo-mucinous Cysts.
1. Much rarer (1 to 10).	1. Very common.
2. Usually bilateral.	2. Usually unilateral.
3. Unilocular.	3. Multilocular.
4. Fluid serous.	4. Pseudo-mucinous.
5. Smaller, size of melon.	5. Very large.
6. Excrescences on cyst wall due to papillary growth inside.	6. Due to over-distension.
7. Epithelium columnar, cubical or ciliated.	7. Always columnar.
8. Implantation metastases occur if ruptured.	8. No metastases, but pseudomyxoma peritonei may rarely occur.
9. Very apt to become malignant.	9. Not nearly so liable to become malignant.
10. Psammoma bodies often found in wall.	10. Not found.

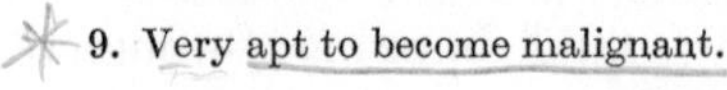

Connective Tissue

Fibroma.—Form 2 per cent. of all ovarian tumours.

1. Usually unilateral, but may be bilateral.
2. Ovary is replaced entirely by the fibroma in most cases.
3. Tumour consists chiefly of white fibrous tissue with irregular spindle cells between.
4. Densely hard, white, smooth.
5. Shape of the ovary is preserved ; size seldom greater than a fœtal head.
6. Pedunculated.
7. Undergoes cystic, hyaline and calcareous change.
8. Often accompanied by ascites and sometimes by hydrothorax.
9. More common after thirty.
10. May become malignant.

Mixed Tissue

Cystic Teratoma (Dermoid).

Theories as to Causation.—

1. Due to fertilisation of one of the primordial ova in the ovary of the developing embryo, so that a second imperfect embryo is formed. The impregnation may be regarded as due to surplus spermatozoa remaining near the morula and fertilising the primordial ovum which is developed early (Shattock).

2. Cell rests—a toti-potent cell being dislocated early and implanted in the ovarian stroma. This cell sooner or later divides actively and gives rise to a teratoma (Bennet).

3. Impregnation of a mature ovum before leaving the Graafian follicle. (But teratoma may occur in infants, virgins and even in fœti.)

Pathology.—

1. Usually unilateral and pedunculated.
2. Usually unilocular, but may contain two to three loculi.
3. Surface smooth and yellow in colour.
4. Ovary is flattened, incorporated in cyst wall, or forms a projection on the wall.
5. Cavity contains sebaceous material and hair, but projecting into the cavity is a solid part consisting of teeth, liver, bone, cartilage, thyroid, etc.—the embryoma—all three layers of the embryo being represented in it; projection is covered by skin.
6. Cyst wall lined by skin near embryoma; in other places it is smooth or covered by granulation tissue with hairs and cholesterin plates embedded in it.
7. Occurs at all ages and grows slowly, rarely becoming larger than a fœtal head.
8. An innocent tumour, but tissues may undergo malignant change.
9. Should rupture occur, implantation growths, but no metastases, occur.
10. Corpora lutea present, which shows that the ovary is still active; this should make one hesitate before removing bilateral tumours.
11. Torsion of the pedicle may occur and the cyst become parasitic. Liable to suppurate after labour. Otherwise usually causes no symptoms and is discovered accidentally.

Endometrial Origin

Endometriomata (see p. 305).

MALIGNANT TUMOURS

Epithelial

Primary—(*a*) **Papillomatous Cystadenoma** and(*b*) **Pseudo-mucinous Cystadenoma.**

1. Cystic carcinoma usually occurs in a papillomatous

cyst, but may occur in a pseudo-mucinous or teratomatous cyst. It may be malignant from the start.

2. Fluid often blood-stained, but may be clear or pus-like.

3. In papillomatous cysts, malignancy may occur only in a small area of the epithelium.

4. Cyst wall eventually perforates and metastases occur.

5. Metastases common in omentum, peritoneum, lumbar and iliac glands, the opposite ovary and tube; carried by lymph or blood-stream, or by implantation.

6. Blood-stained ascites is practically always present.

(*c*) **Solid Carcinoma.**—

1. Less common than cystic.

2. Most common between twenty-five and forty-seven years. Rare after sixty years.

3. May be unilateral or bilateral, probably being unilateral to start with but sooner or later the other ovary is involved.

4. May be smooth and regular or bossed, the bossings being solid or cystic.

5. Rarely larger than a man's hand.

6. May be hard, or soft and brain-like.

7. Usually pedunculated, but torsion is rare due to the presence of adhesions.

8. Encapsuled, but the capsule is perforated early by the growth. The capsule often adheres to adjacent structures through inflammatory change and then the adhesions are invaded by the growth, giving rise to wide diffusion of the growth in the peritoneal cavity.

9. Blood-stained ascites of varying amount is present in over 50 per cent. of cases.

10. Lumbar glands are infected early and metastases in the liver are common.

11. Liquefactive necrosis may produce cystic spaces in the tumour.

12. The tumour may have a medullary or adenomatous structure.

Secondary.—

1. Primary growth usually in stomach, intestine or uterus.

2. When secondary to carcinoma of the stomach or other part of the alimentary tract, it is called Krukenberg tumour.

3. Krukenberg tumours are usually bilateral.

4. May contain cystic spaces.

5. Myxomatous sarcoma-like stroma possessing signet-ring cells.

Connective Tissue

(*a*) **Sarcoma.**—Rarer than cancer.

1. More common at puberty and after menopause.
2. May be unilateral or bilateral and may become very large.
3. Round or oval, smooth, but often bossed.
4. Usually pedunculated and, until large, are encapsuled by the tunica albuginca.
5. May contain areas of necrosis and hæmorrhage.
6. Blood-stained ascites present in 50 per cent.
7. Tumour is not fixed as early as in cancer, due to the presence of the false capsule.
8. Abdominal pain and wasting are early symptoms.
9. Metastases in liver, lungs and lumbar glands are common.
10. Often causes uterine bleeding.

(*b*) **Endothelioma.**—

1. Rare.
2. Rises in endothelium of blood-vessels or lymphatics.

(*c*) **Perithelioma.**—

1. Rare.
2. Rises in connective tissue of vessel walls.

Mixed Tissue

Solid Teratoma.—

1. Rare. Soft. Grows rapidly and reaches large size.
2. Contains cystic spaces.
3. Very malignant.
4. Occurs usually before thirty years of age.
5. Gives rise to increasing abdominal distension and later to pressure symptoms. Pain is usually late and cachexia and debility very late, but ascites is often present early. Menstruation is not affected.
6. Metastases take the form of (*a*) reproduction of primary growth or (*b*) cancer or sarcoma. They are most commonly found in the peritoneum, retro-peritoneal glands, lungs, liver and brain.

LESS COMMON OVARIAN TUMOURS

1. **Brenner Tumour.**—

Appearance is similar to fibroma ; tumour may vary very much in size.

Made up of epithelial cell nests surrounded by fibromatous connective tissue. The cells towards the centre of the nest may undergo cystic degeneration and the cells lining this central cavity may contain glycogen.

The tumour is benign; occurs most frequently after the menopause. There are no specially characteristic symptoms. There is no hormone influence.

2. **Dysgerminoma.**—

Arises from undifferentiated cells and is a neuter tumour. May attain a large size.

Tumour is solid and "rubbery"; is surrounded by a dense capsule. On section, the growth is greyish and shows yellowish areas with necrosis, degeneration and hæmorrhage.

There is often ascites.

The tumour is malignant. Occurs before puberty and in the young woman. There are no characteristic symptoms. There is no hormone influence.

3. **Granulosa Cell Carcinoma.**—

Arises from granulosa cells not utilised for follicle formation.

Tumour may be solid and shows yellowish areas; some tumours may contain many cystic cavities. Ovarian stroma contains clusters of cells resembling granulosa cells; small cavities are often enclosed by these cells, giving a follicular appearance.

May grow to size of melon.

The tumour is malignant and may occur at any age.

The tumour cells produce œstrogen in large amount and this is responsible for the clinical picture.

In young children, secondary sex characteristics become apparent and precocious menstruation will occur.

During reproductive life, the clinical features are not constant, but fit into one of the several pictures of excessive œstrogen production.

After the menopause, the uterus becomes enlarged, the endometrium re-activated and there may be bleeding.

Here there is a very definite hormone influence—due to œstrogen.

4. **Arrhenoblastoma.**—

Arises from male-directed cells in the ovary.

May grow to size of a small melon.

Of firm consistency, these tumours are greyish or yellowish on section and may contain cystic cavities.

This tumour is of low malignancy and occurs most commonly in young women.

Through the hormone influence, defeminising and masculinising characteristics are produced, *e.g.* atrophy of breasts, amenorrhœa, male distribution of the hair, deepening of the voice and hypertrophy of the clitoris.

5. **Adrenal Tumours.**—

May arise from adrenal nests.

They may be benign or malignant and produce a clinical picture similar to the arrhenoblastoma.

Complications of Ovarian Cysts

(*a*) **Torsion of the Pedicle (Axial Rotation).**—

1. *Sudden.*—

(*a*) Commonest in moderate sized cysts which have risen out of the pelvis. (Teratomata in the pelvis are specially liable.)

(*b*) Liable to occur in pregnancy, labour or puerperium.

(*c*) Venous drainage is impaired and tumour becomes congested.

(*d*) Tumour is enlarged and discoloured from vascular engorgement.

Symptoms.—

(1) Acute pain, which becomes easier in time, but never completely abates.

(2) Shock, subnormal temperature and rapid small pulse.

(3) May have vomiting.

(4) Abdomen becomes distended and tender; after initial shock temperature rises slightly. Abdominal movements are restricted.

(5) General and local symptoms tend to improve after a few hours.

Diagnose from: Acute appendix, rupture of a hollow viscus or tubal pregnancy.

2. *Gradual.*—

(*a*) Usually no symptoms, but dull pain may be present.

(*b*) Tumour enlarges and is liable to infection.

Treatment.—Removal of tumour after recovery from initial shock.

(*b*) **Rupture.**—

1. May be spontaneous or due to trauma (at labour, etc.).

2. If spontaneous, is usually due to degeneration in the wall and is very apt to occur in papillomatous cysts ; in some cases it is due to increased tension after hæmorrhage.

3. *Clinical features* depend on the cyst contents :—

(*a*) If serous fluid (usually none)—rapidly absorbed.

(*b*) If pseudo-myxomatous or teratomatous—slight peritoneal reaction is usual, causing adhesions which allow encysting of the contents. Pseudo-myxoma peritonei may occur in former.

(*c*) Papillary or teratomatous—epithelial metastases.

(*d*) Malignant—malignant metastases.

(*e*) Suppurating—acute and rapidly fatal peritonitis.

(*f*) Fatal hæmorrhage may occur due to rupture of vessels.

(*c*) **Inflammation and Infection.**—

1. Often due to axial rotation.

2. Usually occurs in small cysts which are infected from the bowel.

3. Pain and tenderness are present over cyst.

(*d*) **Suppuration.**—

1. If suppuration occurs, fibrinous deposit is thrown out, which fixes tumour and obscures outline.

2. Teratomata are specially apt to suppurate after pregnancy.

3. Severe constitutional and local disturbances.

4. Patient may die owing to septic absorption, or the abscess may rupture externally, internally or into a hollow viscus.

5. Symptoms may become chronic and constitutional symptoms are then slight.

6. Pus often sterile.

(*e*) **Adhesions.**—

1. Due to axial rotation or inflammation.

2. Due to appendicitis, salpingitis, etc.

3. Tumour fixed.

4. Usually cause pain and menorrhagia.

Clinical Features of Cystic Ovarian Tumours

1. **Benign.**—

(1) Usually no symptoms to begin with except gradual enlargement of the abdomen.

(2) Menstruation is not usually affected, but amenorrhœa or menorrhagia may each occur.

(3) Sterility is common, but not constant.

(4) Pain usually denotes a complication, unless it is due to pressure.

(5) Pressure symptoms occur if the tumour is large, *e.g.* varix, dyspnœa, dyspepsia, constipation and slight œdema of both legs.

(6) Retention of urine may occur with cysts impacted in the pelvis thrusting the cervix forwards.

(7) Breasts may enlarge and areolæ form. Fluid may be secreted.

(8) General health deteriorates, face is drawn and emaciation is common—if tumour grows to a large size.

(9) Tumour is elastic and tense ; a teratoma is somewhat doughy.

(10) Does not move with uterus and is separate from it.

(11) If intra-ligamentary, lies at the side of the uterus and pushes the body to the other side.

2. **Malignant.**—

(1) Pain is common and may come on gradually, or suddenly and acutely.

(2) Sudden enlargement of the abdomen is common, due to rapid increase in size of cyst and to ascites.

(3) Menorrhagia and metrorrhagia to begin with, followed later by amenorrhœa. Irregular bleedings often occur in women past the menopause.

(4) Ascites.

(5) Unilateral œdema of legs, especially with a small tumour.

(6) Irregularity of surface.

(7) Fixation of tumour.

(8) Cachexia and wasting.

Diagnosis of Large Cyst in Abdomen.—

From (*a*) Ascites.

Ascites.	Cyst.
1. Fullness in lumbar region, centre flat.	1. Centre full, lumbar region flat.
2. No definite outline.	2. Definite outline.
3. Fluid thrill.	3. Fluid thrill only in a small number.
4. Dull in flanks, resonant at midline.	4. Dull at midline, resonant in flanks.
5. Shifting dullness.	5. Dullness remains at centre.
6. Distance from ensiform to umbilicus more than from umbilicus to pubis.	6. Distance from umbilicus to pubis much the longer.
7. Distance from the umbilicus to the anterior superior spines equal.	7. Longer on one side than the other.

(*b*) Pregnancy (see p. 43).
(*c*) Fibroids (see p. 299).
(*d*) Adiposity—
1. Umbilicus is flush with the skin or protruding when a cyst is present, whereas the depth is increased in adiposity.
2. Dullness over tumour.
3. Definite outline of tumour.

(*e*) Flatulence—abdomen not resonant all over.
(*f*) Hydronephrosis—
1. Per vaginam, both ovaries can be felt in hydronephrosis.
2. Dullness does not pass into loin.

(*g*) Distended bladder—pass catheter.

Treatment of Ovarian Cysts

Ovariotomy. (See p. 368.)

Tapping during laparotomy to decrease size before removal may be carried out in a large benign serous cyst. In other cysts there is danger by tapping of—

1. Implantation metastases.
2. Pseudo-myxoma peritonei.
3. Malignant metastases.

It is usually safer therefore to remove cyst entire if possible.

If the cyst is malignant, then the uterus and opposite appendages should be removed. This may be followed by X-ray therapy.

Other Cysts

1. **Fimbrial Cysts.**—Arise from a collection of tubules which lie along the course of the ovarian fimbria of the Fallopian tube.

May grow to large size.

Unilocular and contain serous fluid. In many women small cysts may be found in relation to the ovarian fimbria and are developed in the homologues of the rete-testis of the male. (Keith.) (Hydatids of Morgagni.)

2. **Parovarian Cysts.**—Arise from the remains of genital tubules, consisting of a duct (Gärtner's) and a number of vertical tubules passing towards the hilum of the ovary.

Those cysts reach their greatest development about the age of thirty-five.

(1) Grow slowly between the layers of the broad ligament; fimbrial cysts attain any size, but the true parovarian cysts never grow to a large size.

(2) Smooth, translucent and thin-walled, being only loosely attached to the peritoneum.

(3) The tube usually lies over the top of the cyst and is elongated; the ovary is separate and distinct; the ovarian fimbria is attached to cyst, but is flattened and spread out.

(4) Unilocular with clear serous fluid or sometimes pseudo-mucin.

(5) Fimbrial cysts are lined by columnar ciliated epithelium, whereas true parovarian cysts are lined by cubical epithelium.

(6) *Differentiate* parovarian *from* true ovarian cysts by—

(*a*) Approximation to uterus, there being just a cleft between the cyst and the cervix.

(*b*) Tend to push the uterus to one side.

(*c*) Move to a slight extent with the uterus.

(*d*) More fixed.

(*e*) Uterus may be extended over the cyst.

(*f*) Has peritoneal covering which must be incised before enucleation.

Treatment.—Removal of cyst and, in some cases, the accompanying tube and ovary.

FALLOPIAN TUBES

1. Benign

Fibromyoma.—

1. Usually small, but may be large.
2. Usually single and may arise from any part of tube.
3. Always unilateral.
4. Subperitoneal commonest and submucous rarest.
5. If large, may undergo degeneration and, by causing obstruction, may be responsible for tubal gestation.
6. May give rise to pain and metrorrhagia.

Papilloma.—Very rare.

1. Probably inflammatory in origin, salpingitis being usually present.

2. Fluid is present in the tube which may be as large as a small melon.

3. Usually in outer two-thirds of tube; adhesions are common.

4. Ostia may be open or shut and fluid is usually gelatinous and yellow.

Clinical Features.—

(*a*) If the abdominal ostium is closed—there may be intermittent discharge (mucoid) from the vagina, associated with pain and disappearance of swelling.

(*b*) If the abdominal ostium is open—fluid will pass into abdominal cavity and give rise to ascites by irritating the peritoneum.

(*c*) If both ostia are closed—a large cyst forms.

Prognosis.—Guarded, as it may be a precursor of malignancy.

Treatment.—Removal.

2. Malignant

(*a*) **Chorionepithelioma.**—

1. May follow uterine or tubal gestation.
2. Most common extra-uterine site after the vagina.
3. Usually occurs in isthmic portion which acquires adhesions; the tumour may eat through into the bowel.
4. Clinical features of tubal pregnancy with or without hæmatocele.
5. May be as large as fœtal head.
6. Usually fatal. Widespread metastases occur in vagina, brain, lungs, spleen, etc.
7. Treated by pan-hysterectomy with removal of appendages.

(*b*) **Malignant Papilloma.**—

1. Inflammation probably predisposing cause.
2. Usually occurs at, or just after, menopause.
3. Starts in mucosa of the middle and outer third of tube.
4. Tube wall invaded by growth which shows active proliferation.
5. Ulceration and necrosis are common.

(*c*) **Adeno-Carcinoma.**—

1. Rarer than papilloma.
2. May be tubular, or consist of alveoli closely packed with cells which are often atypical and resemble sarcoma.

Clinical Features of (b) and (c).—

1. Tube usually sausage-shaped, the inner third being unaffected and looking like a pedicle.
2. Peritoneal surface is shaggy due to adhesions.
3. Fluid is often present in the tube and both tubes are frequently involved.
4. Papillary—cauliflower-like. Adeno—brain-like.
5. Growth erodes tube wall.

Signs and Symptoms of (b) and (c).—

(*a*) Pain in iliac regions or hypogastrium.

(*b*) Blood-stained and watery vaginal discharge, either constant and slight or at long intervals and in gushes. Pain may be due to the extrusion of the discharge.

(*c*) Ascites is common if abdominal ostium open.

(*d*) Tumour may be felt abdominally and per vaginam as a doughy or fluctuant swelling.

Metastases.—Ovary, uterine wall, omentum and retroperitoneal glands.

Prognosis.—Bad—diagnosis made at a late stage.

Treatment.—Pan-hysterectomy with removal of appendages.

Secondary Tubal Cancer.—

1. From body of uterus by direct spread.
2. By implantation on the mucous coat from the ovary.

CHAPTER XX

DISEASES OF THE VAGINA, VULVA AND URETHRA

VAGINA

New Growths

A. *Benign.*

Vaginal Cysts.—Varieties.

1. *Due to Persistence of Embryonic Structures.*—

(*a*) *Gärtner's Duct.*—

(1) Found in the antero-lateral vaginal wall just below the urethral orifice.
(2) Usually single, but, if they are multiple, they are found all in a row.
(3) Not usually larger than a plum.
(4) Contain watery fluid.
(5) No symptoms unless they are large enough to cause feeling of downbearing, protrusion through vulva or dyspareunia.

Diagnosis.—From—

1. Sub-urethral abscess or cyst—pressure decreases size of abscess and causes pus or fluid to come from urethra.

2. Urethrocele.—

(1) Swelling disappears on pressure.
(2) Sound passed per urethram enters cavity.
(3) Frequent and painful micturition.

3. Urethral abscess—discharge of pus on pressure.

4. Cystocele—sound passes into it.

Treatment.—Excision.

(*b*) *Müller's Duct.*—Rudimentary vagina connected with a rudimentary horn, which, if fluid collects, forms a cyst at the side of the functioning vagina.

(*c*) *Misplaced Ureter.*—Found in side wall of vagina and, if punctured, discharges urine.

2. *Due to Trauma.*—

(*a*) From tags of mucous membrane being buried in the stroma.

(*b*) Usually in posterior vaginal wall.

(*c*) Filled with desquamated epithelium or brownish yellow sebaceous material.

(*d*) Small, but often multiple.

(*e*) Rarely cause symptoms unless infected.

(*f*) Treated by excision if necessary.

Fibromyoma.—Rare. Treat by excision.

B. *Malignant*

1. **Chorionepithelioma.**—May be primary or secondary to uterine growth. Appears as a purple nodule, which, if secondary, may be multiple. Bleeds easily on contact.

2. **Carcinoma.**—Rare as a primary growth. Usually found in posterior wall and is usually secondary to cervical carcinoma. Gives rise to slight bleeding and pain in the pelvis.

Treatment.—Radium.

Fistulæ

1. **Vesico-vaginal.**—

(1) Due usually to injury, during labour, by instruments, or prolonged pressure on the anterior vaginal wall by head against symphysis. May occur in advanced cancer of cervix or vagina.

(2) Occurs as a rule in upper half of anterior wall and is very fixed.

(3) Usually is small.

(4) Bladder mucous membrane can be seen prolapsing through, but the margin of the opening in the vagina is lined by white cicatricial tissue.

(5) Urine can be seen trickling through. If fistula cannot be seen inject sterile milk into bladder.

(6) Inflammation of the vulva and vagina and, sometimes, of bladder occurs.

(7) Treated by a plastic operation. (See p. 374.)

2. **Uretero-vaginal** usually occur in the lateral fornices and is due to injury to the ureter in hysterectomy, especially in pan-hysterectomy. May require transplantation of ureter into rectum to effect a cure.

3. **Recto-vaginal**—caused by—

(1) Tear during labour.
(2) Incomplete healing of a complete tear.
(3) Advanced cancer of the cervix or vagina.

If traumatic, treat by plastic repair. In most cases fistula has to be converted into a complete tear before operation can be satisfactorily done. (See p. 372.)

VULVA

1. **Pruritus.**—

Causes.—

LOCAL
- (*a*) Discharges from the cervix or vagina, especially gonorrhœal; those caused by a neglected pessary, vesico-vaginal fistula, etc.
- (*b*) Pediculi, dirt and threadworms (in children).
- (*c*) Chronic ulcers, *e.g.* tuberculous and syphilitic.
- (*d*) Eczema, leukoplakia and kraurosis.

GENERAL
- (*e*) Neurosis.
- (*f*) Diabetes and hyperglycæmia.
- (*g*) Toxæmia during pregnancy.
- (*h*) Deficiency of ovarian hormones with atrophy of external genitalia.

Symptoms.—Irritation and itchiness. At first, worst at night, but if really bad it occurs also by day and causes loss of sleep and may even be responsible for suicide. The labia minora and clitoris are usually the first to be attacked.

Treatment.—Always test urine for sugar.

(1) Remove or treat the cause if it is found.

(2) Analgesic ointments, *e.g.* scuroform, cycloform, nestosyl, anethaine or carbolic (5 per cent.).

(3) Paint with tincture of iodine, 1 per cent., once or twice daily.

(4) X-rays to vulva.

(5) Injection of labia with proctocaine, the solution being injected just underneath the skin and the area involved infiltrated.

(6) Œstrogenic therapy may be tried (as for leukoplakia, see p. 335).

(7) Excision may be required, especially if leukoplakia is present.

(8) Low carbohydrate diet, even if glycosuria not present.

2. **Leukoplakia.**—Four stages. Usually begins at or after the menopause.

Stage 1.—

- (*a*) The parts are reddened, swollen, excoriated and dry.
- (*b*) Proliferation of the epithelium and epithelial processes are present combined with round-celled infiltration.

Stage 2.—

(*a*) The labia minora decrease in size, white patches appear, which coalesce, and may involve all the vulva except the vestibule and the urethral orifice.

(*b*) Plasma cells take the place of round-celled infiltration and hyaline degeneration develops in the superficial layers of the corium.

Symptoms of both stages—pruritus.

Stage 3.—

(*a*) Cracks and ulcers appear; also discharge. Carcinomatous changes may appear in the fissure or ulcer.

(*b*) The epithelial processes disappear, the superficial layers of the corium undergoing fibrosis.

Symptoms.—Pain and soreness due to exposure of the nerve endings.

Stage 4.—

The area becomes white and smooth, the labia minora and clitoris disappear and the disease is quiescent.

Causes no symptoms.

(*N.B.*—Cancer is favoured during the third stage, due to disappearance of the elastic tissue which allows of free epithelial growth. In Stage 4, dense sclerosis checks the epithelial growth and diminishes the risk of cancer.)

Treatment.—

For Stages 1 and 2—

(*a*) Examine urine for sugar to exclude diabetes.

(*b*) It has been found by Swift that in a number of cases leukoplakia is associated with absence of free hydrochloric acid in stomach. A stomach test should be carried out and if hydrochloric acid absent or very deficient, Ac. Hydrochlor. dil. ♏xx–xxx t.i.d. will effect a cure; this may be combined with Vitamin A and D.

(*c*) Œstrogenic therapy, equivalent to 5 mgm. stilbœstrol, twice daily for ten to fourteen days.

(*N.B.*—*If condition does not improve within fourteen days, or recurs, then œstrogenic therapy should not be continued and excision of vulva will be safest treatment.* Several cases of cancer have been seen who have been under treatment with œstrogen without regular examination of area.)

Stage 3—excision, as for epithelioma.

Stage 4—no treatment is required.

3. **Kraurosis.**—Occurs on the labia minora, posterior urethral orifice and periurethral ducts (Skene's); never on the labia majora, perineum or postanal region. Often associated with senile vaginitis. It usually occurs at or after the menopause and is due to deficient œstrogen, allowing cells to atrophy and infection to occur.

Clinical Features.—

1) Irritation, discomfort and often pain.
2) May complain of feeling something coming down.
3) Dyspareunia and often dysuria.
4) Small red areas seen on labia minora and around urethra and often on vaginal mucosa as well.
5) Urethra often exhibits a caruncular condition on posterior lip.

Treatment.—Œstrogenic therapy equivalent to stilbœstrol 5 mgm. twice daily for ten to fourteen days and œstrone pessaries, *e.g.* Kolpon, inserted one nightly from fourth day of treatment onwards; or œstradial benzoate 50,000 I.B.U. can be injected twice weekly and œstrone 1000 i.u. given orally thrice daily for three weeks in place of stilbœstrol.

New Growths

Benign.—Rare. Fibromata, lipomata, papillomata, adenomata and adenomyomata may occur. Treated by excision.

Malignant.—

Epithelioma—the most common. It may occur in the clitoris or on the labia majora. It occurs usually after the menopause and is often preceded by leukoplakia or pruritus.

Signs and Symptoms.—

(*a*) *Clitoris.*—

1. Appears as a hard nodule which rapidly ulcerates.
2. Diffuse infiltration usually involving the inguinal glands.
3. Usually painful, as the clitoris is sensitive.
4. Ulcerates early, giving rise to discharge, which becomes rapidly offensive.
5. More malignant.

(*b*) *Labia.*—

1. May appear as a hard nodule, which ulcerates late, or as a small excavated ulcer with an indurated and everted edge. It starts usually on the inner surface of the labium majus and spreads to the minus. May become cauliflower-like and fungate.

2. There is pruritus to begin with and then pain; very little bleeding unless a large vessel is eroded.
3. There is an offensive discharge, when ulceration occurs.
4. *Treatment.*—Excision of vulva (see p. 375). Glands in groin can be treated by removal, X-ray therapy or radium implants.

Rodent Ulcer, Bowen's Disease and Melanoma.—May occur, but are rare.

Diseases of Bartholin's Glands

1. *Cysts* may occur either in the duct or in the gland, due to inflammatory stenosis of the duct; frequently gonococcal in origin, or due to a calculus.

2. They appear on the posterior surface of the labia majora and may burrow deeply into the posterior labial wall, causing no symptoms other than discomfort.

3. If they are infected, *abscess* results. An abscess may occur without cyst formation, being due in 75 per cent. of cases to gonorrhœa and in the others to streptococci, pneumococci, etc. Gives rise to intense pain, swelling, throbbing, redness and œdema.

4. *Diagnose cyst from*—
   (*a*) Hydrocele of the canal of Nuck.
   (*b*) Inguinal hernia.
   (*c*) Vulval hæmatoma.

Treatment.—*Cyst:* Excision of the gland and duct (p. 375).

Abscess: By opening and treating with spirit and B.I.P. paste (p. 376), or by opening and packing with gauze or worsted to encourage healing from base.

Malignant.—Adeno-carcinoma may arise in Bartholin's gland and may involve the inguinal glands. Very malignant.

Coccydynia

Causes.—

1. Injury during labour.
2. A fall or kick.

} Causing fracture of coccyx with false joint formation.

3. Rheumatism.
4. Neurosis.

Symptoms.—

1. Pain on sitting and on defæcation.
2. Pressure on the coccyx causes pain.

Treatment.—

1. Palliative.
2. Excise the coccyx.

URETHRA

Caruncle.—

1. May be angioma, granuloma, or due to œstrogen deficiency (kraurosis).
2. May be pedunculated (angioma) or sessile (granuloma).
3. Occurs immediately within posterior lip of urethra, but if due to kraurosis may spread to surrounding area.
4. If pedunculated, single and about the size of a large pin head ; if sessile, usually broader.
5. Bright red in colour, especially if pedunculated.
6. Granulomatous caruncles are associated with chronic urinary tract infection (urethritis and cystitis).

Symptoms.—

1. Angiomata cause pain, dyspareunia, dysuria (at times) and bleeding. Exceedingly tender to touch.
2. Granulomata usually cause discomfort, frequency of micturition and slight dysuria, and sometimes bleeding, but may cause no symptoms. Not tender.
3. Those associated with kraurosis cause feeling of something coming down and often extreme discomfort, with possibly some frequency. May be tender to touch.

Treatment.—

1. Angiomata should be excised and base cauterised.
2. Granulomata should be cauterised and urinary tract infection treated. (Very apt to recur.)
3. When associated with kraurosis, intensive œstrogenic therapy will effect a cure without any cauterisation being required.

(*N.B.*—Caruncles may become malignant, or malignant disease secondary to vulva or vagina may affect the urethral orifice. In these cases the whole urethra must be excised with the inguinal glands on both sides.)

Adenomata and carcinomata may arise at the meatus.

Urethritis.—Not so common as in the male. Usually gonorrhœal in origin (see p. 342).

CHAPTER XXI

VENEREAL DISEASES AFFECTING THE GENERATIVE ORGANS

1. Syphilis

A. Primary.—

Appears at the site of innoculation ten to ninety days after infecting intercourse.

May start—

(*a*) As a papule, which gets abraded, leaving a small clean sore, with an indurated base and regular outline. It is insensitive unless there is superadded infection, and oozes serum rather than blood. The area affected is usually œdematous.

(*b*) Atypically, as a septic abrasion in a fissure with tense œdema around and syphilitic lymphangitis.

There is usually an associated indolent inguinal adenitis in either case.

Common Sites.—

1. *The Cervix*, where it passes unnoticed unless careful vaginal examination is made with a speculum. Diagnose from (*a*) an erosion, which is bright red, is not indurated and spreads from the endo-cervix. Spirochætes can be demonstrated in serum obtained by means of a capillary tube if syphilitic; (*b*) cancer, which causes an irregular bleeding and an offensive discharge. Microscopic examination of biopsy is conclusive.

2. *The Vulva.*—

(i) Labia majora. } Where opposition sores often
(ii) Labia minora. } occur.
(iii) Navicular fossa, or posterior part of the introitus, where it commonly originates as a painful fissure and forms a " butterfly " sore.
(iv) Less commonly at the clitoris, urethra or Bartholin orifices.

The vaginal wall is rarely affected.

Diagnosis.—After cleansing the sore with gauze and saline, express serum and examine under dark ground illumination for spirochætes. Blood tests are negative for the first two to three weeks.

B. **Secondary.**—Occurs as—

1. Moist papules, or rash spots which have become rubbed and eroded.

2. Condylomata lata, which are raised, warty, indurated, dirty white growths, moist with serous exudate and degenerating epithelium.

3. Mucous patches, found on the inner surfaces of the vulva, which become abraded to form shallow ulcers.

The inguinal glands are painlessly enlarged as part of a generalised adenitis.

Diagnosis.—Serum is collected from the lesions and in secondary syphilitic lesions; this is swarming with spirochætes. Wassermann and Khan reactions are now strongly positive.

C. **Tertiary.**—

1. Gummata in the labia majora, which break down to form ulcers.

2. Sclerosis vulvæ (late and rare).

Diagnosis.—Blood tests are usually strongly positive and spirochætes are not found in the discharge from tertiary lesions.

2. Chancroid

Incubation period usually one to five days. Due to Ducrey's bacillus.

Features.—

(i) Irregular multiple dirty ulcers with sloughing bases and undermined edges appear on and near the vulva.

(ii) There is acute inflammation around the ulcers with pain and tenderness.

(iii) Inguinal glands are enlarged, matted, painful and tend to suppurate.

Diagnosis.—

(*a*) By clinical features and history.

(*b*) By excluding syphilis (serum for spirochætes and repeated blood tests).

(*c*) By Rienstierna's skin test.

Ducrey's bacillus difficult to isolate in smears taken from underneath overhanging edges of lesions.

Treatment.—Consists in giving one of the sulphonamide

group of drugs (sulphathiazole or sulphadiazine for preference) in dosage 3–5 gm. per day for five days. Streptomycin is also effective.

Locally—cleanliness and mild antiseptic applications are all that are required.

Note.—Serum should always be taken from any vulval sore and examined for spirochætes.

3. Gonorrhoea

A. **Infection.**—

1. It is impossible to say definitely, even if all secretions are negative, that a woman is not infective, as secretions from gland ducts, which cannot be obtained for diagnosis, are produced at sexual intercourse.

2. Coitus just after or during a period is most likely to cause infection, as the secretion then is not so acid and thus the gonococcus may thrive.

B. **Site of Inoculation.**—

1. Urethral meatus and Skene's ducts.
2. Around the external os.

The folds and crypts in both situations form good breeding places and the initial lesions are found in the urethra and cervix.

3. Vagina and vulva are not readily infected (except in little girls below the age of puberty), but the orifices of Bartholin's ducts form good breeding places.

C. **Pathology.**—Incubation period two to ten days.

1. Inflammation occurs with swelling and desquamation of epithelium, gonococci being found between the cells in very early cases. Later the typical gram negative intracellular diplococci are found.

2. The small blood vessels are full of leucocytes, and emigration and phagocytosis cause purulent discharge.

3. Squamous epithelium is more resistant than columnar.

4. Mixed infection, due to staphylococci, streptococci and B. coli, is often superimposed.

5. After a few weeks there is a retrogression and partial cure, which, however, is often incomplete and the disease may become chronic, being sheltered in Bartholin's glands, Skene's tubules, etc.

6. Granulation tissue and white fibrous tissue forms, and the cylindrical epithelium is replaced by squamous.

7. If gonococci are shut up in any closed cavity, they die in a few weeks, being destroyed by the products of their own metabolism, but if there is a slight leak, they may thrive indefinitely.

D. **Complications.**—

1. Uterus, tubes and sometimes peritoneum may be affected.
2. More rarely the bladder and ureter are affected.
3. Metastatic infections may be transferred by the blood giving rise to arthritis, tenosynovitis, iritis, etc., especially if there is a chronic lesion in the genito-urinary tract which acts as a constant source of infection.
4. Septicæmia or pyæmia may result.

E. **Method of Diagnosis.**—

1. Take pus from the urethra on a fine swab, squeezing the canal through the vagina if necessary. Films and cultures are made from this. (The patient should not have passed urine for two to three hours before examination.)
2. Swab the vagina and external os with a dry swab and take smears from the interior of the cervix, again making films and cultures.
3. If the films and cultures are negative, a provocative application to the urethra and cervix of glycerine, or the injection of a provocative vaccine or of neofemergin may be followed in twenty-four hours by positive tests.
4. Wassermann, Khan and gonococcal complement-fixation tests should be done.

F. **Clinical Features.**—May be very acute, but usually not prominent. Often ignored until some complication occurs.

1. *Vulva.*—Inflammation and œdema caused by excessive secretion. Feeling of heat and irritation.
2. *Urethra.*—The lips of the meatus are red and œdematous and pus exudes. Urethritis rarely causes discomfort in the female, but there may be scalding pain on micturition and occasionally hæmaturia or retention.
3. *Bartholin's Glands.*—
   (i) Duct orifices inflamed first, and then the glands are involved.
   (ii) The œdematous mucosa blocks the ducts and the increased secretion is imprisoned.
   (iii) The duct, and sometimes the gland itself, forms an abscess or in more chronic cases a cyst.

4. *Vagina.*—Irritation is caused by the cervical secretion, and lactic acid bacilli disappear as the discharge increases.

5. *Cervix.*—

(i) Acute catarrhal inflammation.
(ii) Mucosa swollen and dull red.
(iii) Pus exudes from the external os.
(iv) Bleeds readily on touching, but is not friable.
(v) Painful to touch.

As the infection spreads to the endocervix and endometrium, backache, abdominal pain and menstrual disturbances occur with profuse, prolonged, painful and irregular periods.

G. **Treatment.**—

1. *General.*—

(i) Rest is not necessary except in complicated cases. Treatment is usually ambulant.
(ii) Penicillin in the form of one intramuscular injection of 1 c.c. = 300,000 units of procaine penicillin will cure practically all acute cases. Complicated cases require repeated injections.
(iii) When there is a possibility of coincidentally acquired syphilis, or for patients showing severe sensitivity to penicillin, one of the sulphonamide preparations (sulphadiazine for preference) may be given in doses of 5 gm. per day for five days. Patient should be instructed to drink freely, and if necessary, a mixture containing potassium citrate should be prescribed.
(iv) A few very resistant or severely complicated cases may require treatment with one of the newer antibiotics such as chloromycetin, or even hyperpyrexia by means of injection of vaccines or the inductotherm cabinet.
(v) Repeated tests are required to prove cure.

2. *Local.*—

(i) Sitz baths, ichthyol pessaries and douching may be advised in certain cases.
(ii) On attendance at the clinic films are taken from the urethra and cervix. The vaginal discharge is examined for yeast or trichomonal infection which may be superimposed and will require local treatment before the patient can be discharged.

3. *Advice to Patients.*—Patients should be told that the discharge is highly infectious, and care must be taken to avoid its transference to some other member of the family or to their own eyes. As the patient may have been infected with syphilis when she acquired gonorrhœa, she should be kept under observation for four and a half months.

4. Vulvo-Vaginitis in Children

Cause.—

1. Organismal, *i.e.* gonococcal, pneumococcal, staphylococcal, diphtheroid, B. coli, etc.
2. Parasitic.—Threadworm, scabies, trichomonas.
3. Traumatic.—Rape, masturbation, insertion of foreign body.
4. Lack of hygiene.

Symptoms.—

1. Irritation and discomfort on walking.
2. Dysuria, which may cause retention and enuresis.
3. Blood-stained pus found on the clothes.
4. Sometimes tenesmus.

Signs.—

1. Whole vulva reddened and bathed in pus.
2. Tender and excoriated.
3. Small red areas found on vaginal walls.
4. Salpingitis very rare. Bartholin glands immature and not affected.
5. Rectum may discharge pus.

Diagnosis.—Films and cultures should be taken from the vulva, urethra, vagina and rectum.

Treatment.—*General.*—

1. Rest in bed until the acute infectious stage is passed.
2. If the causative organism is the gonoccus, then the child should be admitted to hospital and given repeated injections of penicillin, either three-hourly or using the prolonged action procaine penicillin preparations once or twice daily.
3. In the rare cases where penicillin fails or is contraindicated, a course of sulphonamides, or another antibiotic may be used in doses of quarter to half the adult strength.

The mother of the child, or nearest contact should be examined and, if necessary, treated.

Local.—

1. Sitz baths of dilute potassium permanganate or sodium bicarbonate.

2. Local application and irrigation of the vagina with mild antiseptics is now rarely required.

5. Ophthalmia Neonatorum

Definition.—

"Any inflammation of the eyes of an infant accompanied by a discharge from the eyes, commencing within twenty-one days from the date of birth."

It is a notifiable condition. (See p. 387.)

CHAPTER XXII

SEXUAL DISORDERS

1. Sterility

In considering this problem, the husband must not be forgotten, as he may be responsible in 25 per cent. of all cases. The male should therefore be investigated in doubtful cases before the woman is subjected to operative treatment.

Causes (Female).—

1. *Developmental.—*

   (*a*) Atresia of vagina.
   (*b*) Imperforate hymen.

2. *Dyspareunia.—*

   (*a*) Very tight hymen.
   (*b*) Carunculæ myrtiformes.
   (*c*) Vaginismus.
   (*d*) Vulvitis and vaginitis.
   (*e*) Prolapse of ovaries with or without retroversion.
   (*f*) Chronic pelvic inflammation.

      (1) Appendages.
      (2) Utero-sacral ligaments.

3. *Absence of Cervical Insemination.—*

The acid vagina is definitely hostile to sperms, which lose much motility in fifteen minutes and die in one to two hours. Cervical secretion is alkaline and sperms can live in cervix for several days. Therefore, sperms must be ejected near external os. This may be prevented by—

(*a*) Very long and redundant vagina, the mucosa being thrown into folds.
(*b*) Long penis and short vagina—penis entering post-fornix.
(*c*) Cervix up against anterior vaginal wall, with or without retroversion.
(*d*) Elongation of cervix.
(*e*) Prolapse of uterus.

4. *Hostility of Cervical Secretions.*—

Never chemical or bacterial, but may be mechanical due to—

(*a*) Abnormal viscosity of mucus in canal due to excessive secretion.
(*b*) Mucous plug not being removed by precoital excitation—associated with frigidity.

5. *Uterine Causes.*—

(*a*) Tumours filling uterus or blocking entrance.
(*b*) Hypoplasia.
(*c*) Endometritis, preventing nidation.

6. *Tubal Causes.*—

(*a*) Obstruction, due to pressure by tumours.
(*b*) Adhesions, causing blockage of ostia, or acute congestion of tube, kinks or pockets.
(*c*) Hypoplasia with excessive convolution.
(*d*) Chronic congestion, causing adhesions of endosalpingial surfaces or formation of mucous plugs in lumen.

7. *Ovary.*—

(*a*) Non-ovulation—anovular bleeding.
(*b*) Thickening of tunica albugina preventing extrusion of ovum and associated with mittelschmerz.
(*c*) Prolapse of ovary causing dyspareunia or preventing ovum's easy passage to tube.
(*d*) Follicular cysts causing metropathia hæmorrhagica.
(*e*) Persistent corpus luteum.
(*f*) Some neoplasms.
(*g*) Atrophy.

8. *Endocrinal.*—

Anterior pituitary, ovarian or thyroid dysfunction.

9. *Inimicable Partnership.*

Male.—

1. Impotence.
2. Deformities.
3. Insufficient spermatozoa.—Normal about 100,000,000 per c.c. semen. Sterility below 60,000,000 per c.c.
4. Abnormal sperms.—Usually only less than 15 per cent. abnormal, but if incidence is more than 25 per cent. then sterile.

5. Immotility of sperms.—More than 15 per cent. non-motile sperms denote sterility.

6. Non-endurance.—Normally sperms remain alive for twelve to twenty-four hours at room temperature.

Post-coital examination of great value and is usually made one to two hours after intercourse.

Huhner's Test.—Mucous is taken from inside cervical canal with spoon curette within two hours of intercourse; this shows, if sperms are present, normal, motile and in sufficient numbers. (In normal cases two to twenty are found under high power field and most should be motile.) When this is contrasted with normal semen, examination shows if wife or husband is at fault.

Examinations and Treatments.—

1. Perineotomy for congenital atresia, tight hymen and vaginismus, followed by application of glass vaginal dilators in increasing sizes (see p. 376).

2. Endometrial biopsy in premenstrual part of cycle to diagnose anovular bleeding (when there is no premenstrual endometrial reaction) metropathia or endometritis.

3. Insufflation of tubes with air (Rubin's Test). Air is passed into uterus by means of a special cannula, and normally passes into abdomen through tubes at a pressure of 120 mm. Hg. or less. (The air can be heard entering the abdomen with a stethoscope.) If tube is partially blocked, a pressure of 180 mm. may be required and the treatment may be curative, but if 200 mm. is reached without air passing, then no higher pressure should be attempted as it shows that the tube is blocked. In some cases, however, this is due to muscular spasm, and the tube is found to be patent with the injection of lipiodol. (Carbon dioxide may be preferred to air.)

4. Injection of lipiodol through the tubes. This is passed into the uterus through a special cannula by means of a pressure apparatus, or more easily with an ordinary record syringe. Five to six c.c. are passed in slowly at a pressure not exceeding 200 mm. Hg. An X-ray is then taken, which shows the uterus and tubes, if patent, full of opaque substance. Twenty-four hours later a second X-ray of the pelvis is taken, which shows lipiodol mottled throughout pelvis if tubes are patent or if one tube is. This examination is probably more informative than air inflation, as it shows, not only if tubes are open or blocked but, if the latter, where the blockage is, and if any operative interference, such as salpingostomy, is likely to be successful. It would also seem to open up small adhesions

more satisfactorily than air. This, in addition to being a diagnostic procedure, is often curative as well, and the examination is followed within three months by a pregnancy.

5. Attend to general health of husband and wife. Vitamin E to both may be of use. Testosterone for husband if sperm count not satisfactory.

6. Correct any displacement, dilate cervix if stenosed, curette uterus, if endometritis present. Remove any offending tumours.

7. Pregnant mare's serum (F.S.H.) 200 R.U. from tenth to fourteenth day of cycle may produce ovulation in anovular cases, or a large dose, 200 to 500 R.U., may be given intravenously on the day ovulation is expected, *i.e.* fourteen days before next period is normally due. Synapoidin 1 c.c. may be given from tenth to fourteenth day of cycle, the treatment being continued for several months.

2. Dyspareunia

Difficulty in coitus associated with pain.

1. **Primary.**—In women, who have never had painless intercourse.

Causes.—

(1) Clumsiness or inexperience of man.

(2) Fear of being hurt after a first painful coitus.

(3) Tender carunculæ myrtiformes or soreness from hymenal laceration.

(4) Disproportion of penis to vagina.

(5) Prolapsed ovaries—often present with retroverted uterus.

(6) Infections of tubes or ovaries.

(7) Growths of vulva or vagina.

Treatment.—

(1) Treat any local condition. Ung. cocaine (5 per cent.).

(2) If carunculæ or a lacerated hymen be present, advise abstinence till tenderness disappears, for if not, vaginismus may occur.

2. **Secondary.**—After years of painless intercourse or after parturition.

Causes.—

(1) Infection of vulva, vagina or adnexa.

(2) Retroversion with prolapsed ovaries.

(3) New growths of vulva, vagina or cervix.

Pain occurs at the site of the lesion.

Treat cause.

3. Vaginismus

Reflex spasm of bulbo-cavernosi, transversi perinei and levatores ani.

Originally protective, resisting penetration and the stretching of tender spots, but later it becomes nervous, and is accentuated as time goes on.

Treatment.—

1. Cocaine ointment (5 per cent.) locally, and general treatment for neurosis.

2. Stretch the vaginal outlet under anæsthesia, and make the patient wear a glass dilator for two or three hours daily. A Barnes bag may be used instead.

3. Incise the perineum vertically either in the mid-line or at the sides, and stitch up in the transverse. Excise any tender carunculæ. A glass dilator should then be worn for two or three hours daily, the size being increased each day (see p. 376).

CONTRACEPTION

May be advisable for medical, obstetrical, gynæcological, economic or social reasons.

Methods.—(*a*) Chemical. (*b*) Vaginal appliances. (*c*) Intrauterine appliances. (*d*) Male appliances. (*e*) Coitus interruptus. (*f*) So-called safe period.

(*a*) **Chemical.**—

(1) Not entirely satisfactory, as ejaculate may pass directly into cervical canal.

(2) Most potent substances are quinone group, hexylresorcin, formaldehyde, potassium permanganate, plain water (by immobilising sperms). *p*H should be below 3·5 to kill sperms.

Types.—

(*a*) Suppositories.—Not satisfactory.

(*b*) Jellies and pastes.—Useful as lubricants for occlusive pessaries or condoms, or for mass injection into vagina.

(*c*) Foam preparations.—Useful, but expensive; components have to be kept separate in double compartment collapsible tubes before injection into vagina.

Foam tablets, which are quite inexpensive, can also be used, but are not at all certain in action.

(*b*) **Occlusion Pessaries.**—Prevent ejaculate's contact with cervix, but allow semen to be deposited in vagina. Should always be used with a spermicidal jelly.

They permit normal intercourse, being inserted at night and removed in morning.

Types.—

(1) Cervical caps.—Fit closely to cervix and may be harmful as they constrict cervix and prevent free drainage.

(2) Vault pessaries.—Maintain position by contact with vaginal walls, but do not cover vaginal walls.

(3) Diaphragm pessaries.—

- (i) Probably most satisfactory and certainly the easiest to insert.
- (ii) Divide vagina diagonally into two parts : (*a*) an anterior and upper part which includes cervix and anterior vagina, and (*b*) a posterior and lower part, which admits penis, which is then separated from cervix.
- (iii) Has to be fitted accurately and the correct size prescribed.
- (iv) Unsatisfactory for cases of—
  - (*a*) Cystocele and rectocele.
  - (*b*) Marked laxity of vaginal walls.
  - (*c*) Severe constipation.
  - (*d*) Marked erosions with profuse discharge.

(*c*) **Intra-uterine Appliances.**—

Types.—

(1) Stem pessaries (spiral wire or wish bone).—Very dangerous—381 deaths or disorders due to such pessaries have been collected in literature.

(2) Gräfenberg ring.—Consists of gold or silver wire twisted spirally, which is inserted into uterus by special introducer and is removed by same instrument. Probably acts by irritating uterus and causing early abortion. By no means infallible as several X-rays have shown pregnancy with ring in situ in uterus. May cause bleeding, discharge and pain and, by irritation, malignancy at a later date. Not to be recommended.

(*d*) **Condoms.**

(1) Should be used with spermicidal jelly injected into sheath, and also as a lubricant outside.

(2) Sheath must be tested before and after coitus to be sure it is sound and, if found defective after intercourse, a plain water douche should be used immediately.

(3) Should bear date of manufacture and should not be used more than six to twelve months after that date.

(4) May cause impairment of sensation or friction in a dry vagina.

(5) Woman deprived of benefit from absorption of semen if, as some authorities state, such is beneficial.

(*e*) **Coitus Interruptus.**—Should never be practised as definitely detrimental.

(*f*) **Safe Period.**—Fertilisation is unlikely to occur if intercourse takes place more than four days before ovulation.

CHAPTER XXIII

THERAPEUTIC USE OF HORMONES IN OBSTETRICS AND GYNÆCOLOGY

THE following hormones are in common clinical use in gynæcology and midwifery :—

1. Œstrogens (follicular).
2. Progesterone (luteal).
3. Ovulatory (corresponds to anterior pituitary ovulating).
4. Chorionic Gonadatrophin (corresponds to anterior pituitary luteinising).
5. Androgens.
6. Thyroid.
7. Posterior Pituitary—
   (*a*) Oxytocic.
   (*b*) Vaso-pressor.

1. **Œstrogens.**—

(*a*) *Natural.*—

(1) Œstradiol, from sow's ovaries and urine of pregnant mares. (Preparations : Œstradiol benzoate—Progynon B. Oleosum (Schering), Dimenformon (Organon), Œstradiol benzoate (B.W. and Co.), etc. Dosage : 10,000–50,000 I.B.U.)

(2) Œstriol, from placenta. (Preparations : Theelin (P.D. and Co.), Tridestrin (Pabyrn), etc. Dosage : 200–5000 I.U.)

(*b*) *Catabolic-end Product.*—

Œstrone, from urine of pregnant women and mares. (Preparations : Menformon (Organon), Œstroform (B.D.H.), Ovostab (Boots), Progynon (Schering), etc. Dosage : 1000–10,000 I.U.)

(*c*) *Synthetic.*—

Stilbœstrol and its derivatives, stilbœstrol dipropionate, ovendosyn (Menley and James), etc. Dosage : 0·5–5·0 mgm.

Hexœstrol. Dosage : 0·5–5·0 mgm.

Dienœstrol. Dosage : 0·1–5·0 mgm.

Triphenylchloroethylene. Dosage : 0·5–2 gm. (Gynosone) (I.C.I.).

Ethinyl Œstradiol, 0·01, 0·05, 1·0 mgm.

Standardisation.—

1 mgm. Stilbœstrol=approx. 50,000 int. units œstrone.
10,000 int. benzoate units œstradiol benzoate.
400 mgm. triphenylchloro-ethylene.

(Ovendosyn is same strength as Stilbœstrol, but Hexœstrol, just slightly weaker by injection, is only half as strong or less by mouth.) Dienœstrol is approximately the same strength as stilbœstrol when given orally.

(*N.B.*—Stilbœstrol, though used as a standard for dosage, is not advised for use clinically, as it appears to be the most toxic of all the preparations and may cause nausea and sickness. Its derivatives are usually less toxic even in large doses ; so also are the other œstrogens.)

Administration.—

(1) Oral.—(Œstriol, œstrone and synthetic preparations.)
(2) Intra-muscular.—(Œstradiol benzoate preparations.)
(3) Vaginal (pessaries). — (Progynon (Schering), Kolpon (Organon).)
(4) Inunction.—(Natural—ovocyclin ointment (Ciba).
Synthetic—Stilbœstrol ointment (B.W. and Co.).)

Optimum result usually obtained by oral administration and therefore can be easily prescribed. The synthetic preparations are quite cheap.

Common Clinical Uses.—

(1) For menopausal symptoms or after surgical menopause.
Usually a dosage of 0·5 mgm. stilbœstrol daily is sufficient to ward off symptoms of the surgical menopause, but slightly higher doses are required for ordinary menopausal symptoms, 0·5 mgm. twice or thrice daily. The dosage in each case is gradually decreased as time goes on.

(2) To inhibit lactation.
Stilbœstrol 5 mgm. thrice daily for three days, twice daily for two days, and once daily for four days.
Acts by inhibiting the lactogenic hormone in the anterior pituitary.

(3) For senile vaginitis, kraurosis and some cases of leukoplakia.
Stilbœstrol 5 mgm. twice daily for ten to fourteen days ;

or œstradiol benzoate 50,000 I.B.U. twice weekly by injection, and œstrone 1,000 I.U. thrice daily orally for three weeks; combined with œstrone pessaries from fourth to fourteenth days.

Acts by stimulating activity of vaginal and vulval mucosa.

(4) For induction in cases of missed abortion and for primary uterine inertia.

10 mgm. stilbœstrol hourly for eight hours, followed by quinine and post-pituitary induction, if necessary.

For primary inertia, 50,000 I.B.U. œstradial benzoate can be injected hourly or 10 mgm. stilbœstrol every 15 minutes.

(The use of œstrogens in such cases is by no means always followed by success and unfortunately they are still of little use in the induction of labour.)

(5) For uterine hypoplasia and amenorrhœa.

Stilbœstrol, 0·5 mgm. twice or thrice daily for two weeks at a time and repeat for at least three months. For hypoplasia this should be combined with thyroid ½ gr. twice daily over the three months.

A combination of œstrogen and ethisterone such as Menstrogen (Organon) (0·01 mgm. Ethynal œstradiol and 10 mgm. Ethisterone) has been recommended by some authorities.

(6) To promote growth, turgidity and erectility of nipple.

Stilbœstrol ointment used once daily ante-natally and after each feed in puerperium.

(*N.B.*—Stilbœstrol in fairly large doses has benefited greatly some cases of carcinoma of the prostate and possibly of the breast, and has also been used with success to check acromegaly. It is also useful in some intractable cases of chronic mastitis given orally and by inunction.)

(7) In severe spasmodic dysmenorrhœa, 1 to 2 mgm. daily for fourteen days beginning first day of period. Inhibits ovulation.

(8) For metropathia hæmorrhagica and other functional bleeding, 10 mgm. of stilbœstrol daily until bleeding ceases, and then decrease dose by 2 mgm. a day (Novak), or

To stop bleeding—2–5 mgm. stilbœstrol daily.

When bleeding ceases—2 mgm. to complete twenty days.

Fifth day following start of withdrawal bleeding—2 mgm. stilbœstrol for twenty days.

Five days after start of next bleeding—2 mgm. stilbœstrol for twenty days.

Five days after start of next bleeding—2 mgm. stilbœstrol for twenty days; and

Fifteen days after start—20 mgm. ethisterone for ten days.

Five days after start of next bleeding—2 mgm. stilbœstrol for twenty days; and

Fifteen days after start—30 mgm. ethisterone for ten days.

Five days after start of next bleeding—2 mgm. stilbœstrol daily for twenty days; and

Fifteen days after start—40 mgm. ethisterone. (Swyer.)

2. **Progesterone.**—

Given usually by injection (Lutocyclin (Ciba), Progestin (B.D.H.), Proluton (Schering), Luteostab (Boots), Lutren (Bayer), Progesterone (B.W. and Co.), etc.), 1–10 mgm., but can be given orally in ten times the dosage. (Proluton C. (Schering), Progesterol (B.D.H.), Lutocyclin oral (Ciba), Ethisterone (B. W. and Co.), etc.)

Very expensive both by injection and orally.

Uses.—

(1) Habitual Abortion.
2 mgm. twice weekly and dose doubled at suppressed period for at least three months.
Causes uterine relaxation and helps embedding of ovum.

(2) Threatened Abortion.
10 mgm. daily until bleeding ceases, then 5 mgm. for two to three days, followed by 2 mgm. twice weekly as above.
(If ovum has become detached, progesterone often prevents uterine contractions, and ovum will be retained in utero, being passed after several weeks, as a carneous mole.)

(3) Amenorrhœa.
In second half of cycle, in association with œstrogen in first half, 2 mgm. on alternate days.

(4) Dysmenorrhœa.
Two-20 mgm. on alternate days for week before period.

(5) Menorrhagia of Puberty.
5 mgm. daily until bleeding ceases.

(6) Metropathia. Hæmorrhagica.

Four injections of 20 mgm. on alternate days during pre-menstrual week or on first day of bleeding; this should be continued at twenty-eight-day intervals or with the recurrence of bleeding.

3. **Follicle Stimulating (F.S.H.).**—

From pregnant mare's serum. (Preparations: Gestyl (Organon), Serogan (B.D.H.), Antostab (Boots), etc. Dosage: 100–200 I.U. intramuscularly.)

Uses.—

(1) For sterility, due to anovular bleeding or deficient luteinisation.

Two hundred I.U. for three to five injections, the last being given on day ovulation should occur (*i.e.* fourteen days before next period is due). Intravenous injection of 200 I.U. on day of ovulation has been recommended in some cases.

(2) Some cases of dysfunctional bleeding.

As above.

(3) Amenorrhœa and dysmenorrhœa due to under-developed uterus.

One hundred I.U. daily for two to three months, for amenorrhœa.

One hundred I.U. on alternate days for first two weeks of cycle, for dysmenorrhœa.

4. **Chorionic Gonadatrophin.**—

Found in placenta and in human pregnancy urine. Corresponds in action to the luteinising hormone, except that it does not produce luteinisation in the human, but only exaggerates any luteinisation that is present. May also inhibit unknown uterine bleeding factor.

(Preparations: Antuitrin S (P. D. and Co.), (1 c.c.=100 R.U.), Gonan (B.D.H.), Pregnyl (Organon), Prolan (Bayer), Physostab (Boots), Gonadatrophin S. (Pabyrn), etc. Dosage: 100–500 R.U. intramuscularly.)

Uses.—

(1) Menorrhagia of Puberty.

Two hundred R.U. daily until bleeding ceases, and then on alternate days for one week before next period is due.

(2) Metropathia Hæmorrhagica.

Two hundred R.U. for five injections, daily or on alternate days, before period due, for several months.

(3) Habitual abortion.
Two hundred R.U. twice weekly for first four months of pregnancy combined with thyroid extract ½ gr. daily, this dose being doubled at the suppressed period times when patient should be kept in bed.

(4) Sterility due to defective luteinisation.
One hundred R.U. daily from fifteenth to twentieth day of cycle.

(*N.B.*—The synergistic combination of chorionic gonadatrophin and an anterior pituitary hormone (Synapoidin (P. D. and Co.)) is stated to increase ovulation and luteinisation markedly and is given intramuscularly in 0·5 c.c. to 1 c.c. dosage for (*a*) dysfunctional bleeding, daily injections for five days before period, if possible (*b*) some cases of amenorrhœa due to anterior pituitary deficiency, 2 cc. on alternate days for twenty days followed by a ten-days interval, and (*c*) sterility due to anovular bleeding, the injections being given every third day from seventh to fourteenth day of cycle. It may also be of use in helping efficient spermatogenesis in the male.)

5. **Androgens.**—

(Preparations: Testoviron (Schering), Neo-Hombreol (Organon), Virormone (Pabyrn), Testosterone (B.D.H.), Sterandryl (Roussel), Testosterone propionate (B. W. and Co.), etc. Dosage: 10–25 mgms. by injection. Neo-Hombreol M. and Methyl-Testosterone (B. W. and Co.), etc., can be given orally or as linguets.)

Therapeutic Actions.—

(1) Inhibits gonadotrophic hormone activity of Pituitary.
(2) Depresses and decreases œstrogen production.
(3) Inhibits proliferative processes in endometrium.
(4) Inhibits re-activity of uterine musculature.
(5) Decreases flow of blood to uterus and pelvis.
(6) Depresses endometrial bleeding factor.
(7) Suppresses lactation and allays after-pains, but inadvisable for such indications.

Uses.—

Dangerous to use, as it may produce masculinisation even in comparatively small dosage; no more than 150 mgm. should be given in any one month.

Valuable, in intractable cases of—

(1) Dysfunctional bleeding.
25 mgm. being injected thrice during first week, and twice the following week. The future dosage is regulated by its effect, but never more than 150 mgm. should be given at one course. Gradual decrease with lessening of bleeding.

(2) Dysmenorrhœa, especially congestive type.
5 to 10 mgm. being injected on alternate days for a week before and during period, or 10 to 15 mgm. daily by mouth.

(3) Premenstrual mastalgia. 25 mgm. injected twice weekly for a month, and if successful, 10 mgm. orally should be tried next month and gradually decreased until patient will be relieved from symptoms by 5 mgm. daily for two weeks pre-menstrually.

(4) Endometriosis. 10 mgm. orally daily may suffice to relieve pain in mild cases. Larger doses will be required in more severe cases, but 150 mgm. should not be exceeded in any one month.

6. **Thyroid.**—

Ext. Thyroidei, gr. $\frac{1}{2}$–iii daily as required.

Uses.—

(1) Increases activity of all ductless glands.
(2) Prevents excessive concentration of œstrin in endometrium, by increasing elimination in urine.
(3) Helps nidation of ovum.
(4) Helps to stimulate uterine growth.
(5) May cure dysfunctional bleedings, especially menorrhagia of puberty, when due to thyroid deficiency; given alone or in combination with other hormones.
(6) May help sterility by stimulating the anterior pituitary, or by stimulating uterine growth in cases of hypoplasia.
(7) Increases urinary output in oliguria of pre-eclampsia and eclampsia.

7. **Posterior Pituitary.**—(See p. 72.)

CHAPTER XXIV

GYNÆCOLOGICAL OPERATIONS

UTERINE

Supra-vaginal Hysterectomy

1. Open the abdomen in the middle line below umbilicus.

2. Pull up the uterus and clamp the infundibulo-pelvic ligament on one side, or, if the ovary is to be retained, the broad ligament. Cut between the clamps.

3. Clamp the round ligament and cut.

4. Do the same on the other side.

5. Lift the peritoneum over the isthmus with forceps and make a transverse incision through the peritoneum anteriorly, continuing the incision to the round ligaments.

6. Push the bladder down off the upper part of cervix.

7. Apply forceps at each side of the base of the broad ligament, taking a good bite of cervix and keeping close to it to avoid the ureters. These forceps include the uterine vessels. Cut between the forceps.

8. Cut through the cervix and catch hold of the anterior lip with a volsella. (This prevents contamination from the cervix and also controls any adventitious bleeding.)

9. Stitch the cervical opening with interrupted or continuous catgut and hold the ends with forceps as a tractor. (*N.B.*—All needles, volsella, knife, etc., used for the cervix should be thrown away as dirty.)

10. Ligature the uterine arteries, passing the needle first through the lateral wall of the cervix.

11. Ligature the infundibulo-pelvic or broad ligaments, transfixing them with a needle first.

12. Ligature the round ligaments.

13. Cover the raw surface with peritoneum, beginning at one side and including the infundibulo-pelvic and round ligaments in a purse-string suture, to invaginate the cut surfaces; then bring anterior and posterior layers of peritoneum together all the way round and over the cervix (cutting the tractor sutures when reached) till the other ligaments are reached; these are purse-stringed and invaginated as on the other side. (Fig. 32.)

14. Stitch the abdomen in layers.
    (1) Continuous catgut for the peritoneum.
    (2) Interrupted silkworm gut stitches through the skin and anterior rectal sheath (three or four or more as required).

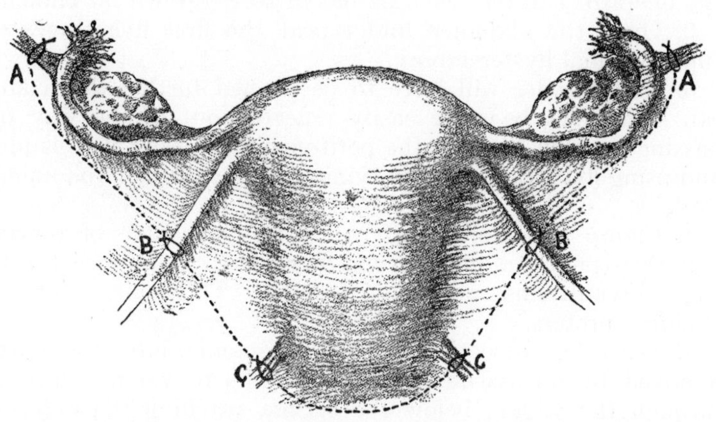

FIG. 32.—S.V. HYSTERECTOMY I. ANTERIOR ASPECT OF UTERUS (diagrammatic).

A, Ovarian vessels; B, Round ligament artery; C, Uterine vessels. Dotted line = incision through broad ligament and peritoneum covering isthmus.

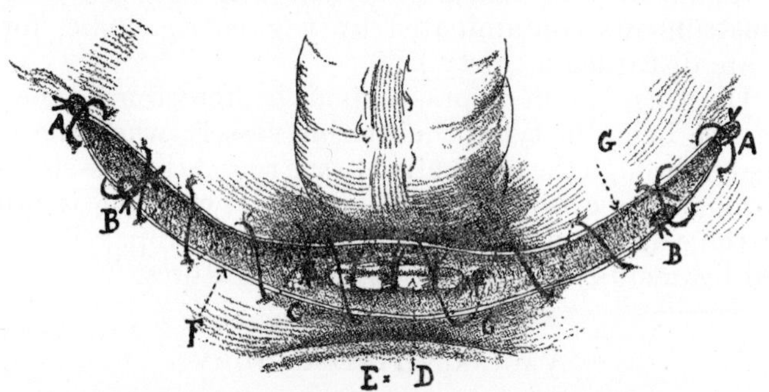

FIG. 33.—HYSTERECTOMY II. PERITONEAL STITCH.

A, Ovarian vessels; B, Round ligament; C, Uterine vessels; D, Cervix (stitched); E, Bladder; F, Anterior layer of peritoneum; G, Posterior layer of peritoneum.

    (3) Continuous catgut for the anterior rectal sheath.
    (4) Tie the silkworm stitches.
    (5) Insert clips for the skin edges.

(*N.B.*—If any prolapse is present, the round ligaments may be stitched to the cervix to support it.)

Pan-hysterectomy

1. Pack the vagina with gauze soaked in Flavazole or Dettol. This cleanses the vagina, raises the uterus and makes the vagina stand out during the operation, so that the operator can tell when he has dissected down far enough.
2. Open the abdomen and repeat the first five stages of supra-vaginal hysterectomy.
3. The bladder will have to be pushed further down and can sometimes be more easily reflected out of the way by passing a stitch through the peritoneum covering the bladder and using it as tractor, or by tying it to the anterior abdominal wall.
4. Clamp the uterine arteries ¼ in. from side of cervix, and then pass straight forceps down each side of cervix to vaginal vault and cut inside clamps. This makes sure of avoiding ureters.
5. When the dissection reaches the vagina, have the gauze removed by an assistant, clamp corners of vagina and cut through the vagina below the cervix, catching the anterior and posterior walls with Allis' forceps.
6. Stitch the edges of the vagina together, taking mattress stitches at the corners where the vessels are found. (*N.B.*—The vagina may be closed or left slightly open for drainage. All instruments contaminated by vagina, *e.g.* knife, forceps, etc., are discarded as dirty.)
7. Do then as in supra-vaginal hysterectomy, the only difference being in tying the uterine vessels, when the needle is passed through the connective tissue round the vessels instead of through the cervix, and the peritoneal covering is brought over the vagina instead of the cervical stump. The utero-sacral ligaments may require separate ligatures.

Vaginal Hysterectomy

1. Make circular incision round the cervix, which is pulled down by volsella.
2. Push up the bladder from the anterior surface of the cervix.
3. Pull the cervix down and, after retracting the bladder, open into the utero-vesical pouch and enlarge the opening out to the sides of the uterus.
4. Pull the cervix forwards and open into the pouch of Douglas.

5. Transfix the utero-sacral ligaments, ligate and divide from uterus.

6. Pull the cervix to one side and, after a transfixing ligature has included the uterine vessels, divide between the ligature and the uterus.

7. Do the same on the other side.

8. Catch hold of the fundus with volsella and deliver it through the utero-vesical pouch or pouch of Douglas.

9. Transfix and divide the round and broad ligaments as in the case of the uterine vessels.

10. The uterus is removed.

11. The peritoneal edges are brought together either with a purse-string suture or interrupted sutures.

12. The broad and utero-sacral ligaments are tied together in the midline.

13. The redundant vaginal mucosa is excised and the edges brought together. Some leave a small opening and insert a drain for twenty-four to thirty-six hours.

14. The pelvic floor is reconstructed if necessary.

Hysterectomy for Cervical Fibroids

1. Open the abdomen and make a transverse incision through the peritoneum and capsule of the tumour. (If the tumour is anterior, be careful of the bladder.)

2. Cut through the capsule down to tumour tissue and work a finger round between the tumour and the capsule, and shell out the tumour.

3. The uterus can now be raised out of the pelvis and a hysterectomy done.

(*N.B.*—If the tumour lies to one side of the uterus, the finger must be kept very close to the tumour during enucleation, so as to separate the ureter along with the capsule.)

Myomectomy

1. Open the abdomen.

2. Make a transverse incision over the tumour and separate it from its capsule as for cervical fibroids, and then enucleate tumour.

3. Stitch the raw surfaces carefully together with deep mattress catgut sutures.

4. Carefully coapt the peritoneal edges of the wound in the uterus with continuous catgut suture.

Dilatation and Curettage

1. Insert a speculum and grasp the anterior cervical lip with volsella.
2. Pass a sound to estimate the length of the uterus and confirm its position.
3. Dilate cervix with graduated dilators, increasing the size each time.
4. Curette the interior of the uterus, passing the curette gently up to the fundus and then bringing it down firmly.
5. The cavity may be flushed out with an aseptic solution.
6. Dry the cavity and apply pure carbolic, iodised phenol, iodine, etc., according to desire. (Some use no medication for the interior of the uterus, relying solely on the curettage.)
7. Pass a wick of gauze into the cavity to act as a drain and pack the vagina loosely.
8. Remove the packing in twelve to twenty-four hours.

CERVICAL

Amputation of the Cervix

(See also the operations for prolapse)

(*Bonney's Method*) (Fig. 34)

1. Dilate the cervix, so that the canal can be defined easily.
2. Put a volsella on the anterior lip and dissect up a flap of mucous membrane with its base above the tear if one is present, the length of the flap being not more than ¾ in.
3. Incise the cervix laterally to the base of the flap.
4. Remove the anterior lip of cervix to the base of the flap.
5. Pass a needle through the apex of the flap and tie it, leaving two equal ends of catgut, each of which is threaded and passed through the entire anterior wall of the cervix from the mucosa to the vaginal surface and there tied, thus covering the raw anterior surface with the flap.
6. Do the same posteriorly.
7. Stitch the lips together laterally.

Cauterisation of Cervix

1. Cervix is dilated as for curettage.
2. Three linear strokes are made with the edge of an electro-cautery into anterior and posterior walls of endocervix up to internal os.
3. Any erosion is cauterised with linear strokes.

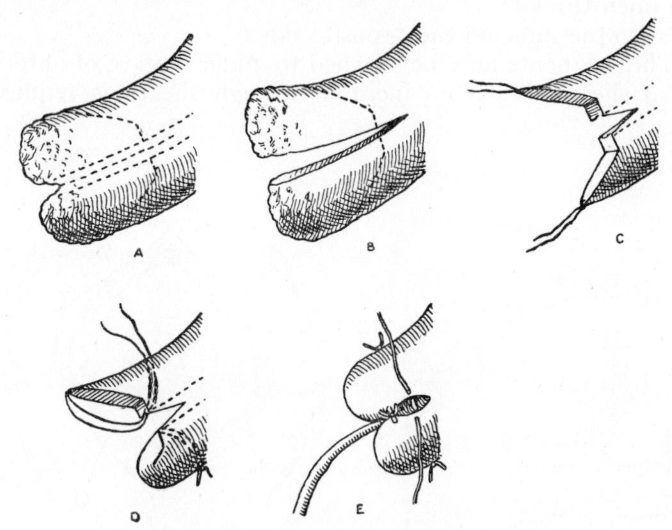

Fig. 34.—Amputation of the Vaginal Cervix.

4. Insert small gauze wick into cervix to keep burnt areas apart. This is removed in twenty-four hours.

ROUND LIGAMENT OPERATIONS FOR RETROVERSION—VENTRO-SUSPENSION

(1) Gilliam (*Mayo's Modification*) (Fig. 35)

1. Make mid-line incision above the pubis.
2. Open the abdomen and pass loop of thread or catgut round each round ligament about $1\frac{1}{2}$ in. from the uterus.
3. Dissect out the anterior rectus sheath and make small incisions through it about 1 in. above and slightly lateral to each pubic spine.
4. Pass a pair of long curved forceps through this incision and then round the lateral margin of the rectus muscle;

then guide the forceps through the internal abdominal ring and then along between the layers of the broad ligament until point is just under suture on round ligament.

5. Pass the point of the forceps through anterior layer broad ligament and seize the suture and withdraw the forceps.

6. Suture the ligament to the anterior rectus sheath with fine linen thread.

7. Do the same on the opposite side.

(The ligaments may be stitched to under surface of anterior rectal sheath, when no incision through sheath is required.

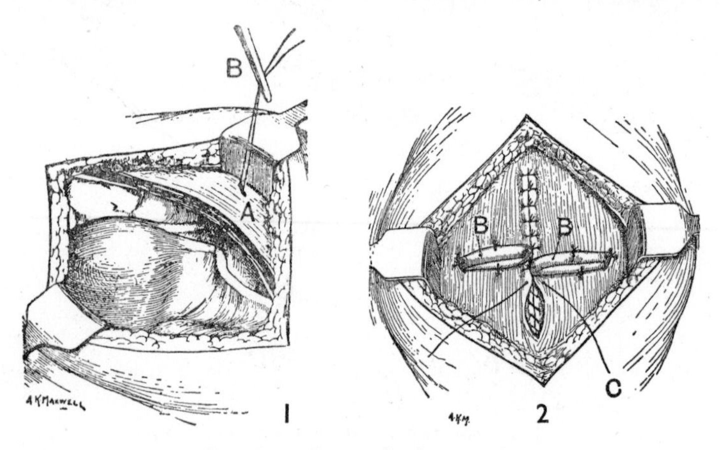

FIG. 35.—GILLIAM'S OPERATION.

A, Rectus sheath ; B, Round ligaments and tractor ligature ; C, Suture of anterior rectus sheath.

This causes less bleeding and probably less post-operative pain.)

8. Stitch up abdominal wound.

Advantages.—

1. Strongest part of the round ligament is used.
2. The pull on the fundus is upward and forward.

Disadvantages.—

1. Internal hernia may develop later. Almost impossible with Mayo's modification.
2. Injury to the deep epigastric artery at the internal ring.
3. Ligament is brought out of its natural course.

(2) Sling (*Baldy-Webster*) (Fig. 36)

1. Open the abdomen in the middle line and bring the fundus forward with elevating forceps.

2. Pass the forceps through the broad ligament just below

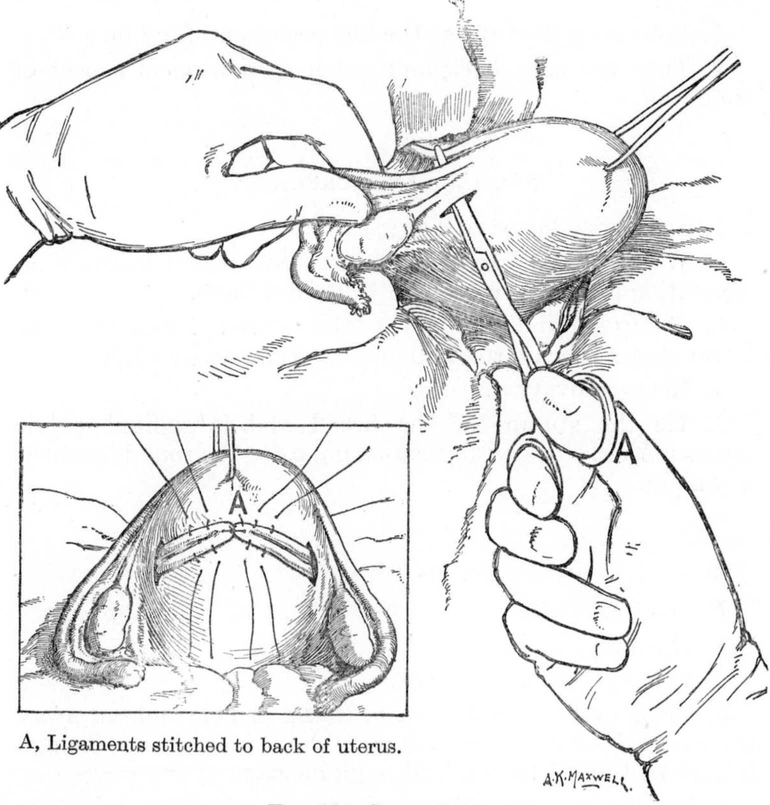

A, Ligaments stitched to back of uterus.

Fig. 36.—Sling Operation.

the ovarian ligament from behind forwards and catch round ligament $1\frac{1}{2}$ in. from uterus.

3. Do the same on opposite side.

4. Scarify the back of uterus fairly high up and stitch the looped round ligaments to the uterus and to each other.

5. Close abdomen.

(*N.B.*—Of great use when ovaries are prolapsed, as they are thus well elevated.)

OVARIAN AND TUBAL

Salpingostomy

For sterility. Only to be done if the tube is comparatively healthy.

1. Split open the tube at the fimbriated end for 2 in.
2. Turn the ends back and stitch to peritoneal aspect of tube wall.

Salpingo-Oöphorectomy

1. Separate adhesions, if any, carefully.
2. Work down posterior wall of uterus in first instance, as separation is usually more easily effected there.
3. Clamp infundibulo-pelvic and broad ligaments, the latter close to the uterus, and make the clamps overlap.
4. Remove ovary and tube.
5. Tie the stumps of the broad and infundibulo-pelvic ligaments and cover with peritoneum, using the round ligament as an aid.

Ovariotomy

For ovarian cysts.—

1. Open abdomen.
2. Free cyst from adhesions.
3. Bring cyst out of abdomen, clamp pedicle and cut away the cyst. If cyst is very large and you are sure it is benign it may be tapped to get it through incision.
4. Tie the pedicle with two ligatures and then cover the tied end of the pedicle with peritoneum.

Resection of Ovary

1. Stretch ovary between Allis' forceps at each end.
2. Cut away diseased portion.
3. Stitch cut edges together with a continuous catgut suture.

VAGINAL AND VULVAL
FOR CYSTOCELE, PROLAPSE, RECTOCELE AND HYPERTROPHY OF THE CERVIX

ANTERIOR COLPORRHAPHY (*Donald*) (Fig. 37)

For cystocele.—

1. Pull down the cervix with volsella.

2. Outline with forceps a diamond-shaped area on the anterior vaginal wall, beginning about ½ in. below urethra.

3. With a knife incise the outline of the area to be removed.

4. Dissect the vaginal mucous membrane, inside the diamond area, from the bladder. (This may be done from above downwards, or below upwards, as desired.) Separate bladder from edges and define fascia.

5. Stitch fascia with interrupted or continuous catgut, or fix bladder up by means of purse string through fascia under mucosa.

6. Stitch the vaginal edges together over the raw area with interrupted or continuous catgut stitches, from below upwards.

ANTERIOR COLPORRHAPHY WITH AMPUTATION OF CERVIX (*Fothergill*)

For cystocele and hypertrophy of the cervix.—

1. Define lower limit of bladder with sound.

2. Measure length of uterine cavity, so as to know how much cervix to remove.

3. Dilate cervix. (Curette uterus if necessary.)

4. Outline the anterior colporrhaphy as before, but instead of one forceps in the centre at the cervix, one is put on each side of the cervix as far out as possible and as high up as the amputation warrants; another forceps is placed on the posterior aspect of the cervix.

5. Make an incision joining the forceps at one side, passing round to the forceps at the back of the cervix and then up the opposite side (Fig. 38).

6. Remove the vaginal mucosa as in an anterior colporrhaphy and push the bladder up from cervix till it is above the amputation level.

7. Incise round cervix with scissors so as to free the cervix from the surrounding tissue, swab peritoneum and pouch of

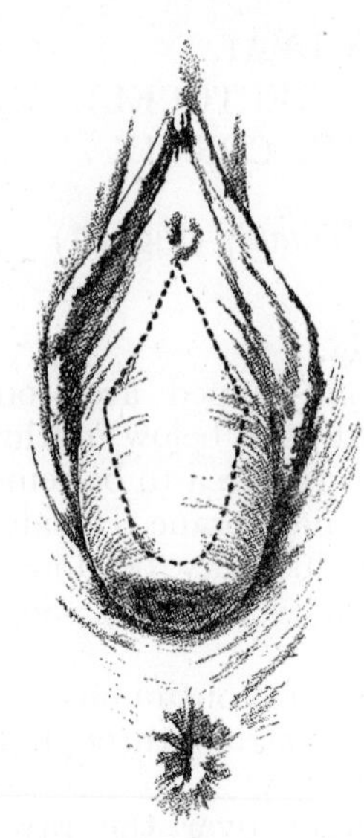

Fig. 37.—Anterior Colporrhaphy Incision.

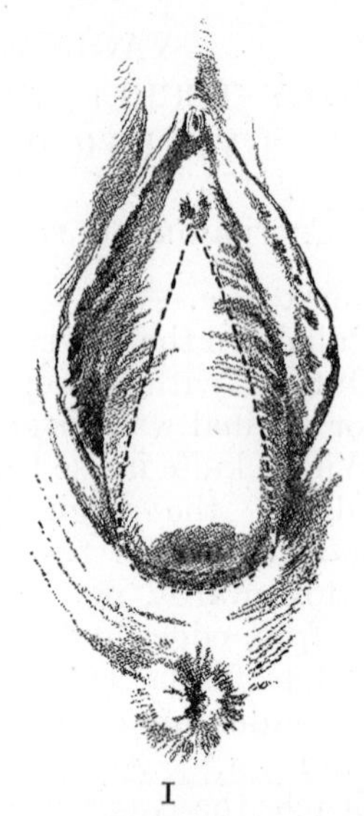

I

Fig. 38.—Anterior Colporrhaphy and Amputation of Cervix.

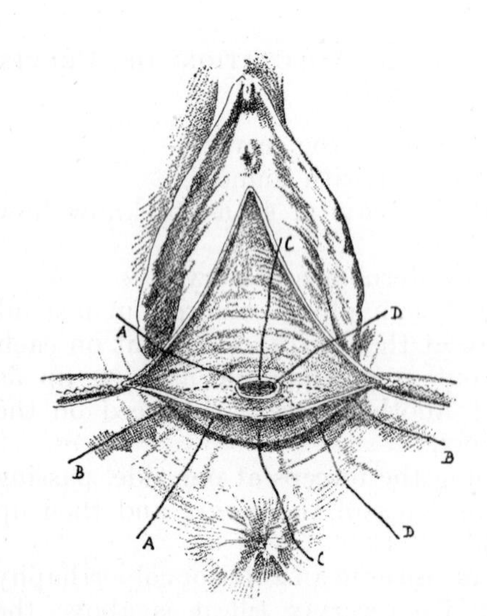

II

Fig. 39.—Anterior Colporrhaphy and Amputation of Cervix.

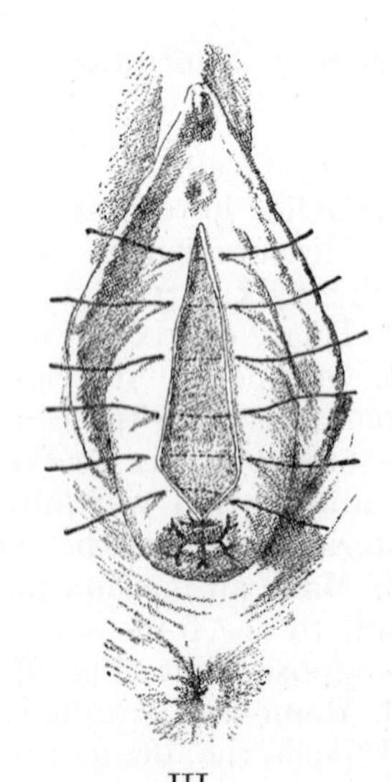

III

Fig. 40.—Anterior Colporrhaphy and Amputation of Cervix.

Douglas off back of cervix; then amputate through cervix, putting a pair of volsella or Allis' forceps on the anterior lip, so as to prevent its retraction when cut through.

8. Stitch the surrounding vaginal mucous membrane to cervical mucosa with catgut sutures, so that the cervical cut surface is covered by vaginal mucosa all round (Fig. 39).

9. Antevert the uterus and stitch the edges of anterior vaginal mucous membrane, the lowermost stitch including the cervix and the transverse cervical ligaments ; the fascia in this case is included with vaginal mucosa (Fig. 40).

10. Pack vagina with gauze and leave packing in for twenty-four to forty-eight hours.

Posterior Colporrhaphy and Perineorrhaphy
(*Donald*)

1. Put forceps at each side of the vulva at the level of the lower ends of the labia minora.

2. Put forceps on posterior vaginal wall at the highest point of the rectocele and outline a triangle with two lateral forceps on vaginal wall in the direction of the vulval forceps (Fig. 41).

3. Incise with a knife the two lateral walls of the triangle and dissect the vaginal mucosa downwards.

4. Continue the lateral incisions in direction of vulval forceps and remove intervening vaginal mucosa by carrying on dissection of upper triangle. (This may all be done at one time, but if the rectocele is large it may have to be done in two or three stages.)

5. Cut away dissected flap, when it comes down to the skin edge.

6. Pass several interrupted catgut sutures through levator ani muscles, the top stitch being as high up as possible. These stitches are tied as the stitching of the vaginal mucosa comes down to level of each deep stitch (Fig. 42).

7. Bring the cut vaginal edges together with interrupted or continuous catgut.

8. Bring perineal body together with interrupted catgut ligatures.

9. Bring skin edges together with buried catgut or Kifa clips.

10. Pack vagina with gauze for twenty-four to forty-eight hours.

Perineorrhaphy

1. Place forceps on each side of the vulva at the level of the lower ends of labia minora.

2. Pull apart and make incision with knife, joining forceps along the junction of the vaginal and skin surfaces.

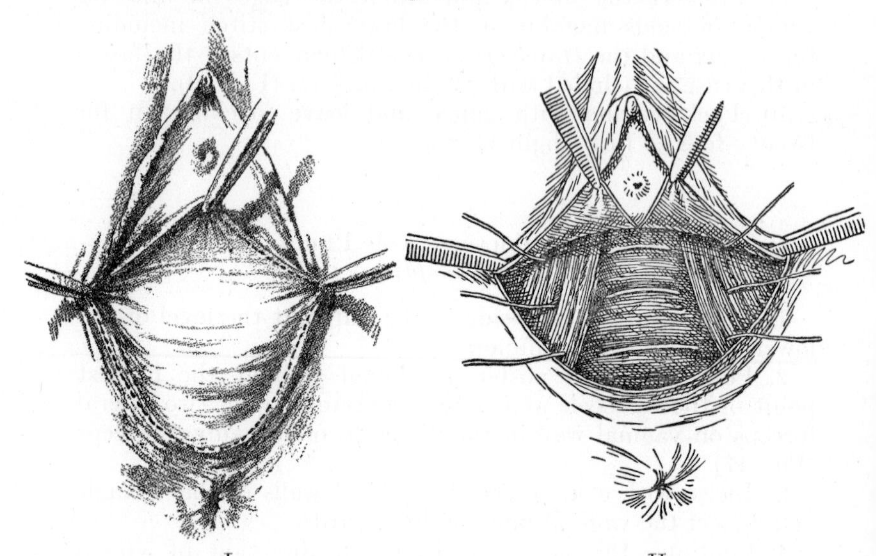

I

Fig. 41.—Posterior Colporrhaphy and Perineorrhaphy. Incision.

II

Fig. 42.—After Removal of Vaginal Mucosa.

3. Dissect the vaginal mucosa upwards and separate the rectum from the vagina with gauze and dissection.

4. Cut away the vaginal flap thus formed in a triangular manner with the apex at top.

5. Stitch up as in a posterior colporrhaphy and perineorrhaphy and pack vagina with gauze.

For Complete Perineal Tear

1. Put forceps at each side of the vulva at the level of the lower ends of labia minora and one at each side of the anus, where a small depression shows cut edge of sphincter.

2. An H-shaped incision is made joining the forceps, the horizontal bar of the H cutting along the recto vaginal

junction, the upper limbs passing to the labial forceps and the lower to the sphincter edges (Fig. 43).

3. Reflect the vaginal flap from rectum until the upper

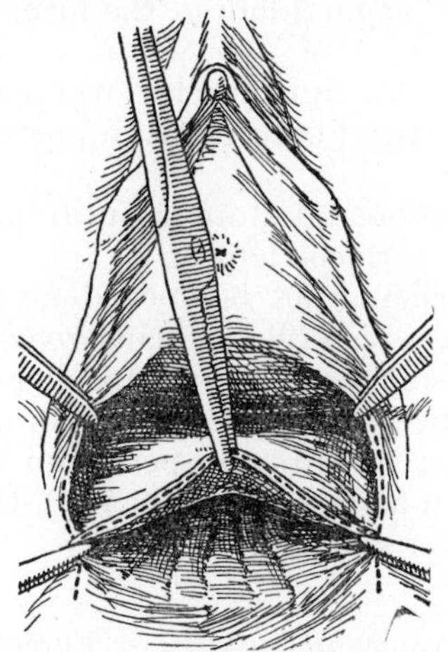

FIG. 43.—OPERATION FOR COMPLETE TEAR OF THE PERINEUM. (First stage.)

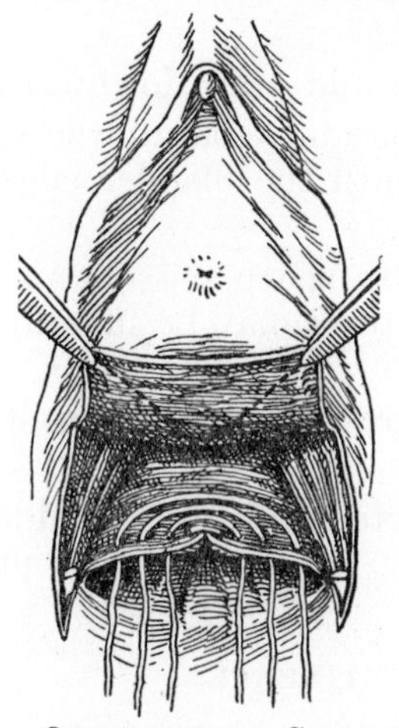

FIG. 44.—OPERATION FOR COMPLETE TEAR OF THE PERINEUM. (Second stage.)

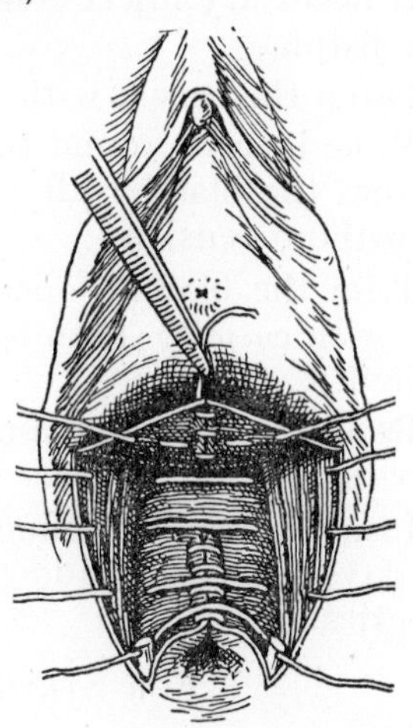

FIG. 45.—OPERATION FOR COMPLETE TEAR OF THE PERINEUM. (Third stage.)

end of the tear is reached; free rectum at sides; tie all bleeding points.

4. Repair the tear in rectum from above downwards with interrupted catgut until skin margin is reached (Fig. 44).

5. Catch the cut ends of the sphincter with Allis' forceps and stitch together with two or three catgut or linen thread ligatures.

6. Cut away the vaginal flap in the form of a triangle with the apex above.

7. Bring the levator ani muscles over rectal stitches with deep, interrupted catgut sutures, as in posterior colporrhaphy (Fig. 45).

8. Stitch the vagina and unite perineal body as in posterior colporrhaphy and perineorrhaphy.

9. The bowels should not be opened for at least five days after operation, liquid paraffin ʒi being given t.i.d. from second day, to ensure a soft motion, and an olive oil enema should be given before bowels are moved by castor oil.

After all perineal repairs the perineum should be treated as a perineum torn at labour (see p. 171), the dressings being done four-hourly for seven to ten days.

For Vesico-vaginal Fistula

1. If necessary inject sterile milk into the bladder, to show up the fistula.

2. Catch the cervix with volsella and draw downwards.

3. Make incision round the fistula and separate the vaginal wall from the bladder all round until the bladder edges will meet without tension.

4. Trim the bladder opening with sharp scissors and then suture with catgut. (Lembert's sutures may be superimposed if desired.)

5. Replace the flaps and suture the vaginal wall with twenty-day catgut.

6. Insert a self-retaining catheter into the bladder for seven days and keep bladder empty. Put patient on urinary antiseptics.

For Stress Incontinence

Many operations have been devised, and until a few years ago repair was attempted by the vaginal route only. Such a method was not always successful, and now several fascial sling operations are employed. These operations should be used only where a previous plastic repair has been unsuccessful. The main points in the technique are as follows :—

Vaginal.—The urethra and bladder base are separated

from the surrounding tissues. The fascial tissues are then approximated with several interrupted sutures (Kelly) over the bladder neck and urethra.

Fascial Sling.—

(i) A strip of external oblique fascia, 2 cm. in breadth, is dissected inwards from each anterior superior spine and pedicled 2 cm. from the mid-line on each side. Those strips are then brought down, posterior to the symphysis pubis, overlapped and stitched together under the urethra, which has been dissected out per vaginam (Aldridge).

(ii) More recently Millin and Read have described a similar operation which is done by the abdominal route alone and is extra-peritoneal. Two fascial strips each 15–18 cm. long, 1 cm. broad and pedicled on either side about 2 cm. medial to the anterior superior spine, are prepared. The recti muscles are separated and the retropubic space opened up. The bladder neck and urethra are identified from above and a tunnel formed, posterior to the urethra, by the Millin-Read forceps. The two fascial strips are passed under the urethra by means of this forceps and stitched together, thus elevating the bladder neck, particularly when the patient exerts herself and uses her abdominal muscles.

Excision of Vulva

1. Make an oval incision from above the mons veneris, along each side of the vulva to the perineum, keeping well clear of the disease and any leukoplakia.
2. Make a second incision around vaginal orifice, the apex being about ½ in. above the urethral orifice.
3. Remove the vulva between the incisions.
4. Ligature vessels and stitch cut edges with catgut, scotia, or thin silkworm gut.
5. The inguinal glands may be removed along with vulva, if cancer is present.

Excision of Bartholin's Gland or Cyst

1. Make an elliptical incision on the skin surface around the swelling.
2. Dissect out the cyst without puncturing it if possible,

3. Ligature bleeding vessels, insert deep mattress sutures and then bring the skin edges together with thin silkworm or scotia gut.

For Bartholin Abscess

1. Incise abscess with knife.
2. Scrape lining with spoon curette.
3. Apply spirit to inside of cavity.
4. Dry thoroughly.
5. Apply B.I.P.P. (bismuth, iodoform, and paraffin paste) to cavity.
6. Remove excess of B.I.P.P. to prevent undue absorption.
7. Stitch skin edges with catgut.

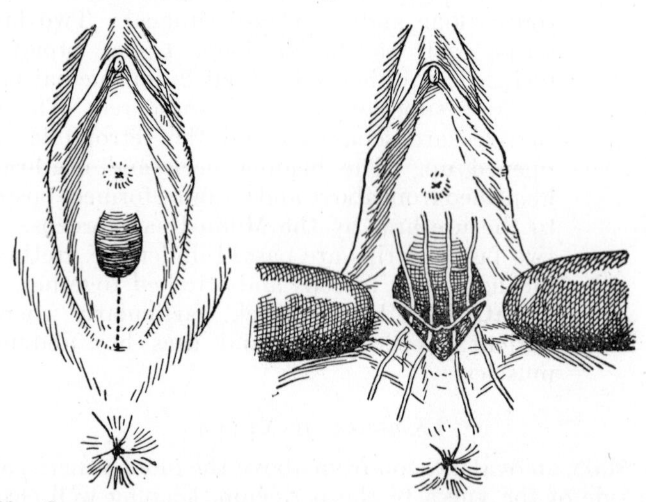

Fig. 46.—Operation for expanding Vaginal Outlet. (First stage.)

Fig. 47.—Operation for expanding Vaginal Outlet. (Second stage.)

For Permanent Stretching of Vulva for Dyspareunia and Vaginismus (Figs. 46 and 47)

1. Incise vulvo-perineal junction vertically in mid-line, the incision being the depth of ½ to ¾ in.
2. Stitch incision with catgut in transverse.
3. Insert a vaginal dilator for two to three hours daily, increasing the size each day.

CHAPTER XXV

THE INFANT

ARTIFICIAL FEEDING OF INFANTS

Cow's milk is the principal substitute for human milk. Goat's milk, which has a similar composition, predominates in some parts of the world.

Comparative Composition of Human and Cow's Milk.

	Protein Percentage.	*Fat Percentage.*	*Lactose Percentage.*	*Salts Percentage.*	*Water Percentage.*
Human milk .	1·5	3·5	7·0	0·2	87·8
Cow's milk . .	3·5	3·5	4·5	0·75	87·75

It is important to realise that the qualitative differences of the principal constituents of cow's milk are more important than the quantitative differences, for instance, human and cow's milk each contain the same amount of lactalbumin, but cow's milk contains six times as much casein as human milk. This great excess of casein in cow's milk is the principal disadvantage of cow's milk in infant feeding, because it forms large indigestible curds in the infant's stomach. Further, although the percentage of fat is the same in the two kinds of milk, the constituent elements are different and the coarser emulsion formed by cow's milk is more difficult to digest.

Modification of Cow's Milk for Infants.

Although some infants can digest whole cow's milk from birth, others cannot do so ; thus diluted milk should be given in the first few months of life.

There are five main objects in modifying cow's milk for infants :—

1. To reduce the excessive amount of casein.
2. To render the casein more digestible.
3. To reduce the amount of fat.
4. To reduce the neutralising effect of the high mineral salt content on the gastric acidity.
5. To raise the amount of sugar to the same level as in human milk.

The first four objects can all be attained by dilution with

water, which is the principal method of increasing the digestibility of cow's milk. If the milk and water mixture is then heated to boiling point, the digestibility of the protein is further improved by making the protein curd in the stomach finer. Momentary boiling does no appreciable harm to milk (only about 25 per cent. of the vitamin C is destroyed) and, in addition to increasing its digestibility, confers on it the benefit of sterilisation.

Dilute with an equal quantity of water at first and then strengthen (two-fifths water) at age of two to three weeks, and in older infants more rapidly according to appetite and age.

Sugar must always be added to cow's milk whether whole or diluted. *The addition of* 1 *oz. of sugar to* 1 *pint of mixture of any dilution increases its sugar content by* 5 *per cent.* Cane sugar is satisfactory for routine purposes, and therefore preferable to other forms as it is cheaper. Brown or Demerara sugar is of use, if baby is constipated. If digestion unsatisfactory, dextrimaltose is better than lactose.

Suitable Forms of Milk for Young Infants.

Fresh cow's milk is now being supplanted to an increasing extent by preserved milk, particularly dried milk. Fresh milk is satisfactory if a high standard of cleanliness is maintained. Keeping is aided by boiling when received or storing in a refrigerator.

Preserved milk is indicated, where storage facilities are poor or the standard of cleanliness is doubtful, in hot climates or where a regular supply is not available. Unsweetened condensed milk and dried milk (half cream for the first three months) are the most suitable forms. Need not commence with equivalent of 50 per cent. dilution, as in the case of fresh milk, for processing increases protein digestibility.

Artificial Feeding in the First Month.

First day.—Water+5 per cent. sugar ad lib. 2 feeds (see p. 81—Breast feeding).

During the first two to three weeks give increasing amounts of the following standard mixture, three-hourly (six feeds) if the birth-weight is under 6 lb. or the baby is a poor feeder, otherwise four-hourly (five feeds) :—

Formula I.—Milk	. .	12 oz.
Water	. .	8 oz.
Sugar	. .	1 oz.

Second day—	1 oz. × 3-hourly (6 feeds) or	1½ oz. × 4-hourly (5 feeds)
Third ,,	1½ oz. × ,, ,, ,,	2 oz. × ,, ,,
Fourth ,,	2 oz. × ,, ,, ,,	2½ oz. × ,, ,,
Sixth ,,	2½ oz. × ,, ,, ,,	3 oz. × ,, ,,
Eighth ,,	3 oz. × ,, ,, ,,	3½ oz. × ,, ,,
Two weeks—	3½ oz. × ,, ,, ,,	4 oz. × ,, ,,

A further increase usually becomes necessary in the third or fourth week. This is the signal for increasing the strength of the standard mixture according to the following formula :—

Formula II.—Milk . . 14 oz.
Water . . 8 oz.
Sugar . . 1 oz.

Two to four weeks.—Formula II—3½–4 oz. × 3-hourly (6 feeds) or 4–5 oz. × 4-hourly (5 feeds).

Calculation of Feeds after the First Month.

Requirements are based on the total amount of breast milk taken per day by healthy infants of corresponding age. The breast milk figures are :—

1 month . .	25 oz.
3 months . .	30 oz.
6 months . .	35 oz.

Give 6 oz. less cow's milk than the appropriate amount of human milk and maintain the daily amount of sugar at 1 oz. and of water at about 8 oz. throughout the period of milk diet. Thus, the latter two constituents are constants and cow's milk is the only variable. (The reason for giving 6 oz. less cow's milk than of human milk is that the 1 oz. of sugar has the same caloric value as 6 oz. of milk, whether cow's milk or human.)

Example.—

An infant of ten weeks normally takes about 28 oz. of breast milk per day.

A suitable cow's milk mixture would be—

Milk . .	22 oz.
Water . .	7 oz.
Sugar . .	1 oz.
Total .	30 oz.

Give five four-hourly feeds of 6 oz.

The caloric requirements of infants vary greatly and some require much more than the theoretical amount stated above—*e.g.* wakeful, lively and fretful babies.

When using fresh milk it is desirable to prepare the appropriate bulk mixture for each day soon after the milk is received, and to warm up the required amount for the individual feeds; in certain circumstances it may be more convenient to prepare each feed separately.

The Addition of Vitamins.

Vitamins A, C and D should always be given to artificially and breast fed infants. Commence at two weeks old with small amount and gradually increase until at two months 2 drachms of cod liver oil (A and D) and ½ oz. of fresh orange juice (C) are being given per diem. If these preparations are taken reluctantly, or cause vomiting or diarrhœa, use concentrated preparations such as halibut-liver oil, 6 drops, or adexolin, 10 drops per diem; both of these contain A and D (calciferol contains only D), and ascorbic acid (vitamin C), giving one 25-mgm. tablet crushed and dissolved in feeds. (*N.B.*—There is great danger of giving too little vitamin D, when dilute preparations such as cod liver oil emulsion, cod liver oil and malt, and virol are used.)

PREMATURE INFANTS

Definition.

Infants, who weigh 5½ lb. (2,500 g.) or less at birth, are classified as premature infants, irrespective of the estimated period of gestation.

Prognosis.

Depends on cause of prematurity (poor in ante-partum hæmorrhage), character of labour and degree of prematurity (weight).

Chief Difficulties.

1. Maintenance of body temperature.
2. Feeding.
3. Protection from infection: effects very serious.

1. Maintenance of Body Temperature.

Temperature is usually subnormal.

The degree of hypothermia corresponds to the degree of prematurity for two reasons: (1) The metabolic rate, and therefore the production of heat per lb., is less in very small infants, because of their poor vitality. (2) The heat loss per lb. is greater in very small infants, because the smaller the infant the greater the surface area per lb.

Temperature may remain about 96° F. to 93° F. for a

week or two in the very premature in spite of all attempts to raise it.

Objects are to diminish heat loss to the uttermost and to increase generation of heat if possible.

Measures taken to minimise heat loss are—

1. Avoidance of bathing with water; instead, anointing with olive oil until weight approaches 5 lb.
2. Provision of air-conditioned nurseries.
3. Provision of air-conditioned incubators.
4. Other measures in default of 2 or 3.

Air temperature should be 80°–90° F. according to degree of prematurity.

Relative humidity should be 65 per cent., a figure which produces a very humid atmosphere.

In the absence of air-conditioning, have the room heated to maximum extent and humidified with a steaming kettle. Also use high-sided cot or box to prevent draughts, hot-water bottles and wrap the infant in cotton wool. (These measures are unnecessary, if atmosphere conditioned.)

Generation of heat may be increased by giving thyroid to raise the metabolic rate.

2. **Feeding.**

Inaugurate very slowly as the immature alimentary tract and liver are not prepared for digestion.

Always give own mother's milk if possible; if there is none available, try to obtain breast milk from another source (this is usually possible in maternity hospitals). Otherwise use sweetened condensed milk, or half-cream dried milk.

Frequency of Feeds.—The practice of not beginning to feed very premature infants until the age of two to four days, because of their precarious condition and the risk of aspiration in the first few days, has recently become popular and is commendable. Once begun feeds should be given three-hourly (eight in twenty-four hours).

Method of Feeding.—Depends on weight, strength and appetite. Majority feed spontaneously from special small feeder (Belcroy) which holds 1 oz., is graduated in drachms, has a small soft teat and a dummy teat at the other end to express milk into the infant's mouth.

If very slow and difficult to feed, or very small, adopt gavage feeding with a fine rubber tube, such as a No. 4 French catheter, until feeding improves.

Larger premature infants of 5 lb. or more can usually

feed themselves at the breast; give seven three-hourly feeds.

Smaller infants should be given the breast on attaining the weight of 4½ lb. if lactation has been kept going.

Size and Concentration of Feeds.—Rules for premature infants cannot be laid down because the weight and vitality vary so much.

Give 5 per cent. dextrimaltose or lactose in sterile water on the first day of feeding, offering 1 drachm per lb. per feed. On the second day give equal parts of this and the selected form of milk, and on the third day of feeding full-strength milk (breast milk, sweetened condensed milk 1 part in 5, or half-cream dried milk 1 part in 10).

After several weeks, when the appetite becomes keen, showing that the digestive organs are functioning well, the appetite is the best guide to the size of the feeds; premature babies at this stage may take 70–80 calories per lb. per day. The volume of full-strength milk should gradually be increased with an increment of 1 drachm per feed every few days. Underfeeding is much less likely to be harmful than overfeeding in the early weeks of a premature infant's life, and a full-strength feed of small volume is less likely to be regurgitated than a weak feed of larger volume.

Additions to the Diet.

1. Thyroid.—Sometimes useful where much apathy and temperature very low. Stimulates metabolism, producing more heat and activity. Give $\frac{1}{10}$ gr. per lb. per day.

2. Iron.—Always give regularly after one month of age to prevent iron deficiency anæmia in latter part of milk period. Give gr. ½–1 ferrous sulph. twice daily as follows:—

℞	Ferrous sulph. . . .	gr. ½–1
	Ac. hypophos. dil. . .	♏ ½
	Dextrose	gr. 15
	Aq. dest.	ad dr. 1

3. Vitamins.—More important in premature than in mature infants. Give double the mature doses (see p. 380).

DISEASES OF THE NEW-BORN INFANT

Morbidity and mortality are much higher in the first few days after birth than at any other period of life. More infants die in the first three days of life than in the remainder of the first month, and as many infants die in the whole of the first month as in the remainder of the first year.

The principal causes of morbidity and death in the first month (new-born) are :—

1. Asphyxia.
2. Intracranial hæmorrhage.
3. Infections.
4. Congenital malformations.
5. Prematurity.
6. Miscellaneous.

Asphyxia

Asphyxiation during labour is the commonest cause of stillbirth and neo-natal death ; practically all the deaths from this cause are concentrated in the first three days of life. Asphyxia arises during pregnancy or labour as a result of interference with the maternal or fœtal circulation (see p. 199). The depressant action of analgesics and anæsthetics on the respiratory centre may inhibit respiratory movements after birth. A slight degree of asphyxia, which does no harm, develops when the placental circulation is impeded during strong labour pains.

Pathology of Asphyxia.—Blood stagnates in venules, blood pressure rises in them, their walls are devitalised because of oxygen lack and some of them rupture causing multiple petechial hæmorrhages and fewer large hæmorrhages.

Petechial hæmorrhages are common under visceral pleura, epicardium and ependyma of cerebral ventricles, also in thymus.

Severe hæmorrhage frequently occurs in the cerebral ventricles, the subarachnoid space (the blood may arise locally or in the ventricles), the lungs, under the capsule of the liver, the suprarenals, etc.

Gasping respiration before birth causes inhalation of liquor containing vernix, meconium and epithelium into the alveoli of the lungs, increasing their bulk ; if respiration can be established after birth, æration of much of lung is difficult or impossible because of inhaled debris, particularly the vernix, which causes the walls of the alveoli to adhere.

Pneumonia usually develops where there is much foreign matter and severe atelectasis is present, and may already have commenced before the infant is born.

Anoxaemia damages the respiratory centre and renders it

hyposensitive to reflex stimuli, diminished blood level of oxygen and increased blood level of CO_2.

Asphyxia *per se* may cause death during or immediately after labour ; its complications, namely hæmorrhage, atelectasis or pneumonia, may prove fatal during the first few days after birth.

Clinical Features and Treatment (see p. 200).

Intracranial Hæmorrhage

There are three common types :—

1. Subdural.
2. Intraventricular.
3. Subarachnoid.

Subdural Hæmorrhage.—Common in both mature and premature infants ; much more common after manipulative delivery. Many babies are stillborn.

Usually arises from a tear in the tentorium cerebelli on one or both sides.

The associated shock and the effects on the brain and lungs are more important than the degree of hæmorrhage.

Clinical signs arise chiefly from irritation of the meninges and brain ; they may be immediate or follow recovery from shock. These " cerebral signs " can be divided into two groups :—

(*a*) Signs of muscular irritability.—Muscular hypertonia producing stiffness of limbs, clenched fists and, in severe cases, arching of back (opisthotonus) ; intermittent localised muscular twitching, generalised convulsions, persistent vomiting.

(*b*) Signs of mental irritability.—Insomnia, anxious expression, piercing cries and restlessness causing purposeless movements of limbs, adder-like protrusion of tongue and jerky movements of eyeballs.

Increased tension of the fontanelle, coma, and inequality and non-reactivity of the pupils indicate severe hæmorrhage, and are grave signs ; they are uncommon. These signs, particularly if associated with unilateral twitching or paralysis, are suggestive of subdural hæmatoma, and are an indication for tapping the subdural space on both sides, through the lateral angles of the anterior fontanelle, to verify the diagnosis.

(*N.B.*—It is important to realise that most infants who

exhibit the "cerebral" signs mentioned, especially the milder forms, have no intracranial hæmorrhage. Trauma of the head (pain), and meningeal and cerebral irritation account for the features, as in cases with intracranial hæmorrhage.)

Treatment of infants showing signs of cerebral irritation is the same whether hæmorrhage is present or not, unless there is a subdural hæmatoma for which prompt neuro-surgical intervention is necessary.

Handle as little as possible and protect from noise and light.

Change and feed in cot; do not feed at breast until a day or two after return to normal.

Give sedative in doses large enough to produce physical and mental relaxation; chloral, in doses of 1 gr. thrice daily or in bad cases 1 or 2 gr. four-hourly, is effective.

Give vitamin K (kapilon or synkovit in aqueous solution, 5 mgm.) intramuscularly to eliminate any hypothrombinæmia, which might accentuate hæmorrhage, if present.

Intraventricular and Subarachnoid Hæmorrhage.—These types of hæmorrhage are much more common in premature than in mature infants. They are often combined and the blood in the subarachnoid space often comes from the ventricles.

Asphyxia is usually the cause of the hæmorrhage, and also of attacks of respiratory failure with cyanosis, which are common in these cases.

Clinical features are not characteristic. The chief are listlessness, limpness, anorexia, coldness, subnormal temperature and cyanotic attacks.

Lumbar puncture will yield blood-stained cerebro-spinal fluid.

Cerebral signs, like those produced by subdural hæmorrhage, are absent.

Treatment consists of application of heat and the giving of oxygen.

Give vitamin K as above (intramuscularly).

Stimulants, such as brandy and coramine, may also be given.

Feed by stomach tube if necessary.

Sequelæ of Intracranial Hæmorrhage.—The severity of "cerebral" signs in the new-born is a poor guide to the immediate prognosis and gives no indication of the likelihood of sequelæ. Very few cases suffer permanent damage. The principal sequelæ are mental defect, hemiplegia and diplegia; mental defect is often associated with the latter two conditions.

Infections

Unlike the other principal causes of morbidity and death in the new-born, the incidence of the various infections is very low in the first few days of life. After the first week the infections are the predominant cause of illness.

The common infections in the first few weeks of life are:—

Staphylococcal skin infections.
Conjunctivitis—Ophthalmia Neonatorum (see p. 387).
Thrush.
Gastro-enteritis.
Nasopharyngitis.
Omphalitis.
Pneumonia.

Septicæmia, meningitis, peritonitis and pyelitis are uncommon. The first three were always fatal before the advent of modern methods of treatment, but the prognosis in septcæmia and meningitis is now fair if the diagnosis is not unduly delayed. Pyelitis responds well to treatment with alkalis, sulphonamide and abundant fluid.

Staphylococcal Skin Infections.—The three common types in order of frequency are pustules, onychia and bullous impetigo. The three less common types are boils, cellulitis, which usually proceeds to abscess formation, and pemphigus.

Regard seriously, as fatal septicæmia occasionally develops.

Onychia is very common and usually affects several fingers. The lesions commence as a small area of inflammation on one or both sides of the nail. The condition soon subsides, as a rule, leaving a small scab in place of the central point of suppuration, but occasionally extensive involvement of the nail-bed with loss of the nail, or septic vesiculation of the adjacent skin, may occur. A soft towel should be used to dry young infants and skin tags at the sides of the nails carefully removed, as the small tears at the base of the tags are the probable portal of infection.

Bullous impetigo has a stronger tendency to occur in epidemics than the other staphylococcal lesions. The epidermal blisters may contain either serous fluid or pus. If untreated, they may rapidly increase in size, and when large areas of skin become affected the condition is known as *pemphigus*.

Treatment of all cases of staphylococcal skin infection, however mild, should be prompt and thorough.

In institutions the first principle is isolation, because of the great tendency for epidemics to arise.

The affected area should be covered with dry lint or gauze to prevent infection of opposing skin surfaces and of other areas by contacting clothes ; this is especially important in the case of the hands, each finger should be bandaged separately and the whole hand kept in a little bag.

In bullous impetigo and pemphigus every vestige of raised skin should be removed.

Apply fomentations to abscesses.

Treat the most trivial staphylococcal skin infections such as small pustules with penicillin cream or an antiseptic protective cream such as cetavlon. All more severe skin lesions are an indication for systemic penicillin, or an alternative antibiotic, in addition to this local treatment.

The oral route is a reliable method of giving penicillin in the new-born, the dose is 30,000–50,000 units in each feed—if breast fed give in a little expressed milk. Procaine penicillin is a convenient preparation which has become popular recently, the dose is 300,000 units (1 c.c.) intramuscularly, daily, of aqueous suspension of procaine aluminium stearate such as "distaquaine." In very acute infections intramuscular penicillin solution, 30,000 units every four hours, is usually preferred.

If a specimen can be obtained and laboratory facilities are available the organism should be tested for resistance to the various antibiotics. If shown to be penicillin resistant, streptomycin, aureomycin or chloromycetin should be substituted. If sensitivity tests cannot be done streptomycin should be preferred in severe staphylococcal infections, owing to the frequency of penicillin resistance in maternity hospitals, or in cases where the clinical response to penicillin is disappointing after two or three days of therapy. The dose of streptomycin is 40 mgm. per lb. per day, given two or three times a day in acute conditions.

Conjunctivitis.—The main cause of conjunctivitis in the first two days of life is the prophylactic silver nitrate instilled into the eyes at birth. This drug sometimes causes an acute reaction with blepharospasm and a profuse serous discharge, but spontaneous recovery occurs within three days.

Infective conjunctivitis may occur at any time after birth, but is uncommon in the first few days of life.

Gonococcal conjunctivitis is much the most serious type. It may arise within a day or two of birth and usually declares itself in the first week. It is generally acute and is a grave condition, which demands immediate diagnosis and thorough treatment, for, if neglected, perforation of the cornea, destruction of the eye and blindness are likely to occur.

Other types of conjunctivitis, which constitute the vast majority of cases, are much less dangerous, but every case of acute conjunctivitis should be regarded as gonococcal until proved otherwise, because of the gravity of the latter type.

The Staphylococcus aureus accounts for most of the cases, but numerous other organisms such as Staph. albus and diphtheroids frequently cause it.

All the strict regulations regarding neo-natal conjunctivitis have been enacted to minimise, and eliminate if possible, serious ocular damage and blindness following gonococcal infection at birth (see p. 345).

Clinical Features.—A copious sero-purulent discharge, œdema, sometimes redness of the eyelids and blepharospasm, which renders inspection of the cornea and lavage of the conjunctival sac extremely difficult.

In mild cases a small serous or sero-purulent discharge is often the only manifestation.

Diagnosis depends on bacteriological examination of conjunctival fluid.

The most accurate method is to spread on a slide a smear of fluid taken from the conjunctival sac with a platinum loop, and examine after staining with Gram. When possible, a blood-agar plate should be cultured directly from the eye, in addition, as organisms often cannot be demonstrated on a slide when sparse, and even when visible, identification may depend on cultural methods.

Treatment.—

(*a*) Prophylactic.—Instillation of an antiseptic into the eyes immediately after birth is obligatory. Silver nitrate 1 per cent. is the most widely recommended, though ½ per cent. is quite strong enough and less painful. (Prophylactic treatment does not necessarily prevent gonococcal and other forms of conjunctivitis.)

(*b*) Curative.—Oral sulphonamide is effective in all types, except staphylococcal conjunctivitis, as it is secreted in the tears and the conjunctival sacs are constantly bathed with it. A suitable oral dose is sulphamezathine ¼–⅛ gm. four-hourly; this is most easily administered in the form of a suspension

In mild cases instil a drop of sulphacetamide (albucid) solution, 15 per cent., into the conjunctival sac before and after each feed.

Since most cases of conjunctivitis in the new-born are staphylococcal it is rational to commence treatment with penicillin. Failure to improve with penicillin or the demonstration of a penicillin insensitive organism are indications for substituting sulphonamide therapy. Streptomycin therapy is occasionally indicated, as in the case of penicillin resistant staphylococcal conjunctivitis.

Penicillin may be given systemically (see Staph. skin infections, p. 387), or locally. The latter method is usually preferred in acute cases, particularly in the early stages of treatment: a drop of aqueous solution, 5,000 units per c.c. is instilled into the conjunctival sac every five minutes for the first hour, and thereafter at gradually lengthening intervals.

Streptomycin is given by intramuscular injection three times a day. The dose is 40 mgm. per lb. per day.

There is no indication for frequent conjunctival lavage when these drugs are given orally; it need be done only when there is a profuse discharge and a few times in twenty-four hours is sufficient. The instillation of a drop of liquid paraffin prevents adhesion of the lids and promotes drainage.

If the above drugs are not available, the régime of former years must be followed, namely, frequent lavage with boracic lotion or sterile water (hourly in acute cases) and the instillation of silver salts (20 per cent. argyrol) four or eight-hourly; the latter must be washed out of the conjunctival sac after fifteen minutes—not with saline.

Thrush.—Oral thrush is common in young infants, particularly in institutions and in the bottle fed. It is caused by the fungus Monilia albicans. It is more common in infants born of women with vaginal thrush, but infection is usually caused by an imperfect nursing routine.

Thrush seldom develops before the end of the first week.

The lesions may appear in any or all parts of the buccal cavity or on the tongue; they are small, whitish, adherent spots, but, if untreated, the lesions may become confluent.

Infants are not adversely affected in mild cases, but develop anorexia and fail to thrive if it is severe.

It may invade the œsophagus, and even the stomach and intestine. These complications cause severe illness, and the vomiting is likely to cause broncho-pneumonia.

Death from thrush is not rare, therefore take seriously all cases of thrush, however mild, and treat carefully.

Treatment is both prophylactic and curative. In institutions immediate isolation and barrier nursing are essential measures to prevent cross-infection, as the organisms are passed in the stools, and the infant's hands and clothes are contaminated.

Local treatment with gentian violet 1 per cent. in aqueous solution is effective, if applied twice a day for a few days, and then once daily until after all the lesions have vanished. More frequent application of gentian violet may cause local sloughing.

Gastro-enteritis.—Much the most serious of the more common neo-natal infections, for the mortality is very high unless treatment is prompt and skilful.

A variety of organisms may cause the disease, but it is now widely believed that B. coli neopolitanum and other forms of atypical B. coli are responsible for the majority of cases.

In institutions, usually occurs in epidemics, which fortunately are infrequent; over-crowding and lack of a barrier nursing régime enable epidemics to arise.

Clinical Features.—The illness seldom develops before the end of the first week and the infant is nearly always bottle fed.

The first signs are sudden loss of appetite, diminished vitality, a tired expression and pallor.

Diarrhœa develops soon after but may be delayed for a day or two; the stools are watery and yellow, like urine, in acute cases, and may be uncountable.

Signs of dehydration usually appear by the second day and progress rapidly. The weight falls abruptly.

Fever and vomiting are generally present, but may be absent.

Abdominal colic is common and causes piercing cries; abdominal distension develops later in severe cases.

The metabolic disturbance caused by the loss of water and electrolytes from the alimentary tract constitutes the main danger of the disease.

Treatment should be commenced as soon as a provisional diagnosis is made.

Immediate isolation and very strict barrier nursing are imperative in all suspected cases, for the consequence of dilatory methods is almost inevitably an epidemic of gastro-enteritis—the most dreaded of all visitations in infants' institutions.

Milk must be withheld completely until the appetite returns. Water electrolytes and some calories should be supplied by giving Hartmann's solution and 10 per cent. glucose in equal proportions ad lib. at two or three-hourly intervals. When the appetite returns gradually introduce a weak milk mixture. Oral feeding should be discontinued and parenteral fluid therapy substituted in very acute cases and where there is severe vomiting or anorexia. Hartmann's solution and 10 per cent. glucose in equal parts is a suitable solution for intravenous administration, and Hartmann's solution and 5 per cent. glucose in equal parts for subcutaneous use. The addition of hyaluronidase to the latter trebles the amount which can be given at one time by accelerating absorption.

A sulphonamide, such as sulphamezathine $\frac{1}{4}$ gm. six-hourly, should always be given. Well absorbed sulphonamides are now preferred to slowly absorbed ones such as sulphaguanidine, in this disease, because parenteral infection, especially respiratory, is a very common feature. Penicillin should also be given in severe cases as a prophylactic measure against staphylococcal infections.

Nasopharyngitis.—Infection of the upper respiratory tract is not uncommon in the new-born.

It can usually be traced to the mother or a member of the staff who has a " cold."

Isolate to prevent an epidemic from air-borne infection; exalted virulence in an epidemic is likely to cause laryngitis, bronchitis and broncho-pneumonia.

No special treatment is indicated in nasopharyngitis, but sulphonamides and penicillin are called for when the infection passes down the respiratory tract.

Omphalitis.—Serious infection of the umbilicus causing septicæmia, peritonitis or a severe local inflammation of the adjoining abdominal wall is uncommon nowadays, because of the careful aseptic precautions taken with umbilical dressings.

Mild degrees of omphalitis are still common; the infection is usually mixed, but the Staph. aureus and hæmolytic streptococcus are the principal infecting organisms.

The signs of infection are a sero-purulent discharge, slight bleeding and the development of an excrescence of granulation tissue.

Treatment.—Remove any granulation tissue, as it prevents healing.

If a pedunculated polypus has formed apply a tight ligature and it will separate in a day or two; or grasp with Allis' forceps and rotate until it separates.

If sessile, and above methods impracticable, apply a caustic such as copper sulphate daily, until it has disappeared.

In all cases instil an antiseptic such as methylated spirit or penicillin powder twice daily.

Instruct mother always to open up the umbilicus to maximum extent, wash, dry thoroughly and powder at bath time.

Pneumonia.—Usually broncho-pneumonia.

Former grave prognosis now much improved with new antibiotic agents.

Vast majority are secondary to asphyxia with inhalation and atelectasis, cerebral hæmorrhage with atelectasis, or prematurity with inhalation of regurgitated feeds.

Digestive Disorders

Common in first weeks of life because the complicated process of digestion does not begin until after birth. Digestion consists of chemical and mechanical processes. Most of the neo-natal digestive disorders are mechanical, namely, over-distension with fluid or gas and inco-ordination between contracting viscus and relaxing sphincter.

Swallowed Air.—Commonly known as "wind." If baby not relieved of this by eructation after feed, distending effect may cause vomiting, colic or diarrhœa.

Vomiting.—Very common in infants and often due to minor causes.

Little attention need be paid to it if it occurs at intervals of a few days, particularly if the infant is thriving.

Persistent vomiting should always command attention and its character be studied. The principal *causes* of vomiting are—

1. Jerky handling after feeds.
2. Retention of swallowed air causing over-distension.
3. Over-feeding causing over-distension, particularly in breast-fed infants, when there is an ample milk supply. Treat by reducing length of feed to a few minutes, and, if necessary, by expressing 1 to 3 oz. of milk before each feed.

4. Cerebral irritation caused by birth trauma is often associated with persistent vomiting. Treatment is directed to the nervous disorder and the vomiting usually subsides quickly.
5. Congenital obstruction of the alimentary tract in various situations should always be borne in mind as a possible cause of vomiting in the early days of life.
6. Unsuitable or badly tolerated cow's milk feeding may cause vomiting. The feeds should be modified to facilitate digestion.
7. Allergy, such as idiosyncrasy to cow's milk may cause severe vomiting.
8. Gastro-enteritis is usually accompanied by vomiting.
9. *Pyloric stenosis* should always be considered as a possible cause of vomiting, when a baby, who has made good progress, commences to vomit at the age of a fortnight or in the following few weeks. The vomiting soon becomes persistent and is abnormally forcible. The infant seems well and is hungry, but will soon lose weight. The stools are constipated. The patient is generally a boy.

   Diagnosis depends on these features, the presence of exaggerated gastric peristalsis and the presence of a palpable pyloric tumour.

   Treatment is surgical except in mild cases.
10. *Pyloric spasm* is often confused with pyloric stenosis, but, unlike the latter, the vomiting usually dates from the first week.

    The weight is maintained, there is no constipation, no exaggerated gastric peristalsis and no palpable pylorus. The patient is usually a girl.

    Treat by giving antispasmodic drugs (eumydrin), sedatives (chloral), and feeds thickened with partly malted starch (Benger's Food) if the infant is bottle fed.

Diarrhœa.—It is normal for breast-fed infants' stools to be unformed; this is especially so in the early weeks of life. The stools of infants fed on cow's milk are much firmer, and may be formed, because of the higher protein content of cow's milk. The principal *causes* of diarrhœa are :—

1. Retention of swallowed air causing distension.
2. Over-feeding, causing distension.

3. Indigestion of cow's milk formula. More often caused by unsuitable feeding, particularly an excess of sugar, than by intolerance of cow's milk. The stools are loose, green and curdy, and the infant fails to gain weight.
4. Gastro-enteritis.

Constipation.—True constipation does not occur in breast-fed babies, but is fairly common in those fed on cow's milk.

Only a small proportion of infants alleged to suffer from constipation are so affected ; they usually have an infrequent passage of normal motions and require different treatment from those with true constipation.

The principal causes of infrequent motions with a normal consistence are under-feeding, anal spasm and anal fissure ; it is not uncommon for healthy contented breast-fed infants to have phases of infrequent defæcation, when a normal stool may be passed without difficulty once every two or three days.

The features of anal spasm, which is fairly common, are severe straining during the passage of a normal motion and spasm of the sphincter ani detected on examination with the little finger. Treatment consists of digital dilatation every second day for a week or two.

True constipation may be rectified by giving Demerara sugar in the feeds and increasing the amount of fruit juice, but mild aperients are usually necessary. Milk of magnesia and petroleum emulsion in doses of 1 to 3 drachms a day, as indicated, are the most suitable.

Anorexia.—In the absence of other illness and faulty feeding this is usually caused by sluggish liver function. A period of relative starvation assists the resumption of normal function. Feed on sterile water containing 5 per cent. dextri-maltose for one to three days, then introduce weak feeds and gradually strengthen.

Dehydration Fever

Infants who obtain little at the breast in the first few days may develop a sudden high fever unless the deficient fluid intake is compensated by giving additional fluid.

Clinical Features characteristic.

The temperature rises suddenly and may reach 103° F. or 104° F., the lips and mouth are parched, the infant is very thirsty and restless, the urine is scanty and highly coloured and the napkin may be stained red by uric acid crystals.

Treatment simple ; it consists of the liberal and frequent administration of fluid. Plain boiled water and water with 5 per cent. sugar should be given alternately ad lib. every hour or two. An alkali such as sod. citrate, 5 gr., every two hours reduces the acidity of the urine. Such measures rapidly bring down the temperature and normal health is restored in twelve to forty-eight hours.

Jaundice

The principal causes are :—

Icterus neonatorum (physiological jaundice).
Prematurity.
Icterus gravis (hæmolytic disease of the new-born).
Congenital obliteration of the bile ducts.
Infection.

Icterus Neonatorum.—A considerable minority of infants develop a mild degree of icterus sometime between the latter part of the second day and the fifth day. It usually disappears in two or three days, but when more severe, it may last for a week or longer.

It does not interfere with health in the typical mild case, and such cases constitute the vast majority, but when severe, there is lethargy and anorexia owing to poor liver function, and normal progress is checked.

No treatment is called for except in severe cases and they should be given water with 5 per cent. sugar for one to three days to rest the liver and allow a return of the appetite.

It is generally believed that icterus neonatorum is caused by the inability of a sluggish liver to excrete sufficiently rapidly the large amount of bilirubin, which is produced by the destruction of superfluous erythrocytes after birth. In these circumstances the icteric index rises in the blood and jaundice develops.

Prematurity.—Icterus neonatorum is much more common in premature infants and is usually more severe and persistent. This is presumed to be due to relative immaturity of the liver.

Icterus Gravis.—This is the commonest manifestation of hæmolytic disease of the new-born (erythroblastosis fœtalis). (See Hæmolytic disease of the new-born p. 396.)

Congenital Obliteration of the Bile Ducts.—The features of this rare condition are progressive jaundice, commencing in the latter part of the first week, and the passage of white or cream-coloured stools and bile-stained urine. Death occurs after a few months. Operation offers only a remote hope of cure, since the bile-duct atresia is generally intra-hepatic.

Jaundice may develop in congenital syphilis, septicæmia.

Hæmolytic Disease of the New-born

Immunology.—This fœtal and neo-natal disease is caused by immunisation of the mother by specific fœtal red cell antigens, which she herself lacks, and which are inherited by the fœtus from the father. Immune antibodies thus formed in the circulation of the mother are transferred to the circulation of the fœtus, through the placenta, and hæmolyse the antigenic fœtal red cells.

Although several blood groups have been shown to be associated with this disease, immunisation to one or other of the antigens forming the **Rhesus Factor** accounts for the vast majority of cases—particularly immunisation to the Rhesus positive or " D " antigen.

It is convenient, therefore, to describe hæmolytic disease of the new-born in relation to the Rhesus factor, remembering that the same principles apply to immunisation by the A.B.O. system, for instance.

Immunisation may be produced by the introduction into the mother's circulation of Rhesus incompatible blood by (*a*) pregnancy (*b*) injection—subcutaneous, intramuscular or intravenous—at any time. Immunisation by transfusion usually produces more severe hæmolytic disease than immunisation by pregnancy; the disease rarely occurs in a first pregnancy unless the mother has previously received blood by transfusion or injection. **It is important to realise that the majority of Rh− women with Rh+ husbands have an uneventful obstetrical career; only about 5 per cent. of Rh− women ever develop antibodies in pregnancy.** Rh immunisation is much more likely to follow transfusion with incompatible blood; 50 per cent. of individuals develop antibodies in these circumstances. Even intramuscular injection of blood is a potent stimulus.

Once established, immunisation is permanent. Rhesus incompatible blood should therefore never be given to a female by any route, even in the neo-natal period.

The Rhesus Factor.—The severity and incidence of the disease in any particular family is related to the genetic pattern of the Rhesus factor. There are six Rhesus antigens in the red cells designated C, D, E, c, d and e; each is capable of producing its corresponding antibody. These antigens are contained in three pairs of closely linked allelomorphic genes—C, c; D, d; and E, e;—inherited according to Mendelian principles. Thus a single Rh chromosome will carry the gene for C or c, etc., but not both. Combinations of one antigen from each of these three pairs give rise to eight Rhesus sub-types: CDe, cde, cDE, cDe, cdE, Cde, CDE and CdE in that order of frequency, and the components of each group occur close together on the same chromosome.

The nucleated cells of each individual (except the sex cells) carry two Rh chromosomes, one from each parent, and the presence or absence of the D gene determines whether a person is Rhesus positive or Rhesus negative. Thus if a chromosome carrying the D gene is inherited from both parents, the constitution of the individual will be DD (Rh+) homozygous. If a D gene is inherited from one parent, and a d gene from the other, the constitution will be Dd heterozygous, but such an individual can transmit either a positive or negative gene. If a d gene is inherited from both parents, the constitution will be dd (Rh−) and, of course, homozygous —thus Rh− individuals must always be homozygous for the d antigen.

In Hæmolytic Disease.—In the vast majority of cases of hæmolytic disease, the mother is Rhesus negative (dd), the father Rhesus positive (DD or Dd) and the fœtus Rhesus positive. In any case where sensitisation has occurred, therefore, it is important to know the genotype of the father, since if he is homozygous (DD) all his children will carry the D antigen and will be affected by the anti-D formed in the mother's blood, whereas if he is heterozygous (Dd) there is an even chance that his children will be Rhesus negative (dd) and therefore unaffected. At present it is usually impossible to test directly for the presence of the d antigen, so that to determine whether a person is homozygous or heterozygous to D depends on the presence or absence of the various other antigens.

Clinical Applications.—Systematic Rhesus testing of all women attending antenatal clinics is a valuable aid to the detection of possible iso-immunisation, and thus to the treatment of its effects on the fœtus. The detection of immune antibodies may be the first indication of the probable occurrence of hæmolytic disease of the new-born, and in addition, it affords a useful safeguard against the accidental immunisation of women by the transfusion of Rhesus incompatible blood. Thus, any woman found to be Rhesus negative should be given a written and verbal record of the fact, as a warning against the use of blood of unknown Rhesus group should she ever require a transfusion. This precaution is even more imperative in the case of a woman known to have Rhesus antibody in her blood, since a first transfusion of Rhesus positive blood in these circumstances may be followed by an immediate serious reaction.

In addition, in cases of known or suspected Rhesus sensitisation in pregnancy, the genotype of the husband should be determined. It may be a valuable aid to diagnosis to use the cells of husband or surviving children when testing the mother's serum for antibodies.

Apart from the first examination, tests for antibodies are likely to yield the best results if carried out at the following intervals during pregnancy. (1) Before the fifth month. (2) Between the twenty-eighth to thirtieth week. (3) Between the thirty-fourth to thirty-sixth week. (4) In the second week of the puerperium.

Prognosis.—The interpretation of the serological results, in relation to the severity of the disease, is not fully understood. The prognostic value of the antibody titre in the mother's serum has proved disappointing. High titres early in pregnancy usually signify a poor fœtal prognosis, but the contrary is not necessarily true, and a continuously low titre may be followed by the birth of a severely affected infant. In general, a sharp fall in the antibody titre after the thirtieth week, or a steady rise to a high level near term are bad prognostic signs. A rising antibody titre does not prove that the infant is affected since it may be Rh— and normal—so-called anamnestic response. In the present state of knowledge no single finding can be regarded as of paramount importance, and the best results are obtained by an assessment of all the known facts—serological and clinical.

Whenever there is a possibility of an infant being affected by hæmolytic disease, either on clinical or serological grounds, the mother should be confined in hospital. Arrangements should be made: (1) For the prompt supply of compatible blood for both mother and baby, if necessary (this usually means Rhesus negative blood). (2) For carrying out the following observations on the cord blood of the infant immediately after birth: hæmoglobin; erythrocyte, erythroblast and reticulocyte counts; serum bilirubin; Coombs' Test; Rhesus test.

Clinical Features.—The principal clinical types of hæmolytic disease are :—

Anæmia hæmolytica.
Icterus gravis.
Hydrops fœtalis.
Intra-uterine death with maceration.
Miscarriage.

Anæmia hæmolytica is the least severe type ; there is no jaundice, and spontaneous recovery from the anæmia is the rule.

Icterus gravis, which is much the commonest type, is more serious and about one-quarter of the affected babies die within a few days of birth, while about 10 per cent. of the survivors have a permanently crippled nervous system (kernicterus).

Easy to diagnose because jaundice is either present at birth or it develops on the first day and it rapidly becomes very severe ; anæmia does not usually become severe for several days. The development of characteristic "cerebral" signs reveals the presence of cerebral degeneration (kernicterus).

Hydrops fœtalis is associated with a large pale œdematous placenta and the infant is either stillborn or only survives for a few minutes. The cases in which intra-uterine death with maceration occurs are also associated with a large pale placenta, but the fœtus may not show much œdema.

The fundamental pathology is the same in all types. Erythroblastæmia ; erythropoiesis in the liver and spleen and perhaps in the kidneys and other tissues ; great enlargement of the spleen, which can often be palpated.

Treatment.—The former practice of inducing labour at the thirty-sixth week, to curtail the infant's exposure to Rhesus antibody when there was reason to anticipate a severely affected infant, has been discontinued, since the incidence of the dreaded kernicterus is now known to be greater in premature infants.

An exchange transfusion with compatible Rhesus-negative blood should be given within a few hours of birth when the cord blood hæmoglobin is below 95 per cent. (normal 120–130 per cent.). The procedure, which occupies several hours, should be entrusted to experienced hands. (For details refer to works on the subject.) The objects of replacement transfusion are to remove antibody, to avoid the harmful effects caused by the products of hæmolysis and to maintain a high level of hæmoglobin. The hope that the procedure would prevent kernicterus has not been realised though its frequency and severity may have been reduced. Following replacement transfusion only slight jaundice, if any, develops, and further transfusion is seldom necessary.

In milder cases not requiring an exchange transfusion a simple transfusion (15 c.c. per lb.) should be given if, in the course of the first few weeks, the hæmoglobin falls below 50 per cent. Spontaneous recovery from a less severe degree of anæmia will occur.

Breast feeding is not contra-indicated, as was formerly believed.

Satisfactory management of hæmolytic disease of the new-born depends on close integration of obstetric, pædiatric and blood transfusion services.

Hæmorrhagic Disease

(Pathological Hypoprothrombinæmia)

Spontaneous hæmorrhage in the first five days of life is not very uncommon. In the great majority of cases it is a manifestation of prothrombin deficiency in the blood, but in others it may be a manifestation of some form of hereditary hæmorrhagic diathesis such as hæmophilia.

All infants show a phase of physiological hypoprothrombinæmia in the first few days of life, when the infant is deprived of its placental source of maternal vitamin K (the precursor of prothrombin) and has not yet acquired an adequate supply from the mother's milk because of the small amount available at that time.

In cases where the mother's diet in pregnancy has been lacking in foods rich in vitamin K, notably milk and green vegetables, the blood prothrombin level in the early days of life may fall very low (pathological hypoprothrombinæmia) and hæmorrhagic disease may develop.

Clinical Features.—Spontaneous, persistent oozing of blood from mucous surfaces. The alimentary tract is much the commonest site, but bleeding may occur from the respiratory and urogenital tracts, and from the umbilicus. Melæna is more common than hæmatemesis, and the stools may be black or red ; tarry stools are sometimes confused with meconium.

Treatment.—More simple and effective since the introduction of synthetic vitamin K a few years ago, which may be given orally or intramuscularly. The latter method is preferable as the dose required is smaller and the effect more rapid; 5 mgm. synkavit or kapilon will raise the prothrombin index to a high level and control the hæmorrhage in an hour or two. (Aqueous solutions have displaced oily solutions to eliminate tissue necrosis and abscess formation.)

Transfusion of blood is always immediately effective.

Prophylactic administration of vitamin K to the mother within twelve hours prior to the birth of the baby, or to the baby immediately after birth, effectively prevents the disease, for it even precludes the development of the physiological hypoprothrombinæmia. It should be a routine procedure in cases of complicated delivery and prematurity, so as to preclude prothrombin deficiency as a possible cause of defective coagulability of the blood in case of hæmorrhage arising from trauma or anoxia.

APPENDIX

THE USES OF X-RAY IN OBSTETRICS AND GYNÆCOLOGY

OBSTETRICS

Diagnosis of Pregnancy.—From the sixteenth week onwards, the fœtal bones are sufficiently ossified to allow of a positive diagnosis of pregnancy.

Hydatidiform Mole.—Where the uterus is the size of a four-months' pregnancy, or bigger, absence of fœtal parts is suggestive of hydatidiform mole.

Lithopædion.—This condition, where the fœtus has died in utero and become infiltrated with lime salts, can be recognised.

Intra-uterine Fœtal Death.—If not in labour, collapse of the vault and overlapping of the cranial bones indicate fœtal death. (Spalding's sign.)

Fœtal Abnormality.—Should always be suspected in hydramnios and X-ray examination should therefore be carried out. Anencephaly can be recognised easily by the absence of skull vault and hydrocephalus by enormous enlargement of the head and great width of sutures. In some cases spina-bifida can be demonstrated.

Presentation and Position.—The presentation can be judged with accuracy and, if a breech presents, X-ray shows whether the legs are, or are not, extended. By taking antero-posterior and lateral radiographs, the position too can be ascertained.

Pelvic Mensuration and Shape.—Where contraction or abnormal shape of the pelvis is suspected, X-ray examination may be most helpful. This applies to the false pelvis and to all levels of the true pelvis.

Descent of Head during Labour.—In trial labours to see if head is descending satisfactorily.

Fœtal Maturity.—A fairly accurate idea as to the stage of pregnancy, or age of the fœtus, can be obtained. This applies more to the later months, when a study of the centres of ossification seen, indicates the approximate time of delivery or, on the other hand, whether the fœtus is post-mature. This may be of medico-legal importance.

Placenta Prævia.—The position of the placenta may be demonstrated by a " soft tissue " X-ray. This method is not always successful, however, and it may be necessary to inject into the bladder 2 oz. of a 10 per cent. solution of sodium iodide or air. If no part of the placenta lies in the lower segment, the space between the bladder shadow and that of the fœtal skull should not exceed 1 cm.

GYNÆCOLOGY

Malignant Disease.—X-ray therapy may be used, in conjunction with radium or operation, in malignant disease of the vulva, cervix, uterine body or ovary.

Artificial Menopause.—This may be brought about by X-rays, mainly through the action on the ovaries. In cases of metropathia hæmorrhagica, for example, where the patient is approximating the menopause and where more conservative treatment has failed, an artificial menopause may be produced in this way. Small fibroids may be treated in a like manner, if operation is contra-indicated.

Pruritus.—This condition can, in some cases, be relieved by X-rays.

Tubal Patency.—Intra-uterine injection of lipiodol, with X-ray examination at the time and twenty-four hours later, will show whether the tubes are patent. If obstructed, the site of the block is shown.

Uterine Abnormalities.—Where there is some doubt clinically, X-ray examination, following the intra-uterine injection of lipiodol, will demonstrate congenital uterine abnormality, *e.g.* uterus bicornis unicollis.

Fibromyoma.—Following intra-uterine injection of lipiodol, a filling defect is seen in cases of submucous fibroid. Interstitial fibroids may straighten the uterine wall, enlarge or cause alteration in shape of the cavity. A calcified fibroid will show up clearly with X-ray.

Dermoid Cysts.—May be diagnosed when teeth are present.

INDEX

Cervical spondylitis

MO/-
17 11 56